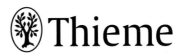

General Pathology and Internal Medicine for Physical Therapists

Gabriele Steffers, MD
Former Lecturer
School of Physical Therapy
Friedrichsheim University Orthopedics Clinic
Frankfurt, Germany

Susanne Credner, MD
Private Cardiology and Angiology Practice
Frankfurt, Germany

288 illustrations

Thieme
Stuttgart · New York

Library of Congress Cataloging-in-Publication Data is available from the publisher.

This book is an authorized translation of the 1st German edition published and copyrighted 2006 by Georg Thieme Verlag, Stuttgart. Title of the German edition: Allgemeine Krankheitslehre und Innere Medizin für Physiotherapeuten.

Translator: Gertrud G. Champe, Surry, Maine, USA

Illustrator: Martin Hoffmann, Thalfingen, Germany

© 2012 Georg Thieme Verlag,
Rüdigerstrasse 14, 70469 Stuttgart, Germany
http://www.thieme.de
Thieme New York, 333 Seventh Avenue,
New York, NY 10001, USA
http://www.thieme.com

Cover design: Thieme Publishing Group
Typesetting by medionet Publishing Services Ltd.,
Berlin, Germany
Printed in China by Everbest Printing Co., Ltd

ISBN 978-3-13-154321-9
eISBN 978-3-13-164431-2

Preface

With the German version of our book already in its second edition, we were very pleased that our book also aroused interest in the English-speaking world, and that Angelika-M. Findgott of Thieme Publishers arranged for an English translation.

Our hope for *General Pathology and Internal Medicine for Physical Therapists* is that it will make the entry into the world of medicine easier for physical therapy students and give them a foundation for all the fields of special pathology. We explain the mechanisms that make us sick, describe important signs of disease and consider their possible origin. The first part of the book concludes with basic ideas regarding diagnostic and therapeutic procedures.

In the second part of the book, we look step by step at the most important disease patterns for internal medicine. For a clearer understanding, the physiological basis is discussed first. Internal medicine is an important discipline for physical therapists, since internal diseases are encountered in every area of medicine. Even though their work concentrates on the motor apparatus, they will have to take the underlying diseases of their patients into account.

With this book, we hope to provide future physical therapists with a guide throughout their study of clinical pathology, a reference work for their practical training, and, finally, a useful tool as they prepare for the examination. Even later, in practice and for their everyday clinical work, they will often be able to use the book as they deal with questions of internal medicine. What is more, students of other health care professions will also be able to profit in the same way from the content of this book, both during their training and later in their professional work.

We thank the team at Thieme Publishers for an excellent collaboration, most particularly Angelika-M. Findgott and Anne Lamparter, without whom this book would not have been possible.

Finally, we wish all physical therapy students enjoyment in reading this book and much satisfaction in a well-grounded education as well as great success in their examinations and professional lives!

Gabriele Steffers, MD
Susanne Credner, MD

The Authors

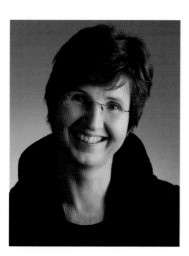

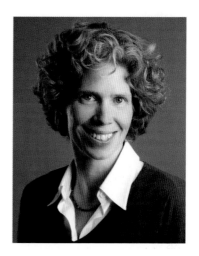

Gabriele Steffers, MD, is a physical therapist and physician. For more than 10 years, she was a full-time lecturer at the School of Physical Therapy of the Friedrichsheim University Orthopedics Clinic in Frankfurt/Main, Germany. There she developed and implemented a teaching plan that relates the fundamental subjects of visceral anatomy, physiology, and general pathology to internal medicine. At the same time, among other professional activities, she taught at a college for osteopathic medicine and wrote a pediatrics textbook.

Susanne Credner, MD, is a specialist in internal medicine and cardiology. For 12 years, she worked at the hospital of the Johann Wolfgang Goethe University in Frankfurt/Main and at the Offenbach Hospital, Germany, before practicing preventive medicine for 2 years. She is currently a member of a practice specialized in cardiology and angiology.

Contents

List of Abbreviations

AAA	abdominal aortic aneurysm	CML	chronic myeloid leukemia
AAT	alpha-antitrypsin	CMV	cytomegalovirus
ACE	angiotensin-converting enzyme	CNS	central nervous system
ACR	American College of Rheumatology	COLD	chronic obstructive lung disease
ACTH	adrenocorticotropic hormone	COPD	chronic obstructive pulmonary disease
ACVB	aortocoronary venous bypass	CPAP	continuous positive airway pressure
ADH	antidiuretic hormone	CRC	colorectal cancer
AED	automatic external defibrillator	CRH	corticotropin-releasing hormone
AFP	alpha-fetoprotein	CRI	chronic renal insufficiency
AIDS	acquired immune deficiency syndrome	CRP	C-reactive protein
ALL	acute lymphocytic leukemia	CRT	cardiac resynchronization therapy
AML	acute myeloid leukemia	CSA	cyclosporin A
ANA	anti-nuclear antibodies	CVC	central venous catheter
ANCA	anti-neutrophilic cytoplasmic antibodies	CVI	chronic venous insufficiency
ANS	autonomic nervous system	CVVH	continuous venovenous hemofiltration
APC	activated Protein C	DBP	diastolic blood pressure
APL	anterior lobe of the pituitary gland	DCM	dilatated cardiomyopathy
ARDS	acute respiratory distress syndrome	DEET	diethyl-meta-toluamide
ARF	acute renal failure	DMARDs	disease-modifying antirheumatic drugs
ARVC	arrhythmogenic right ventricular cardio-myopathy	DNCG	disodium cromoglicinate
		DVT	deep vein thrombosis
AS	ankylopoietic spondylarthritis, Bechterew disease	DXA	dual X-ray absorptiometry
		EBV	Epstein–Barr virus
AT III	antithrombin III	ECG	electrocardiogram
AV	atrioventricular	EF	ejection fraction
BAL	bronchoalveolar lavage	EP	electrophysiological
BC	blood count	ERCP	endoscopic retrograde cholangiopancrea-tography
BGA	blood gas analysis		
BP	blood pressure	ESR	erythrocite sedimentation rate
BMI	body mass index	ESSG	European Spondylarthropathy Study Group
BMT	marrow transplantation		
BS	blood sugar	ESWL	extracorporeal shock wave lithotripsy
c.i.s.	carcinoma in situ	FAP	familial adenomatous polyposis
CABG	coronary artery bypass grafting	FEV_1	forced expiratory volume in the first second
CAD	coronary artery disease		
CAPD	continuous ambulatory peritoneal dialysis	FNH	focal nodal hyperplasia
		FRC	functional residual capacity
CDC	(US) Centers for Disease Control and Prevention	FSH	follicle-stimulating hormone
		GFR	glomerular filtration rate
CF	cystic fibrosis	GN	glomerulonephritis
CID	chronic inflammatory intestinal disease	GVHD	graft versus host disease
CK	enzyme creatine kinase	Hb	hemoglobin
CKD	chronic kidney disease	HbA1c	hemoglobin A1c
CLL	chronic lymphocytic leukemia	HCM	hypertrophic cardiomyopathy

Hct	hematocrit	OSAS	obstructive sleep apnea syndrome
HDL	high-density lipoprotein	PAD	peripheral arterial disease
HIV	human immunodeficiency virus	PEG	percutaneous endoscopic gastrostomy
HLA	human leukocyte antigen	PIP	proximal interphalangeal
HNCM	hypertrophic nonobstructive cardio-	PPL	posterior lobe of the pituitary gland
	myopathy	PSS	progressive systemic sclerosis
HNPCC	hereditary nonpolypous colon cancer	PTA	percutaneous transluminal angioplasty
HOCM	hypertrophic obstructive cardiomyopathy	PTCA	percutaneous transluminal coronary
HP	*Helicobacter pylori*		angioplasty
HPV	human papillomas viruses	PTH	parathyroid hormone
HSV	herpes simplex virus	PTT	partial thromboplastin time
HTX	heart transplantation	RA	rheumatoid arthritis
ICD	implantable cardioverter defibrillator	RAAS	renin–angiotensin–aldosterone system
Ig	immunoglobulin	RAST	radioallergosorbent test
IM	intramuscular, into the muscle	RCM	restrictive cardiomyopathy
INR	international normalized ratio	RV	residual volume
IRV	inspiratory reserve volume	SC	subcutaneous, under the skin
ISWL	intracorporeal shock wave lithotripsy	SCLC	small-cell lung cancer
ITP	idiopathic thrombocytopenic purpura	SCT	stem cell transplantation
IV	intravenous, into the vein	SLE	systemic lupus erythematosus
JRA	juvenile rheumatoid arthritis	SSS	sick sinus syndrome
KTX	kidney transplantation	STD	sexually transmitted disease
LDL	low-density lipoprotein	STH	somatotropin; somatotropic hormone
LED	disseminated lupus erythematosus	SBP	systolic blood pressure
LH	luteinizing hormone	T_3	triiodothyronine
LTX	lung transplantation	T_4	thyroxine
MCH	mean corpuscular hemoglobin	TB	tuberculosis
MCP	metacarpophalangeal	TBE	tick-borne encephalitis
MCTD	mixed connective-tissue disease	TC	total capacity
MCV	mean corpuscular volume	TEA	thrombendarteriectomy
MEN	multiple endocrine neoplasms	TEE	transesophageal echocardiography
MIS	minimally invasive surgery	TRH	thyrotropin-releasing hormone
MRSA	methicillin-resistant *Staphylococcus*	TSH	thyroid-stimulating hormone
	aureus, or colloquially "multiresistant	TTE	transthoracic echocardiography
	Staph. aureus"	TX	transplantation
MSH	melanocyte-stimulating hormone	UICC	Union for International Cancer Control
NASH	nonalcoholic steatohepatitis	UTV	urine 24-hour volume
NBM	nil by mouth	VC	vital capacity
NHL	non–Hodgkin lymphoma	VF	ventricular fibrillation
NIPD	nightly intermittent peritoneal dialysis	VIP	vasoactive intestinal polypeptide
NSARD	nonsteroidal antirheumatic drug	VLDL	very-low density lipoprotein
NSCLC	non–small-cell lung cancer	VT	ventricular tachycardia
NYHA	New York Heart Association	vWS	von Willebrand syndrome
OGTT	oral glucose tolerance test	VZV	varicella zoster virus

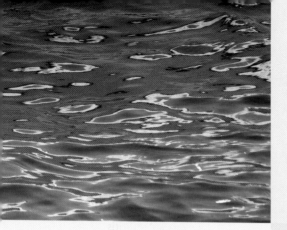

Part 1
General Pathology

The first part of this book deals primarily with the answers to four questions:

1. Why do people get sick in the first place?
2. What causes can be at the root of the various symptoms?
3. What are the diagnostic possibilities?
4. What are the basics of treating diseases?

The answers developed step by step provide a foundation for understanding internal medicine and the other areas of special pathology.

1 Basic Principles

Health and Illness

■ Health

The World Health Organization (1946) defines health as a state of complete physical, mental, and social wellbeing, not merely as the absence of illness and frailness.

■ Illness

Consequently, illness designates a disorder of life processes that changes the whole organism or its parts in such a way that the affected person is subjectively, clinically, or socially in need of help.

■ Scientific Approaches to the Explanation of Health and Illness

There are different ways of looking at the maintenance and loss of health as well as at the origin and course of diseases. These views are reflected in a variety of research directions; here, we will present the biomedical model and the model of salutogenesis.

Biomedical Model

The biomedical model is a classical pathogenetic explanation that places the *causes of disease* in the foreground. Illness is understood as basically a disturbance of physiological or biochemical processes of the organism, whose scope is determined by comparison with normal values such as laboratory results, blood pressure, or body weight. In the biomedical model, a person is either healthy or sick.

Model of Salutogenesis

The Israeli-American medical sociologist Aaron Antonovsky (1923–1994) criticized the purely pathogenetic point of view and, with his model of salutogenesis (*salus*, Latin: wellbeing) pointed the

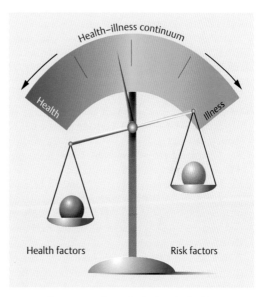

Fig. 1.1 The position of an individual on the health–illness continuum is determined by the current constellation of health and risk factors.

way to another approach. The salutogenic approach puts primary importance on the *causes of health* and the central question is not *What causes illness?* but rather *What maintains health?*

According to Antonovsky, all individuals are exposed to numerous stresses and risk factors, which they can counter with their own stress-reducing and protective factors. The result is a health–illness continuum with gradual transitions from health to illness (**Fig. 1.1**).

Fundamental Epidemiological Concepts

Originally epidemiologists studied only epidemics. Today, however, epidemiology is a science concerned with transmittable and nontransmittable diseases and their consequences in the population. This kind of study requires methods derived from the fields of statistics, demographics, and the clinical sciences.

In this chapter, we will explain concepts used by epidemiologists to report the results of their study.

- *Morbidity:* This concept reports the number of persons suffering from a certain disease out of 100 000 inhabitants at a certain point in time. Morbidity provides information about the frequency with which a population group contracts a certain disease within a certain period of time.
- *Mortality:* Mortality expresses the death rate. It reports how many individuals out of 100 000 inhabitants in a specific population have died as the result of a specific disease within a certain period of time.
- *Lethality:* This concept gives the percentage of patients who have died of a certain disease out of the total group of patients with that disease. Thus the lethality gives information about how life-threatening the disease under study is.
- *Incidence:* Incidence gives the number of new cases of a certain disease within a certain period of time. The *incidence rate* gives the number of new cases per unit of time in relation to the number of persons exposed.
- *Prevalence:* This concept defines the number of cases or frequency of the disease or characteristic under study at a certain point in time (point prevalence) or within a certain time period (period prevalence). The *prevalence rate* gives the number of affected patients or the frequency of the characteristic in relation to the size of the group under study.
- *Average life expectancy:* This gives the period of time after which 50% of all persons in a specific population group, e.g., women, have died.

Causes of Illness

Etiology

Etiology is the study of the causes at the root of diseases or malformations. These can be divided into exogenous and endogenous factors (**Fig. 1.2**):

- Exogenous factors represent a threat from outside. Damaging environmental factors are called noxae and can be influenced to a greater or lesser degree.
- Endogenous factors such as genetic inheritance cannot be influenced. They often determine a person's disposition to certain diseases.

Causal Pathogenesis

Causal pathogenesis describes the conditions under which diseases arise. It takes into account the interaction between causes of illness on the one hand and disposition and resistance on the other.

- Disposition means the inborn or acquired susceptibility to certain diseases.
- The ability of an organism to fight disease triggers is called resistance.

General Reaction Types of Cells and Tissues

The organism's chief responses to many endogenous and exogenous causes of illness are:

- Adaptation through hypertrophy, hyperplasia, or atrophy
- Inflammation
- Necrosis
- Regeneration or fibrosis

■ Adaptation Reactions

Cells that do not die as a result of damage react with changes in structure and functional metabolism that result either in increased activity, such as hypertrophy and hyperplasia, or in a decrease in activity, such as atrophy.

Hypertrophy

Hypertrophy is enlargement of cells or of an organ through enlargement of cells. Examples of physiological forms of hypertrophy include:

- Muscle hypertrophy through strength training
- Uterine hypertrophy in pregnancy

Examples of pathological forms include:

- Left ventricular hypertrophy in aortic valve stenosis (p. 111) or arterial hypertension (p. 117)
- Hereditary hypertrophic cardiomyopathy (p. 113)
- Congenital pyloric stenosis (pyloric spasm)

▮ *Hypertrophy: Cell enlargement.*

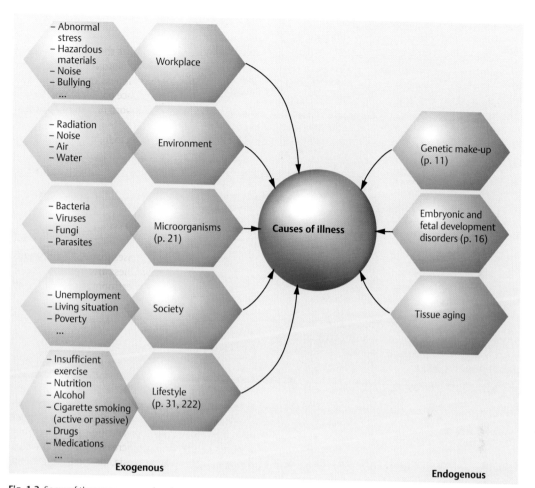

Fig. 1.2 Some of the exogenous and endogenous causes of illness.

Hyperplasia

Hyperplasia is organ enlargement due to an increase in the number of parenchymal cells, e.g.:
- Hormonally caused endometrial or prostate hyperplasia
- Thyroid gland hyperplasia (goiter, p. 234)

▍ *Hyperplasia: Cell proliferation.*

Atrophy

Atrophy is a decrease in the number of parenchymal cells with reduction of organs and tissues. Atrophy is an adaptation reaction to decreased activity, load, blood supply, nutrition, or endocrine stimulation. Muscle atrophy resulting from inactivity, lying in bed or paralysis, and the atrophy of old age is physiological.

Examples of diseases with organ atrophy include:
- Osteoporosis with loss of bone substance beyond the age-dependent physiological extent (p. 225)
- Alzheimer disease with premature aging of the brain and loss of intellectual capacity

■ Inflammation

Definition

Inflammation is the organism's complex defense reaction against local tissue damage. This local reaction is intended to limit the effect of the damage and keep the area of damage to a minimum. The local inflammatory reaction can be accompanied by a more or less marked reaction of the entire organism.

The suffix *–itis* is used when speaking of inflammation in an organ or tissue.

Table 1.1 Triggers of inflammatory reaction

Factor	Important examples	Page
Physical, chemical, and immunological factors	• Physical triggers: – Mechanical influences such as pressure – Thermal influences such as heat and cold – Actinic influences (radiation) such as UV radiation	
	• Chemical triggers, e.g.: – Acids – Alkalis	
	• Immunological triggers: – Allergens – Autoantigens in autoimmune diseases – Foreign antigens after organ transplantation	27 29 69
Microbiological factors	• Bacteria • Viruses • Fungi • Parasites	21

Triggers

An inflammatory reaction can be triggered by microbiological or physical, chemical, or immunological factors (**Table 1.1**).

> Inflammation does not always include an underlying infectious process!

Inflammatory Reaction

An inflammatory reaction is a complex interplay of the reactions of:
• The blood vessels
• Certain blood cells and plasma components
• The connective tissue

Inflammation Mediators

Tissue damage releases countless signal substances that have local and systemic effects. Important inflammatory mediators are histamine, prostaglandins, and kinins.
• *Histamine* is primarily stored in the mast cells; when it is released, it stimulates dilation of the blood vessels, an increase in permeability of the vessel walls, and itching.
• There are different *prostaglandins* that, for example, are waiting in the capillary endothelium to spring into action. In addition to having a vasodilator effect, they are pain mediators.
• The *kinin system* consists of a series of plasma proteins that have an action similar to that of prostaglandin when they are activated.

Systemically, the mediators elicit a leukocyte washout and fever.

Exudation

The action of the mediators causes increased circulation in the inflamed area. Blood plasma and inflammatory cells pass through the more permeable walls of the vessels. This phenomenon is called exudation and its purpose is to:
• Dilute toxins
• Destroy infectious agents through infiltration of defensive leukocytes
• Limit dissemination of noxae by slowing blood flow

Signs of Inflammation

Local Signs of Inflammation

The five cardinal symptoms of inflammation, which can be expressed to different degrees, are:
• Reddening (rubor)
• Swelling (tumor)
• Excessive warmth (calor)
• Pain (dolor)
• Functional limitation (functio laesa; **Fig. 1.3**)

Systemic Signs of Inflammation

The total organism reacts in different ways to local inflammatory processes:
• Loss of appetite
• Increased need for sleep
• Fall in blood pressure
• Fever

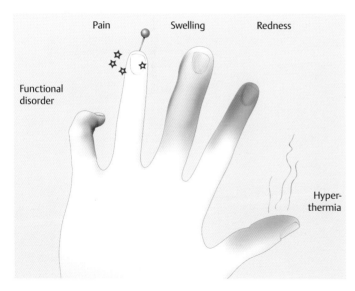

Pain   Swelling   Redness

Functional
disorder

Hyper-
thermia

Laboratory Values

Nonspecific indicators of inflammation in the blood are:
- Leukocytosis, i.e., increased leukocyte level in the blood
- Acute phase proteins such as C-reactive protein (CRP)
- Elevated sedimentation rate

Forms of Inflammation

Acute Inflammation

Five different forms of inflammation can be distinguished on the basis of the exudate (**Fig. 1.4a–e**):
- In a *serous inflammation*, the exudate consists of the fibrinogen-free, protein-rich fluid of the blood serum. It can be triggered by bacteria and viruses, as well as by chemical and physical influences.
- A *seromucous inflammation* at the mucosa-lined surfaces of the respiratory and gastrointestinal tracts is also triggered by bacteria, viruses, chemical or physical irritants. The exudate consists of serum, mucus, and sloughed-off mucosal epithelium.
- In *fibrinous inflammation*, fibrin-containing exudate is produced. A cause might be toxin-producing bacteria such as those that cause diphtheria (p. 270) or mechanical trauma.
- In a *purulent infection*, the exudate consists chiefly of leukocytes of the neutrophilic granulocyte type and of cell debris. Purulent infections are almost always induced by pyogenic pathogens such as streptococci and staphylococci (p. 273). Abscess,

phlegmon, and empyema are special forms of purulent infection (**Fig. 1.5a–c**).
- – An *empyema* is a collection of pus in an anatomically preexisting cavity, e.g., intra-articular space, pleura, pericardium, or gallbladder.
- – An *abscess* is usually caused by staphylococci creating a new body cavity by tissue destruction. The collection of pus in this cavity is called an abscess. Subsequently, granulation tissue creates an abscess membrane.
- – A *phlegmon* is a purulent infection that spreads diffusely in loosely fibrous connective tissue. It usually originates as a streptococcal infection such as erysipelas (p. 274).
- In a *hemorrhagic infection*, the exudate contains large amounts of erythrocytes. Thus, for example, bacterial toxins produce vessel damage that permits the escape of erythrocytes.

Another form of acute infection is *necrotizing infection*, in which tissue loss or death dominates the picture.

Chronic Infection

A chronic infection arises when the infectious irritant persists over a period of weeks, months, or years. It can be organ-specific, as in chronic hepatitis (p. 192), or systemic, as in diseases of the rheumatic spectrum (chapter 13). In the late phase, there may be cicatrizing (scarring) tissue destruction.

One form of chronic infection is granulomatous disease, in which macrophages form nodules several millimeters in size called granulomas. Examples of granulomatous disease are sarcoidosis (p. 162), tuberculosis (p. 268), and foreign body granulomas.

Type of inflammation	Exudate

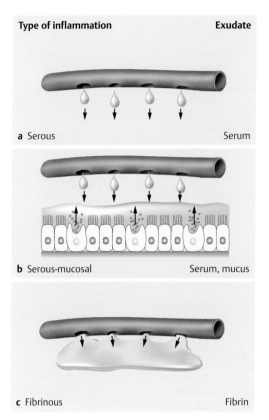

a Serous — Serum

b Serous-mucosal — Serum, mucus

c Fibrinous — Fibrin

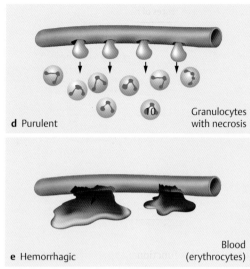

d Purulent — Granulocytes with necrosis

e Hemorrhagic — Blood (erythrocytes)

Fig. 1.4a–e Forms of inflammation classified by exudate.

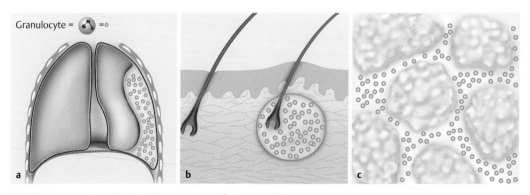

Granulocyte = ⬤ = ○

Fig. 1.5a–c Forms of purulent infection: **a** empyema; **b** abscess; **c** phlegmon.

▓ Necrosis

Definition

Necrosis is cell or tissue death in living organisms.

Causes

Necrosis occurs when noxious influences overcome the adaptive powers of cells or tissues. Necrosis can be the result of an infectious reaction (**Table 1.1**) or ischemia (lack of oxygen).

> *An ischemic necrosis is called an infarct, such as myocardial infarction (p. 101).*

Regeneration or Fibrosis

Depending on the specific tissue affected, necrosis can be followed by complete regeneration or by sub-

Table 1.2 Consequences of necrosis

Tissue type	To be found in	Repair
Regenerative tissue	• Cells of the hematopoietic system • Cells of the lymphatic system • Epidermal epithelium • Mucosal epithelium • Glandular epithelium	Complete regeneration
Stable tissue	• Cells of connective and supportive tissue • Endothelium • Smooth muscle cells • Liver cells	Complete regeneration
Postmitotic tissue	• Skeletal muscle cells • Cardiac muscle cells • CNS ganglion cells	Incomplete regeneration (fibrosis)

stitution of nonfunctional connective tissue, called fibrosis, or by incomplete regeneration (**Table 1.2**). Scars, sclerosis, wheals, calluses, and cirrhosis are forms of fibrosis.

Disease Progression

■ Acute

Acute diseases usually progress intensely over a period of a few days to weeks. A cure with complete recovery is often possible. A fulminating disease usually leads to death in a very short time.

■ Chronic

Chronic diseases progress over periods of months to years.
• Chronic-continuous diseases persist at a certain level of illness.
• In chronic-relapsing diseases, phases with and without signs of illness alternate, e.g., bronchial asthma (p. 153).
• In a chronic progressive disease, the symptoms increase as the disease progresses.

■ Death

The termination of all functional processes essential for life is designated as death. A distinction is made between clinical and biological death. After the first heart transplantation, the additional concept of brain death was defined.

Clinical Death

Definition

Clinical death is defined as the standstill of breathing and the cardiac–circulatory system.

Ambiguous Signs of Death

The clinical signs of death are ambiguous:
• Respiratory arrest
• Cardiac–circulatory arrest
• Unconsciousness
• Muscular atonia
• Absence of reflexes
• Absence of pupillary reaction
• Pale skin
• Falling body temperature

The decisive factor is whether reanimation can succeed within the resuscitation time limit. Of all the organs, the brain has the shortest resuscitation time limit at 3–5 minutes (**Fig. 1.6**).

Biological Death

Definition

Clinical death is followed by biological or final death with irreversible termination of all organ function.

Sure Signs of Death

Biological death is expressed by sure signs of death that occur in the following order:
1. Postmortem lividity (livor, hypostasis), which results 20–30 minutes after death from settling

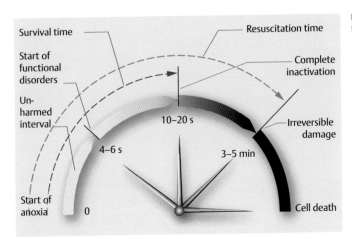

Fig. 1.6 Impact of a lack of oxygen on brain function and resuscitation time.

Survival time — Resuscitation time

Start of functional disorders — Complete inactivation

Un-harmed interval

10–20 s

4–6 s

3–5 min

Irreversible damage

Start of anoxia   0

Cell death

of the blood in lower (dependent) regions of the body.

2. Rigidity (rigor mortis) that begins 2–4 hours after death and is fully developed after 6–8 hours, resolving spontaneously after 2–3 days. It is explained by the decomposition of adenosine triphosphate (ATP), so that actin–myosin cross-bridges can no longer be decoupled.

3. Autolysis through the body's own enzymes and decomposition through bacterial activity.

Brain Death

Definition

Because pulmonary and circulatory function can be maintained for a long time by intensive care measures, the concept of *brain death* has been introduced. This defines the advent of death as the irreversible absence of all brain functions. Clinical signs are:

- Coma
- Absence of spontaneous respiration
- Both pupils fixed
- Absence of brainstem reflexes

Brain death may be declared when two independent examiners have confirmed the findings and the signs have existed for at least 12 hours. To shorten the observation time, additional examinations, such as an EEG, are performed.

Consequences

Confirmation of brain death permits interruption of intensive care and—if it is the previously stated wish of the deceased or their family—harvesting of organs for organ transplantation (p. 69).

2 Types of Diseases

Genetically Determined Diseases

■ Chromosomal Aberrations

Chromosomally determined diseases are the result of either an abnormal number of chromosomes or a defective chromosomal structure. Chromosomal aberrations occur frequently during formation of gametes. It is suspected that:

- About 10% of all diagnosed pregnancies end in a miscarriage that was caused by a chromosomal defect.
- About 0.5% of all live births exhibit a chromosomal aberration.

The changes can usually be recognized with a light microscope (**Fig. 2.1**). Diagnosis is based, for example, on lymphocytes or cells that were harvested during prenatal diagnosis through amniocentesis.

Numerical Chromosomal Aberrations

The Normal Genome

The genome describes the number of chromosomes in every cell nucleus, which is species-specific. Every cell in the human body (except for the enucleate red blood cells) has 46 chromosomes or *23 chromosome pairs*, in which a distinction can be made between:
- 22 autosomal chromosome pairs, the autosomes and
- one sex or gonosomal chromosome pair, the gonosomes. Female cells contain two X chromosomes; male cells contain one X and one smaller Y chromosome (**Fig. 2.1**).

So that the number of chromosomes does not double from generation to generation, the *diploid genome* described here must be halved during cell formation. This requires a special form of cell division called meiosis. Meiosis is also called reduction division, since the diploid genome is reduced to a *haploid genome*. In fertilization, the nuclei of the ovum and the sperm cell merge, so that a diploid genome is restored.

> *Meiosis: Diploid genome → haploid genome*
> *Fertilization: 2 × haploid genome → diploid genome*

Fig. 2.1 Karyogram of a boy with free trisomy 21 (Sitzmann 2002).

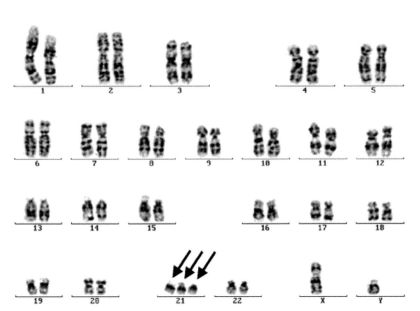

Pathophysiology

In numerical chromosomal aberrations, the number of chromosomes deviates from that of the regular genome. The cause is an error in meiosis called *nondisjunction*. A chromosome pair does not separate and the chromosomes are incorrectly distributed in the daughter cells. After fertilization, the affected chromosome is then either single (monosomy) or triple (trisomy). Nondisjunctions occur with increasing frequency as the parents age. Any chromosome can be affected by incorrect distribution. **Table 2.1** summarizes the most frequent monosomies and trisomies.

> *Nondisjunction:*
> → *Chromosome absent or doubled in the gamete*
> → *Monosomy or trisomy after fertilization*
> *Monosomy of the autosomes is not compatible with life.*

Structural Chromosomal Aberrations

Transformations within a chromosome, or between different chromosomes, change their structure while the amount of genetic material usually remains the same.

Translocations

In a translocation, whole chromosomes or parts of chromosomes are shifted onto other chromosomes. A *balanced translocation* exists when the amount of genetic information corresponds to that of a regular genome. The carrier of a balanced translocation is therefore clinically unremarkable. However, meiosis can give rise to gametes in which one section of a chromosome is absent or doubled.

During fertilization, unbalanced translocation results in monosomy or trisomy of the affected chromosome sections (**Fig. 2.2**).

Fragile X Syndrome

In this syndrome, one X chromosome is fragile. Since in girls the defective chromosome can be counterbalanced by another X chromosome, only boys will be symptomatic. Fragile X syndrome is also known as Martin–Bell syndrome and, after trisomy 21, is the second most frequent cause of mental retardation.

Table 2.1 Important symptoms of clinically relevant monosomy and trisomy

Affected chromosomes	Monosomy	Trisomy

Gonosomes	Turner syndrome (45, XO):
	• Congenital characteristics such as:
	  – Pterygium colli (webbed neck)
	  – Hair growing low on neck
	  – Cubitus valgus
	  – Lymphedema on dorsa of hands and feet
	• Absence of ovaries
	• Consequences of absent sex hormones such as:
	  – Primary amenorrhea (no menstrual periods)
	  – No secondary sex characteristics
	  – Sterility
	• Short stature
		Klinefelter syndrome (47, XXY):
		• Somatomegaly (abnormally large size)
		• IQ 10–15 points under that of siblings
		• Small testicles
		• Sterility
		• Consequences of low testosterone such as:
		  – Sparse body hair
		  – Osteoporosis (p. 225)

Autosomes	Not compatible with life	• Down syndrome (trisomy 21; **Fig. 2.1**):
		  – Congenital characteristics, e.g., oblique eye fissures
		  – Muscular hypotonia
		  – Cognitive retardation
		  – Short stature
		  – Possible organ dysplasia, e.g., congenital heart defects (p. 115)
		  – Elevated risk of leukemia (p. 247)
		  – Susceptibility to infection
		• Patau syndrome (trisomy 13):
		  – Microcephaly (small skull)
		  – Lip–jaw–gums cleft
		  – Micro- or anophthalmia (small or absent eyes)
		  – Organ dysplasia
		  – High mortality rate as early as in the first month of life

Microdeletion Syndrome

In a deletion, sections of a chromosome are absent. Usually the piece lost is so small that it cannot be detected with the light microscope, but only by means of special techniques.

Examples of Microdeletion Syndrome

- *Di George syndrome:* The defect on chromosome 22 occurs at a frequency of 1:5000. Since the thymus is absent, the chief problem for patients is weakness of defense reaction as a result of defective T lymphocytes that are normally formed in the thymus.
- *Cat cry syndrome:* The defect on chromosome 5 occurs at a frequency of 1:25000. Deformity of the larynx causes the characteristic cry. In addition, the microdeletion leads to microcephaly and mental retardation.

■ Monogenetic Inheritance

Definitions

A mutation in a specific gene, inherited strictly according to Mendel's laws, is the basis of monogenetically inherited diseases. In describing hereditary pathways, the following terms are frequently used:

- *Homologous chromosomes* are chromosomes that correspond to each other.
- The carrier of two identical genes at the same locus on homologous chromosomes is called *homozygous.*
- The carrier of two genes of different qualities at the same locus on homologous chromosomes is called *heterozygous.*
- If a characteristic is inherited *dominantly*, the information need only be present on one gene in order to manifest itself.

Fig. 2.2 Translocation of chromosome 21 to chromosome 14 and the possible consequences for the next generation.

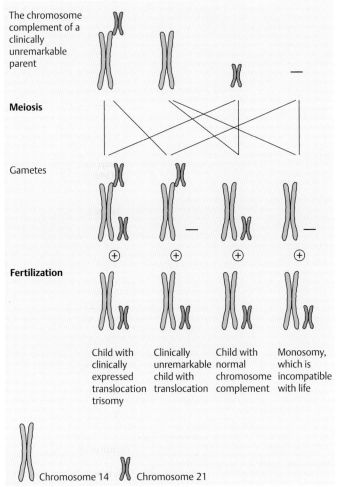

The chromosome complement of a clinically unremarkable parent

Meiosis

Gametes

Fertilization

Child with clinically expressed translocation trisomy

Clinically unremarkable child with translocation

Child with normal chromosome complement

Monosomy, which is incompatible with life

Chromosome 14   Chromosome 21

2

- If a characteristic is inherited *recessively*, the information must be present on both genes in order to manifest itself.

In view of the fact that genetic information can be present on autosomes or gonosomes and can be dominant or recessive, four hereditary pathways can be distinguished in monogenetic inheritance:
- Autosomal dominant
- Autosomal recessive
- X-linked recessive
- X-linked dominant

Autosomal Dominant

For an autosomal dominant trait, one mutated gene on an autosomal chromosome is sufficient for manifestation of the disease. The affected person is usually heterozygous. In homozygous persons, the hereditary illness is usually particularly severe, so the homozygous type is very rare. Very often, couples in which one partner is heterozygous for a disease and the other is healthy seek genetic counseling. **Figure 2.3** shows the consequences for the following generation:
- The diseased person passes the mutated gene to half of their offspring. For each child, the disease risk is 50%.
- In all generations, both sexes are affected with equal frequency.
- If the disease allows the patient to reach reproductive age and fertility has not been compromised, affected persons can occur in every generation.
- If there is no family history, the illness is due to a new mutation.

Examples of Autosomal Dominance in Hereditary Diseases
- Familial adenomatous polyposis (FAP, p. 189)
- Huntington chorea, which appears between the ages of 30 and 50 years and is associated with muscular hypotonia, hyperkinesia and progressive dementia
- Some forms of osteogenesis imperfecta, also called brittle bone disease

Autosomal Recessive

For an autosomal recessive disease to become clinically manifest, the changed gene must be present on both autosomes. Thus a patient is homozygous and usually has heterozygous parents who are clini-

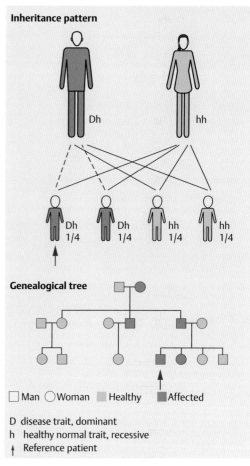

Inheritance pattern

Genealogical tree

☐ Man ◯ Woman ▨ Healthy ▪ Affected

D disease trait, dominant
h healthy normal trait, recessive
↟ Reference patient

Fig. 2.3 Autosomal dominant inheritance

cally unremarkable (**Fig. 2.4**). Characteristics of this inheritance pathway are:
- Only carriers of homozygous genes become ill.
- The disease risk for children of heterozygous parents is 25%; 50% of the children are healthy carriers of the trait and 25% of the children do not have an altered gene.
- Daughters and sons are affected with equal frequency.
- Patients do not occur in every generation.
- Patients are more often children of parents who are related.

Many metabolic diseases are autosomal recessive, e.g.:
- Mucoviscidosis (p. 161)
- Alpha$_1$-antitrypsin deficiency, which can lead to emphysema (p. 149) and to liver cirrhosis (p. 192)
- Galactosemia, a relatively rare disease of carbohydrate metabolism with serious consequences.

Inheritance pattern

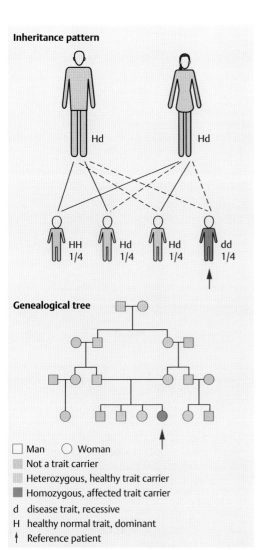

Fig. 2.4 Autosomal recessive inheritance

Man   Woman
Not a trait carrier
Heterozygous, healthy trait carrier
Homozygous, affected trait carrier
d   disease trait, recessive
H   healthy normal trait, dominant
↑   Reference patient

Inheritance pattern

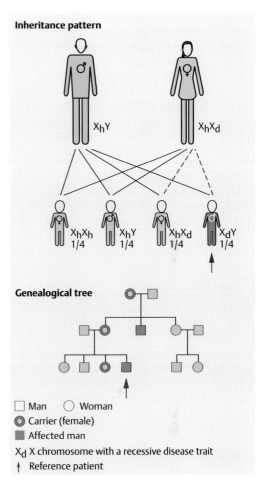

Man   Woman
Carrier (female)
Affected man
X_d X chromosome with a recessive disease trait
↑ Reference patient

Fig. 2.5 X-linked recessive inheritance.

Because of an enzyme deficiency, galactose, a component of the milk sugar lactose, cannot be broken down. The accumulation of galactose in the liver, kidneys and brain can be lethal.

- Phenylketonuria, an enzyme deficiency in which the amino acid phenylalanine can no longer be transformed into tyrosine. The main consequences of phenylalanine accumulation and tyrosine deficiency are cerebral seizures, psychomotor retardation, and pigment disorders.

X-Linked Recessive

This inheritance pathway is also called *gonosomal recessive*. A female carrier of a trait can compensate the tendency to the disease on one sex chromosome completely with the other normal X chromosome and as a result, she is healthy. But since a man cannot compensate the mutated gene on his X chromosome with his Y chromosome, he will become ill. **Figure 2.5** shows the rules of X-linked recessive inheritance:

- The disease is found almost exclusively in men. Hypothetically, the disease can occur in a girl if she is the daughter of a patient and a trait carrier.
- A heterozygous, clinically unremarkable individual with the trait is called a carrier. She passes on the disease to her sons with a probability of 50%; 50% of her daughters will also be carriers.

- A man who is affected cannot pass the disease on to his sons, since they will receive a Y chromosome from him. His daughters receive the X chromosome with the abnormal gene and are carriers.
- Patients are more often children of parents who are related.
- The disease can also arise from a new mutation.

Examples of Diseases That Are Passed On by Gonosomal Recessive Inheritance
- Hemophilia A and B (bleeders' disease; p. 253)
- Duchenne muscular dystrophy, which leads to atrophy of striated muscle and thus to progressive paralysis. Since no causal treatment is known, affected patients die at the age of about 20 years from the consequences of respiratory paralysis and heart failure.
- Red–green color blindness

X-Linked Dominant

X-linked dominant inheritance, that is also called gonosomal dominant, is rare. Since the gene of only one X chromosome needs to be altered for the hereditary disease to manifest itself, both sexes can be affected. Boys, who do not have an intact gene to compensate the mutated one, are usually very strongly affected and generally die very early.

Examples of Diseases That Are Passed On by Gonosomal Dominant Inheritance
- Rett syndrome with cerebral atrophy, short stature, and vitamin D-resistant rickets
- Alport syndrome with renal insufficiency and loss of hearing

■ Multifactorial Diseases

Multifactorial diseases are frequently familial. They result from the interaction between:
- Genetic tendency in which several gene loci are involved and
- Environmental factors

In addition to physical characteristics such as height, weight, hair color and intelligence, many diseases are multifactorially determined, e.g.:
- Obesity (p. 222)
- Diabetes mellitus (p. 215)
- Atopic dermatitis (eczema) (p. 27)
- Arterial hypertension (p. 117)
- Schizophrenia

Rules of Thumb for Genetic Counseling
- If one parent or one child is affected, the risk of repetition in another child is 2%–5%.
- If two relatives in the first degree are affected, the risk of repetition in another child is 10%–15%. Relatives in the first degree are parents and siblings.

Disrupted Prenatal Development

Normal Development

Normal prenatal development lasts for 280 days (±10 days). This is equal to 40 weeks of pregnancy, or 9 calendar months, or 10 lunar months of 28 days each. A pregnancy can be divided into three phases:
- The development of the blastocyst covers the period from fertilization to implantation and lasts about 15 days.
- Embryonic development begins with implantation and ends with the 8th week of pregnancy. The first 3 months of pregnancy, or the first trimester, are often simply called the embryonic period (**Table 2.2**). During this time, all organ systems are laid out. **Figure 2.6** illustrates organogenesis and shows that a distinct period of time is specified for each "construction phase."
- The fetal phase lasts from the 9th week of pregnancy to birth, or for the second and third trimesters. During this time, the organism grows and some organs already begin to function.

Table 2.2 Simplified overview of prenatal development and its disturbances

First trimester	Embryonic phase: organogenesis	• Miscarriage • Embryopathy
Second trimester	Fetal phase: growth and differentiation	• Miscarriage • Stillbirth • Premature birth • Fetopathy
Third trimester		

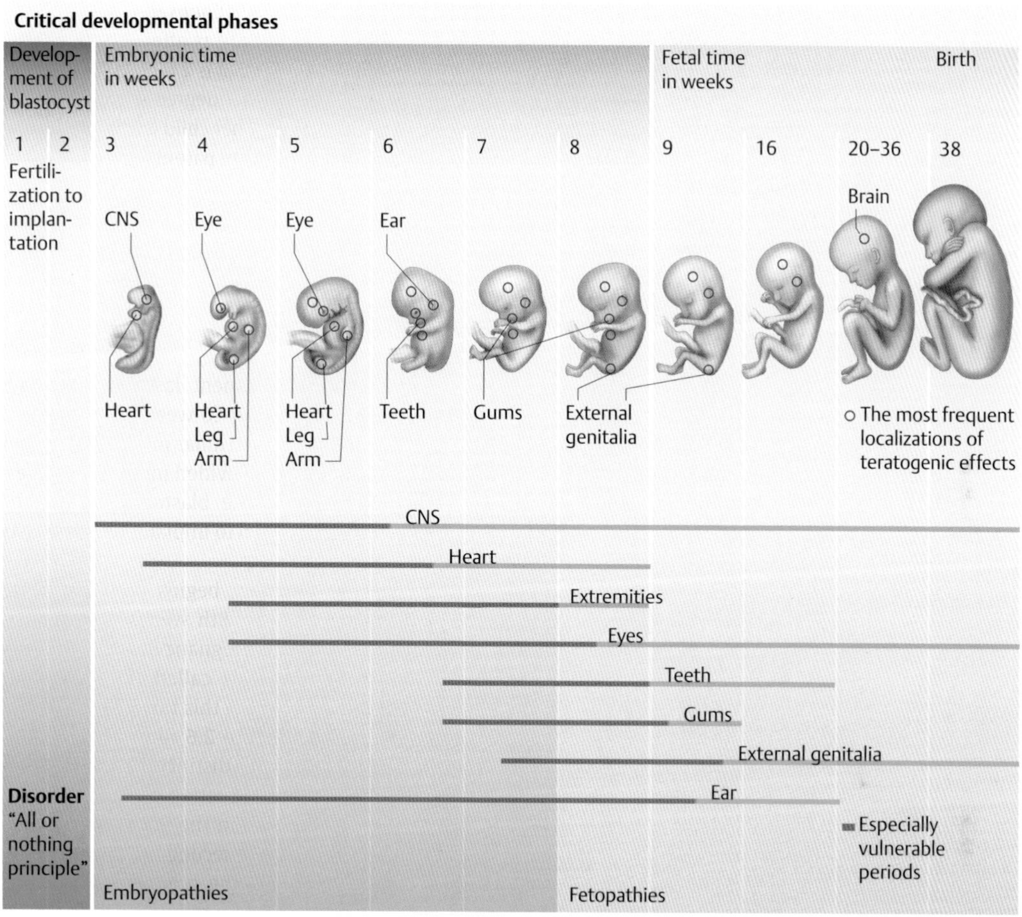

Critical developmental phases

Fig. 2.6 Embryonic and fetal development.

Harmful Influences

Numerous physical, chemical and biological influences as well as illnesses of the mother can damage embryofetal development. Possible consequences are disruption of growth, disruption of function, or malformations or death of the fetus. Exogenous factors that can lead to malformations are called *teratogens*.

- The primary physical teratogen is radiation, for instance X-radiation.
- Important chemical teratogens are alcohol, nicotine and medications such as Contergan (thalidomide) (**Fig. 2.7**).
- Maternal infections can be transmitted to the child by diaplacental transmission, during birth or through the mother's milk. **Table 2.3** summarizes the effects of the most important prenatal infectious diseases.

- Other influences on embryofetal development are diabetes mellitus (p. 215) and blood group incompatibility.

"All-or-nothing" Principle

Before implantation, the all-or-nothing principle operates. That is, that in the first 2 weeks of pregnancy, teratogens either lead to an early miscarriage or create no lasting damage, so that the embryo continues to develop normally.

Embryopathies

Disruptions of organogenesis lead either to intrauterine embryonic death or to malformations, called embryopathies. Their localization and expression

Table 2.3 Consequences of the chief prenatal infections

Illness	Transmission pathway	Consequences	Page

Rubella	Diaplacental	• Rubella embryopathy (Gregg syndrome) with:
		  – CNS involvement
		  – Congenital heart defects
		  – Inner ear involvement
		  – Eye involvement
			17

Cytomegaly	• Diaplacental
	• Perinatal
	• During nursing
		• First trimester: miscarriage
		• Second and third trimesters: fetopathy with:
		  – CNS involvement
		  – Pneumonia
		  – Enlargement of liver and spleen
		  – Anemia
		  – Loss of hearing
			278

Toxo-plasmosis	Diaplacental	• Fetopathy with:
		  – Encephalitis, intracerebral calcification and hydrocephalus
		  – Chorioretinitis, i.e., inflammation of the retina and choroid
		  – Hepatosplenomegaly, i.e., enlargement of liver and spleen
		  – Myocarditis
		  – Interstitial pneumonia
		• Possible miscarriage or stillbirth
			284

Syphilis	Diaplacental	• Congenital syphilis with:
		  – Changes in skin and mucosa
		  – Pneumonia
		  – Meningitis and hydrocephalus
		  – Osteomyelitis and
		  – Deafness as early symptoms
		  – Late symptoms like saddle nose, deformities of teeth and skeleton have become rare.
		• Possible miscarriage or stillbirth
			281

Hepatitis B	Perinatal	Chronic hepatitis B with danger of liver cirrhosis and liver carcinoma in 90% of infected children	192
HIV	• Perinatal • Rarely diaplacental and during nursing	• Failure to thrive • Enlargement of lymph nodes, liver and spleen • Neurological symptoms • Relapsing infectious diseases • AIDS appears earlier than in adults	283

depend on the time of the damage as well as on the type and intensity of the teratogens.

Examples of Embryopathies
• Rubella embryopathy (**Table 2.3**)
• Thalidomide embryopathy (**Fig. 2.7**)

Fetopathies

Damaging influences in the second and third trimesters lead to fetopathies. These are characterized by:
• Delayed growth
• Disrupted differentiation
• Inflammatory changes
  and sometimes also
• Miscarriage, death, or premature birth

One example is toxoplasmosis fetopathy (**Table 2.3**).

In some cases, embryopathy and fetopathy are difficult to distinguish from each other, for example, embryofetal alcohol syndrome (**Fig. 2.8**).

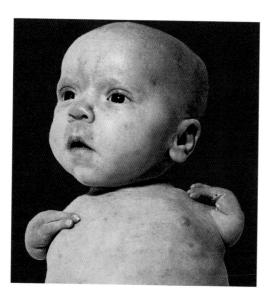

Fig. 2.7 Thalidomide embryopathy: Between 1958 and 1963, use during pregnancy of the sedative thalidomide, which was originally considered unproblematic in the Western industrialized nations, led to malformations of extremities. (Riede 2004.)

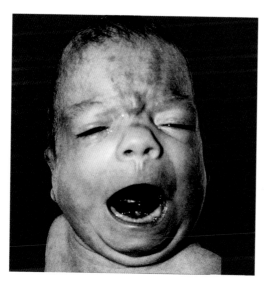

Fig. 2.8 Facial dysmorphy in embryofetal alcohol syndrome, with oblique and drooping eyelids, shortened nasal bridge, narrow lips, and small chin; the children are also notable for low birth weight and delayed cognitive and sensorimotor development. (Riede 2004.)

Infectious Diseases

■ Basic Concepts

Infection and Infectious Diseases

Although these two terms are often used interchangeably in colloquial speech, they are differentiated in medical language:

- The concept of *infection* describes the transmission, adhesion, penetration, and multiplication of microorganisms such as bacteria and viruses in the human body.
- It is only when symptoms appear that the term *infectious disease* is used.

Whether an infection will be clinically silent or have the course of a manifest infectious disease depends on the immune status of the infected person and the pathogenicity (virulence) of the microorganism:

- Microorganisms that trigger an infectious disease in every person infected for the first time are designated as *obligate pathogens.*
- In Europe and North America, however, *facultative pathogens* play a greater part. These trigger signs of disease largely in older or immune compromised patients. A disease triggered by a facultative pathogen is called an *opportunistic infectious disease.* If this disease is contracted in a hospital, it is called a *nosocomial infectious disease.*

Chain of Infection

The concept of chain of infection describes the pathway of a pathogen or of an infectious disease:

- The source of infection
- The transmission pathway
- The host, which can become a source of infection

Sources of Infection and Modes of Transmission

Exogenous Infection

Animate and inanimate pathogen reservoirs can serve as sources of infection.

- Animate sources of infection are human beings and animals.
- Examples of inanimate sources of infection are air, water, food, implements, and textiles.

The microorganisms can be transmitted directly or indirectly from the source of infection to the host. Indirect transmission can take place, for instance, through contaminated hands, intermediate hosts and inanimate sources of infection such as air conditioners. The chief direct and indirect modes of transmission are summarized in **Table 2.4**.

Endogenous Infection

Endogenous infections are triggered by microorganisms residing in the body. For instance, intestinal flora can lead to urinary tract infections. Tuberculosis (p. 268) or herpes zoster (shingles, p. 277) are caused by endogenous re-infection by their microorganisms.

Portals of Entry

In an infection, the microorganism must enter the host organism. The chief portals of entry are:
- (Smallest) skin or mucosal injuries
- Intact mucosa
- Insect stings (such as those causing borreliosis or malaria)

Some microorganisms can even be transmitted from mother to child before birth through the placenta. (**Table 2.3**).

Course of an Infectious Disease

- During the *infectious phase* the microorganisms penetrate into the organism.
- During the *incubation period* between infection and the first signs of disease, the pathogens multiply. Most infectious diseases have an incubation period of a few days to 3 weeks. Deviations outside these limits are possible.

> *The infected person can already be a source of infection during the incubation period.*

- After the incubation period comes the *disease phase.* The symptoms depend on the type of infectious disease as well as on the resistance of the patient and range from only slight impairment to life-threatening disease.
- Some infectious diseases result in a long-lasting *immunity* that protects the affected person against repeated illness due to the same pathogen. This fact is made use of in active inoculation.

Spread of an Infectious Disease

Epidemic

An epidemic is a time- and place-limited clustering of infectious disease. An epidemic results when only a few people are immune to obligate pathogens and the pathogens spread rapidly from person to person, e.g., an influenza epidemic.

Table 2.4 Direct and indirect paths of transmission of infections and infectious diseases

Transmission	Transmission pathway;		Examples	Page
Direct	Contact or smear infection	Fecal–oral	• Salmonellosis • Hepatitis A	271 192
	Droplet infection	Airborne	• Pneumonias • Tuberculosis • Chickenpox	155 268 276
	Blood	Hematogenous	• Hepatitis B and C • HIV	192 283
	Water and nutrients	Alimentary	• Salmonellosis • Hepatitis A	271 192
Indirect	Contaminated hands of medical personnel		Almost everything	
	Inanimate sources of infection, e.g., air conditioners, nebulizers		Pneumonias	155
	Intermediate hosts		• Malaria • Tick-borne diseases • Tapeworms	285 279

Pandemic

In a pandemic, the infectious disease is not limited to one location but spreads over a continent or the whole world.

Endemic

In an endemic, the pathogen is widespread in one region and always present. In this region it is particularly children and visitors who fall ill, since the older local residents have already become immune as a result of previous infection.

■ Microorganisms

In this section we will discuss *bacteria* and *viruses* in detail and compare them (**Table 2.5**). Finally, the most important *fungi* and *protozoa* which are pathogenic for humans will be introduced.

Bacteria

Structure

Bacteria are microorganisms about 0.3–2 µm in size. **Figure 2.9** shows the typical basic structure of *prokaryotes*. This differs from the structure of eukaryotic cells of higher organisms in the following points:

- The nuclear membrane is lacking, so that the genetic information lies in the cytoplasm as "naked" strands of DNA. The genome of the bacterial cell is termed a *nuclear equivalent* or *nucleoid*.
- In addition to the nucleoid, many bacteria have circular DNA structures in their cytoplasm termed *plasmids*. Plasmids are very important as

carriers of virulence factors and characteristics of resistance to antibiotics.
- Cellular organelles such endoplasmic reticulum, Golgi apparatus, and mitochondria are absent. The enzymes required for metabolic processes are components of the cytoplasmic membrane in bacteria.
- In contrast to animal cells, bacteria have a *complex cell envelope* that gives the microorganisms their rigid shape and mechanical protection. This cell envelope is the attack point of some antibiotics.
- Some bacteria also have:
  - Capsules that protect against phagocytosis and thus represent a virulence factor
  - Flagella, whose propellerlike action enables the bacteria to move forward
  - Pili—short, rigid structures acting as adhesion organelles that facilitate colonization of the host organism

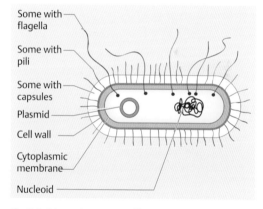

Some with flagella
Some with pili
Some with capsules
Plasmid
Cell wall
Cytoplasmic membrane
Nucleoid

Fig. 2.9 Schematic structure of bacteria

Table 2.5 Important differences between bacteria and viruses

Criteria	Bacteria	Viruses
Size	• 0.3–2 µm • Visible with the light microscope	• 25–250 nm • Visible only with the electron microscope
Structure	• Prokaryotes • Capable of metabolism	• No cellular structure • Incapable of metabolism • Need a host cell
Diagnosis	• Direct proof of a pathogen • Can be grown on culture medium	• Serology: indirect proof of pathogen by means of antibodies formed • Can only be grown in cell cultures
Therapy	• Usually causal treatment with an antibiotic	• Usually symptomatic therapy

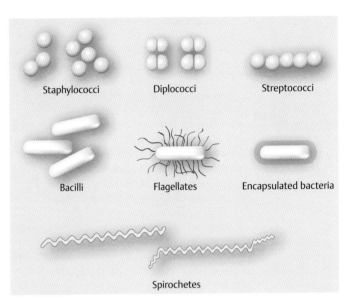

Fig. 2.10 Typical bacterial shapes

Staphylococci

Diplococci

Streptococci

Bacilli

Flagellates

Encapsulated bacteria

Spirochetes

Classification

Bacteria can be divided into different groups, chiefly on the basis of the following characteristics:

- External shape (**Fig. 2.10**)
- Ability to form spores
- Need for oxygen

Basic Forms

- *Cocci* (Greek denoting rounded shape) are spherical bacteria with a diameter of about 1 µm. Depending on the grouping, a difference is made between:
  - Diplococci, which exist in pairs
  - Staphylococci, in which the spherical bacteria form large clumps (p. 273)
  - Streptococci, in which the spherical bacteria form chains
- In *bacilli*, one axis is much longer than the other. At their poles, bacilli can be either pointed, rounded or almost rectangular.
- There are *screw-shaped bacteria* with turns of different diameters.

Spores

When nutrients are lacking or under other adverse external conditions, certain bacteria can form spores, which are cell forms with extremely low metabolism. Spore formation begins with constriction of the cell membrane. The DNA-containing portion is "wrung out" and the considerable water loss leaves a resistant, lasting form of the genome behind. This is resistant to desiccation, strong heat, radiation, and chemicals and can survive for decades. Under favorable conditions, the form capable of reproduction develops again.

Need for Oxygen

- *Aerobic* bacteria require oxygen to produce energy from glucose and other carbohydrates.
- *Anaerobic* bacteria are oxygen-independent. They produce energy by fermentation.

Reproduction

Bacteria reproduce asexually by binary fission. One mother cell produces two daughter cells that subsequently themselves divide. In this way, a number of identical cells arise from a single cell of origin and are termed stem cells or clone.

Reproduction Rate

The reproduction rate depends on the composition of the culture medium and the incubation temperature. Most medically relevant bacteria have a temperature optimum of between 36 and 43 °C.

Under optimal conditions, the doubling time can range from 15 minutes (e.g., for *Escherichia coli* and *Staphylococcus aureus*) to 20 hours for tuberculosis pathogens.

Reproductive Stages

If a small quantity of bacteria is placed in a culture medium and incubated, the number of microorganisms changes in a characteristic pattern (**Fig. 2.11**).

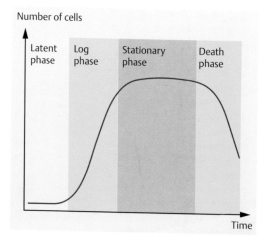

Fig. 2.11 Bacterial growth curve

- *Latent phase:* At first, in spite of favorable conditions, the number of organisms remains constant. To be able to use the available nutrients, the bacteria must first synthesize the necessary enzymes.
- *Logarithmic or exponential phase:* The rate of reproduction has reached its maximum and does not change.
- *Stationary phase:* Growth comes to a standstill, i.e., the size of the population does not change. Growth is limited by a lack of nutrients and the accumulation of metabolic products.
- *Death phase:* The number of bacteria decreases. The causes of this decrease are largely unknown.

The natural course of a disease reflects these phases.

Diagnosis

Materials used for microbiological examination are:
- Body fluids such as blood, urine and cerebrospinal fluid
- Stool
- Secretions with increased production, e.g., sputum
- Smears, e.g., wound smears

To avoid contamination, the material must be collected with care, adhering to hygiene standards. In addition, the appropriate transport and storage mode must be selected so that the microorganisms do not die or reproduce; possibilities include interim storage in a refrigerator or warming cabinet.

Testing Procedures

- Bacteria, like fungi and protozoa, are visible in stained and unstained preparations under the light microscope. Observation of the *native preparation* immediately after sample collection provides a first orientation concerning the causal pathogen. However, microscopic examination of the native preparation is often unsuccessful because of a low bacterial count, so that first the organism must multiply in culture medium.
- To grow a *bacterial culture*, the study material is transferred to a suitable nutrient medium and placed in an incubator. Under these circumstances, the microorganisms multiply rapidly on solid nutrient and form visible colonies that can then be studied further.
- *Identification of antigens* without previous culturing of pathogens is gaining increasing practical importance. For some bacteria, there are already quick tests that can identify the microorganism within minutes.

Antibiogram

After the microorganism has been identified, an antibiogram is prepared. In this sensitivity test, it is determined whether the addition of certain antibiotics inhibits the growth of the bacteria. The result of the test permits targeted antibiotic treatment.

Therapy

The causal treatment of an infectious disease is administration of an antibiotic.

Viruses

Structure

A virus particle is termed a *virion*. It is between 25 and 250 nm in size and has an extremely simple structure (**Fig. 2.12**).
- *Nucleic acid*, the carrier of genetic information, is always present. Viruses contain either DNA or RNA.
- The nucleic acid is surrounded by a *capsid*. The building blocks of this protective coat are the capsomeres.
- An additional outer *shell* occurs in only a few viruses.

There are no cell organelles, so that viruses exhibit no cell structure. They are "vagabond genes" that require host cells for their metabolic processes and reproduction.

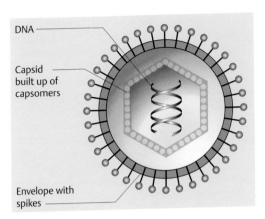

DNA

Capsid built up of capsomers

Envelope with spikes

Fig 2.12 Schematic structure of a virion.

Classification

Currently accepted virus systematics is built on four classification criteria.

- DNA and RNA viruses are distinguished according to the *type of nucleic acid.* The nucleic acid can be present as a double or a single strand. Usually virus DNA is present as a double strand while virus RNA is present as a single strand.
- Under the electron microscope, it is possible to recognize the *shape of the capsid,* which may be cylindrical, spherical, or icosahedral. (An icosahedron has 20 faces.)
- A *shell* may be absent or present.
- *Enzymes* such as polymerases may be absent or present.

Reproduction

Virus replication proceeds according to the same mechanisms as those for metabolic function. The virus particle channels its genetic information into the nucleus of the infected cell, thus delivering to it the complete program of synthesis for future generations of viruses. Production of them is taken over by the host cell's machinery. The replication cycle of viruses can be subdivided into the following phases (**Fig. 2.13**):

- In *attachment,* the virion adheres to the host cell. Many viruses exhibit an organ tropism. This means that they bond only with very specific target cells, e.g., hepatitis viruses attack liver cells exclusively (p. 192). In this phase, the virion is still free at the surface of the cell and can be attacked by antibodies.
- In the *penetration* phase, the virus particle penetrates into the host cell.

- The *eclipse* phase encompasses the replication stages, during which no complete virus particles are visible in the infected cell. First the virion sheds its capsid (uncoating). The exposed nucleic acid is integrated into the host cell and serves as a blueprint for the virus that is implemented by the organelles of the infected cell.
- After the *assembly* of the individual virus building blocks, complete virus particles, capable of producing infection, emerge from the host cell. *Virus release* takes place through ejection or lysis of the host cell.

The host cell can perish during virus replication. The symptoms of the infectious disease result from cell death and the immune response of the individual, e.g., fever.

Diagnosis

Direct demonstration of the virus is diagnostically difficult because:

- Being very small, viruses can only be seen with the electron microscope.
- Viruses do not have their own metabolic process, so they cannot be cultured on nutrient medium but only in cell cultures.

Serology

Because of the difficulties listed above, in practice viral infection is demonstrated indirectly by determining the *antibodies* that are formed.

Therapy

Virustatics that inhibit the multiplication of viruses exist for only a few types of viruses. Usually, viral diseases are treated symptomatically.

▍ *Most viral diseases cannot be treated with antibiotics.*

Fungi

There are more than 100 000 species of fungi, of which about 100 species are human pathogens. However, their pathogenicity is usually low, so that they are facultative pathogens that can only lead to an infectious disease if the host's local or generalized resistance in low. A fungal disease is called a *mycosis.*

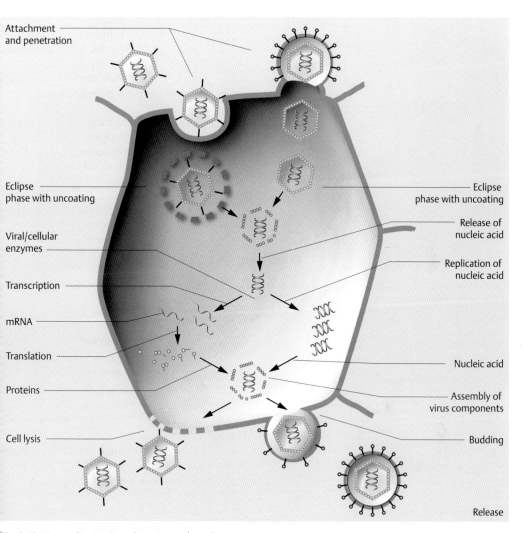

Attachment
and penetration

Eclipse
phase with uncoating

Viral/cellular
enzymes

Transcription

mRNA

Translation

Proteins

Cell lysis

Eclipse
phase with uncoating

Release of
nucleic acid

Replication of
nucleic acid

Nucleic acid

Assembly of
virus components

Budding

Release

Fig. 2.13 Virus replication (two alternative pathways).

Structure

Fungi are eukaryotes; they may be unicellular or multicellular. Medically relevant unicellular fungi are about 10 times larger and more highly organized than bacteria but less well organized than plant or animal cells.

• In contrast to plant cells, fungi have no chlorophyll, so that they cannot carry on photosynthesis but must rely on carbohydrate-containing nutrients brought in from the outside.

• In contrast to animal cells, fungi have a cell wall that gives them their rigidity and immobility. Asexual reproduction takes place by budding.

Classification

Fungal human pathogens are classified as dermatophytes, yeasts, or molds.

• *Dermatophytes* cause mycoses of the skin and cutaneous appendages, i.e., hair and nails.

• *Yeasts* cause mycoses of the skin and mucosa. The most important members of this group are the *Candida* species that can lead to the typical white coating on mucosa (**Fig. 2.14a, b**).

• The most important members of the molds are the *Aspergillus* species that in cases of severely compromised resistance can attack internal organs, causing, e.g., *Aspergillus* pneumonia.

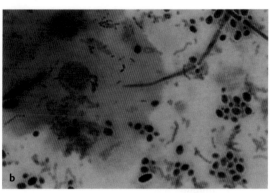

Fig. 2.14a, b Thrush (Jung 1998). **a** White deposits (which can be scraped off) on reddened, painful, and easily injured oral mucosa. **b** Microscopic image of scrapings from the oral cavity with Gram stain.

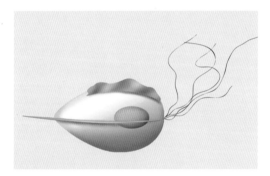

Fig. 2.15 *Trichomonas vaginalis*

Protozoa

Protozoa are animal unicellular organisms that can move about with flagella (**Fig. 2.15**). Since they prefer evenly warm surroundings, they are usually found in equatorial regions as the cause of tropical diseases such as malaria (p. 285) and amebic dysentery.

In the European and North American latitudes, only toxoplasmosis (p. 284) and trichomoniasis play a role. Trichomoniasis is a vaginal inflammation (vaginitis) caused by *Trichomonas vaginalis*.

Disturbed Immune Reactions

The organism has a variety of *defense mechanisms* available to ward off harmful substances, e.g.:
- The acid mantle that protects the skin
- The mucosal barrier of the gastrointestinal tract and the bronchial system
- Certain proteins and enzymes, e.g., the complement system, C-reactive protein
- Various leukocytes and lymphocyte species that, among other functions, act as scavenger cells

In addition, there is a *specialized defensive system,* the actual immune system, that develops targeted antibodies against potentially harmful substances foreign to the body. The bearers of the immune system are the lymphocytes, which develop from stem cells in the bone marrow and, during the embryonic phase, settle in the lymphatic organs of the body, such as the spleen, lymph nodes, and intestinal wall.

B lymphocytes have the capability of forming specific antibodies against substances foreign to the body. Other lymphocytes mature in the thymus gland and are therefore called *T lymphocytes*. They learn to differentiate between substances proper to the body and substances foreign to the body. Substances foreign to the body are recognized as antigens which trigger an immune response. Depending on their surface markers and their function, T-lymphocytes are classified as:

- *T helper cells* that recognize foreign substances and transmit information to the B lymphocytes, which then produce specific antibodies. T helper cells produce mediator substances that activate generalized resistance, e.g., scavenger cells.
- *T killer cells* can recognize, attack, and destroy foreign cells (e.g., after transplantation) or cells that have become foreign (e.g., virus-infected or denatured cells).
- *T suppressor cells* suppress an overshoot in activity of the T helper cells.
- *Memory cells* remember a foreign substance once it has invaded the body so that at a later secondary encounter they can immediately react by producing antibodies that will fend off the disease. This mechanism forms the basis of immunization, wherein weakened or killed pathogens stimulate our body to an immune response. The memory cells and the resulting antibodies subsequently offer protection against natural infection with these pathogens.

The *antibodies* formed by the B lymphocytes (immunoglobulins, Ig) are proteins and can be differentiated according to their structures.
- IgM antibodies are formed as the first response to an antigen stimulus.
- In the second step, IgG antibodies are formed and remain present for months to years.
- IgA antibodies are formed chiefly in mucosa and provide a protective barrier there, e.g., in bronchi and the gastrointestinal tract.
- IgE antibodies mediate allergic reactions.

Antibodies bind to the foreign material (antigen), forming an antigen–antibody complex that activates a cascade of inflammatory and cell reaction with the objective of neutralizing the antigen.

This necessary reaction can generate an illness-causing reaction if the body's own tissues are damaged by the inflammatory and cell reactions. The following inappropriate immune reactions will be discussed in this chapter:
- Allergies
- Autoimmune diseases
- Immune deficiency syndromes

■ Allergies

An allergy is a hypersensitivity reaction to foreign substances. The organism responds to the secondary contact with an already-known antigen or allergen with an overshooting immune reaction.

Individuals inclined to this type of hypersensitivity reaction of skin and mucosa are said to be atopic. Atopic diathesis (tendency) is multifactorial, i.e., determined by the interplay of several genetic and environmental factors (p. 16). About 25% of the population in Western industrialized countries suffer from at least one disease in the atopic spectrum. These include:
- Allergic rhinitis (hay fever)
- Urticaria (hives)
- Allergic bronchial asthma (p. 153)
- Atopic dermatitis (eczema)

In 1949, Coombs and Gell described four immunopathological reactions that serve to improve understanding of hypersensitivity reactions.
- Type I and type IV reactions explain allergic processes.
- Type II and type III reactions explain autoimmune processes in which the hypersensitivity reaction is directed against the body's own structures (p. 29).

Type I Reaction

Pathological Mechanism

The type I reaction, also called the IgE-mediated immediate reaction, is based on a genetic predisposition and evolves in three phases (**Fig. 2.16**).
- *Sensitization phase:* The immune system responds to certain antigens (allergens) by producing an abnormally high number of specific type IgE immunoglobulins (antibodies). These attach to the surface of mast cells.
- *Secondary exposure to allergens:* On renewed contact, the specific allergen can bridge two neighboring IgE molecules so that the mast cell releases mediator substances such as histamine.
- *Anaphylactic reaction:* Within minutes, the released mediator substances cause constriction of the respiratory passages as well as local and systemic vasodilatation with increased capillary permeability, resulting in edema (p. 47).

▌ *The type I reaction is an immediate reaction.*

Clinical Examples

The following clinical pictures are brought about by the type I reaction described above:
- Rhinitis allergica (hay fever)
- Urticaria (hives), which can also be caused by physical and other irritants

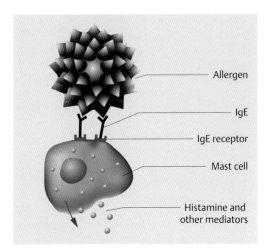

Fig. 2.16 Type I allergic reaction.

- Quincke edema (**Fig. 2.17**)
- Allergic bronchial asthma (p. 153)
- Anaphylactic shock (p. 54)

Diagnosis

Differential diagnosis is based on a detailed self and family history that may point to familial tendency, the time and duration of the complaint, and possible allergens.

In addition to the history, skin tests and laboratory studies are carried out in the symptom-free interval, in order to identify the allergen.

- In the *prick test,* a drop of allergen extract is applied to the inner arm and the skin is scratched through the drop with a lancet. If a wheal forms after 10–20 minutes, the prick test is positive.
- For the *intradermal test,* a small amount of allergen solution is injected into the dermis. This test is performed when there is a suspicion of allergy to penicillin or insect venom, both of which can also trigger an immediate allergic reaction.
- After sensitization has been confirmed by a prick or intradermal test, *provocation tests* directly at the affected organ can show that this allergen actually triggers the illness, e.g., conjunctival, nasal or inhalation provocation.
- The *total IgE* in the blood is only informative to a limited extent, since there are also other diseases that exhibit elevated IgE values.
- The *radioallergosorbent test* (RAST) can detect specific IgE antibodies against numerous allergens. This test documents sensitization, but the clinical significance for the patient remains in doubt.

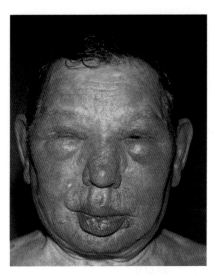

Fig. 2.17 Quincke edema. There is a danger of air hunger due to swelling of respiratory pathways. (Jung 1998.)

Therapy

If the identified allergens can be removed from the patient's environment, the patient will be free of complaints without further treatment. If these decontamination measures have only limited effectiveness, drug therapy or hyposensitization can be considered.

Drugs

- Disodium cromoglicinate (DNCG) stabilizes the mast cells and thus prevents histamine from being released.
- Antihistamines block the histamine receptors and prevent the action of histamine.
- Glucocorticosteroids also have an antiallergic effect (p. 77).

Hyposensitization

Hyposensitization is applied chiefly in case of allergic bronchial asthma and hay fever if the causal allergen cannot be completely avoided. The treatment is effective in 70% of individuals allergic to pollen, whereas only 50% of patients with allergies to dust mites or mold profit from it.

Over a period of 3 years, the identified allergen is injected subcutaneously in rising concentrations. This is intended to stimulate the production of IgG antibodies that capture the allergen upon subsequent exposure and thus avoid the type I reaction.

Type IV Reaction

Pathological Mechanism

The type IV reaction is mediated by sensitized T lymphocytes. On subsequent antigen exposure, these cells release mediator substances called lymphokines, which can sensitize other cells of the immune system such as macrophages and neutrophilic granulocytes (microphages) (**Fig. 2.18**). A tissue-damaging inflammatory reaction results. This damage is manifested by a type IV reaction after 24–72 hours, so that it is called a delayed reaction.

▪ *The type IV reaction is a delayed reaction.*

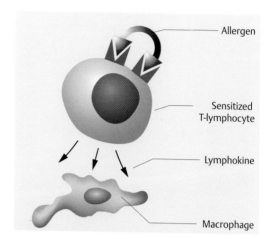

Fig. 2.18 Type IV allergic reaction.

Clinical Examples

- Contact allergies of the skin (**Fig. 2.19**)
- Tuberculin test (p. 268)
- Transplant rejection (p. 69)

Diagnosis of Contact Allergies

- Detailed medical history
- Clinical picture
- Epicutaneous test: Test strips with potential allergens are pasted onto the back. The skin reactions are read after 24, 48, and 72 hours (delayed reaction) (**Fig. 2.20**).

Therapy

- Removal of allergens to the greatest extent possible
- Application of glucocorticosteroids to the skin changes during the acute episode

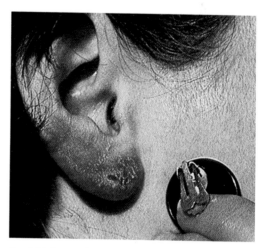

Fig. 2.19 Contact dermatitis in a patient with nickel allergy. (Riede 2004.)

▪ Autoimmune Diseases

Synonyms

- Autoaggressive diseases
- Autoimmunopathies

Overview

The immune system can differentiate the body's own structures from foreign structures, so that under normal circumstances the body does not attack itself. This autoimmune tolerance is suppressed in autoimmune diseases: Lymphocytes produce autoantibodies against the body's own antigens. An antigen–antibody complex results that elicits an inflammatory reaction and thus damage to cells and tissues. Depending on

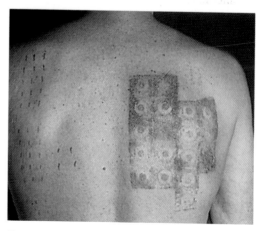

Fig. 2.20 Skin test after 24 hours: numerous positive reactions. An additional allergy to the test tape prevents accurate reading. (Jung 1998.)

Table 2.6 Overview of important autoimmune diseases

Group	Examples	Page
Systemic autoimmune diseases	• Systemic lupus erythematosus	261
	• Rheumatoid arthritis	256
	• Progressive systemic sclerosis	262
	• Dermatomyositis	264
	• Vasculitis	265
Organ-specific autoimmune diseases	• Endocrine organ tissue:	
	– Type 1 diabetes	215
	– Basedow disease	235
	– Hashimoto thyroiditis	236
	– Addison disease	241
	• Exocrine organ tissue:	179
	– Type A gastritis with pernicious anemia	
	• Other:	253
	– Immunothrombocytopenia	
	– Multiple sclerosis	
	– Myasthenia gravis	

the nature of the autoimmune disease, this process can be organ-specific or systemic (**Table 2.6**).

Diagnosis

- Medical history and clinical data
- Identification of antibodies in blood and biopsy material

Principles of therapy

Treatment depends on the disease picture.
- If endocrine organs are affected, hormone substitution is sufficient to treat the resulting deficient function.
- If a system is involved, such as the central nervous system, the immune system must be suppressed with drugs. Side-effects of immunosuppression are susceptibility to infection and increased risk of tumors.
- In rare cases, plasmapheresis can become necessary. In plasma exchange therapy, the patient's plasma, in which the autoantibodies are found, is replaced with a protein-containing solution. This therapy is applied cautiously because other important proteins, such as regularly produced antibodies and clotting factors, are also removed.

▣ Immune Deficiency Syndromes

Immune deficiency syndromes are disease pictures in which the response of the nonspecific or specific immune system to an antigen stimulus is insufficient or absent.

Causes

Leukopenia

Leukopenia is the fall of the total leukocyte count to below 5000/µL. The affected cells are usually the neutrophilic granulocytes (p. 242) that function in the immune system as scavenger cells. Causes are a disorder in cell formation or increased cell turnover.

The disorder in cell formation is caused by damage to the bone marrow that can be caused, for instance, by:
- Medications, e.g., cytostatics
- Chemicals, e.g., benzol
- Radiation, e.g., in oncological therapy (p. 67)
- Infiltration of the bone marrow by malignant tissues

Leukocytes can be destroyed by certain medications and autoimmune processes (p. 29).

B Cell Defects

B cell defects can be congenital or acquired and can affect the B lymphocytes themselves or their products, the immunoglobulins (Ig).
- The most important example of a congenital disorder is *isolated IgA deficiency*, which occurs at a frequency of 1:600. Since IgA occur predominantly in secretions of the respiratory tract or the gastrointestinal tract, where they form a protective barrier, individuals with this disorder suffer from frequent infections of the respiratory and gastrointestinal tracts.
- Immunoglobulins are proteins. Therefore, a *lack of proteins* caused by reduced intake or increased loss, e.g., in kidney disease or burns, can lead to an

acquired immune deficiency. Lymphomas spring-
ing from B lymphocytes can be the cause of an
acquired B cell defect (plasmocytoma, p. 252).

T cell defects

T cell defects are rare; they can also be congenital
or acquired.

- An example of a congenital T cell defect is the
Di George syndrome, in which the thymus is
not formed, so that the T lymphocytes are not
imprinted.
- Acquired disorders are due to viral diseases such
as HIV infection (p. 283), medications such as glucocorticosteroids (p. 77) and other immune suppressants, and T cell lymphomas.

Consequences

In addition to an increased risk of infection, patients
with immune deficiency have an increased risk of
tumors, since neoplastic cells are not recognized
and eliminated by the immune system.

Arteriosclerosis

Arteriosclerosis can be ascribed mainly to the
lifestyle of people in the Western industrialized
nations. It is often called "civilization disease" and
represents more than 50% of the causes of death.

Arteriosclerosis is a thickening and stiffening of
the vessel walls of the arteries, i.e., the arteries of
the high-pressure system (p. 85). Since the altered
vessels have a diameter of more than 2 mm, arteriosclerosis is also called macroangiopathy.

Pathogenesis

Figure 2.21a–e shows the structure of a vessel wall
and, in simplified form, how arteriosclerosis arises.

- At the beginning of the process, the intima is
damaged. The smallest endothelial injuries and
local inflammatory processes can be the triggering event.
- As a result of the endothelial defect, the intima
becomes porous and lipids find their way into the
vessel wall.
- The lipids are followed by macrophages, i.e., scavenger cells that intend to eliminate the lipids in
the vessel wall.
- At the same time the macrophages stimulate the
cells of the media, which now synthesize collagen

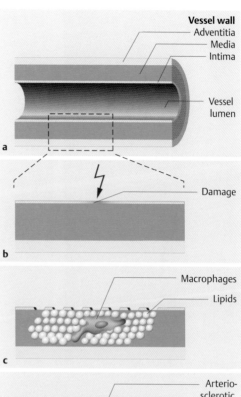

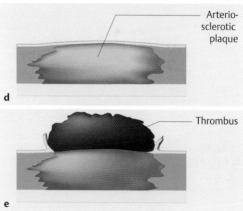

Fig. 2.21a–e Simplified depiction of vessel wall changes in
arteriosclerosis. **a** Longitudinal section through a vessel and
schematic structure of the vessel wall. **b** Damage to intima.
c Lipids enter the vessel wall through the porous intima,
macrophages follow. **d** Production of collagen and formation
of arteriosclerotic plaque. **e** Plaque rupture with subsequent
thrombus formation.

threads and lead to an arteriosclerotic plaque in
the vessel wall through the production of connective tissue. This stiffens the vessel wall and narrows the lumen of the vessel as the plaque grows
(**Fig. 2.22a, b**).

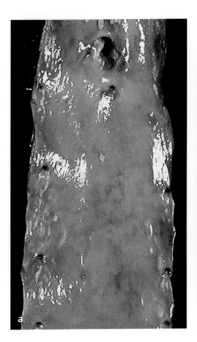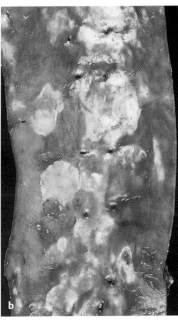

Fig. 2.22a, b Intact and arteriosclerotic vessels compared (Riede 2004). **a** Smooth intima of an unchanged aorta. **b** Aorta with pronounced arteriosclerotic plaques.

Table 2.7 Vascular risk factors

Risk factors unable to be influenced	Risk factors that can be influenced	Page

• Genetic disposition:
  – Coronary artery disease, myocardial infarction or stroke in first degree male relatives before the age of 55, in first degree female relatives before the age of 65
• Age:
  – Men older than 45
  – Women older than 55
	• Main risk factors
	  – High blood pressure
	  – Diabetes mellitus
	  – Lipid metabolism disorder
	  – Cigarette smoking
	• Other risk factors
	  – Obesity
	  – Lack of exercise
	  – Psychosocial risk factors like negative stress and low social status
	  – Changes in the clotting system
	  – Chronic inflammatory states
	  – Glucose metabolism disorders (pre-diabetes)
		117
		215
		220
		
		222

Risk Factors

The complex events that produce arteriosclerosis have not yet been elucidated in detail. What is certain is that various different risk factors play a decisive role. The most important risk factors currently known are listed in **Table 2.7**.

Consequences

Table 2.8 summarizes the possible consequences of arteriosclerosis.
- Coronary artery disease is the manifestation of arteriosclerosis in the coronary arteries.
- The blood vessels supplying the brain may also be affected. In that case, stroke and multi-infarct dementia are possible consequences.

Table 2.8 Possible consequences of arteriosclerosis

Clinical picture	Page
• Coronary artery disease (CAD)	98
• Myocardial infarction	101
• Cerebral arterial disease	123
• Stroke	
• Peripheral arterial disease (PAD)	123
• Acute occlusion of a limb artery	126
• Acute occlusion of a mesenteric artery (acute abdomen)	50
• Aortic dissection	127
• Aortic aneurysm	127

- Peripheral arterial occlusive disease is caused by an arteriosclerotic process in the arteries of the extremities.

Progressive changes in the arteriosclerotic sections of the vessels can present an acute threat for the patient.

- Plaque rupture can occur, in which the intima over the arteriosclerotic (unstable) plaque breaks up. The endothelial damage activates platelets and clotting, a thrombus is formed that occludes the vessel, e.g., in the case of a cardiac infarction (**Fig. 2.21e**).
- If parts of this thrombus are dislodged, a distal thromboembolic vessel occlusion can result.
- Bleeding into the plaques and into the vessel walls leads to dissection.
- Formation of a pouch in the weakened vessel wall is called an aneurysm.

Collateral Circulation

If blockage of a main blood vessel progresses very slowly, collateral vessels can create functional bypass circulation (**Fig. 7.2**). This is made up of blood vessels that branch off a main blood vessel and, running alongside it, supply the same target area. They arise from existing connections between two arteries that under physiological conditions make little or no contribution to blood supply. The opening up of such a natural bypass takes place when there is a chronic lack of oxygen in the area supplied.

> *Patients can make use of this effect, for instance, by promoting collateral vessels in peripheral artery disease through walking exercise (p. 123).*

Tumors

■ Overview

The term "tumor" can also be expressed more colloquially as a "lump"; it describes a growth of tissue that is not natural, regardless of the cause.

> *More specifically, the term "tumor" designates an abnormal tissue growth formed by an independent, excessive division of the body's cells.*

This formation made up of new tissue is also called a *neoplasm*. The structure and function of the lump vary to different degrees from those of the originating tissue. A tumor continues to grow even when the originating tissue is no longer functional. On the basis of the clinical course, it is possible to distinguish:

- Innocent or benign tumors
- Virulent or malignant tumors
- Semimalignant tumors

Benign Tumors

Benign tumors are usually separated from surrounding tissue by a connective tissue capsule. Since they grow slowly, displacing other structures, they often remain unnoticed for some time. Sometimes they can hardly be distinguished histologically from the mother tissue. Benign tumors do not move to other parts of the body; that is, they do not form metastases (**Fig. 2.23a**).

> ■ *Benign tumors grow by simple expansion.*

Malignant Tumors

Malignant tumors grow quickly and penetrate surrounding tissue aggressively, destroying it with their invasive growth (**Fig. 2.23b**). Since malignant tumors can also penetrate into lymph and blood vessels, distant colonies can be formed. The different pathways for metastasis are explained on page 34. On microscopic examination it can be seen that the tumor tissue hardly resembles its tissue of origin.

> ■ *Malignant tumors grow invasively and destructively, and they metastasize.*

Benign and malignant tumors are compared in **Table 2.9**.

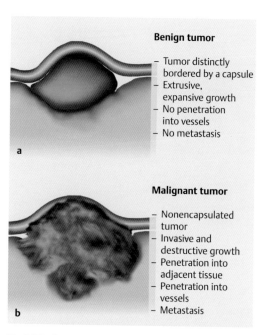

Benign tumor
- Tumor distinctly bordered by a capsule
- Extrusive, expansive growth
- No penetration into vessels
- No metastasis

a

Malignant tumor
- Nonencapsulated tumor
- Invasive and destructive growth
- Penetration into adjacent tissue
- Penetration into vessels
- Metastasis

b

Fig. 2.23a, b Morphological and biological features of benign and malignant tumors compared.

Table 2.9 Important differences between benign and malignant tumors

Differences		Benign tumors	Malignant tumors
Pathological anatomical	Growth form	Expansive, space occupying	• Infiltrating • Invasive, destructive
	Tumor capsule	Present	Absent
	Mitosis rate and cell content	Low	High
	Cell size and shape	Uniform	Heterogeneous
	Nucleus size and shape	Uniform	Heterogeneous
	Tissue type	Mature, differentiated	Usually immature, undifferentiated
	Necroses	Seldom	Frequently
Clinical	Patients' age	Primarily young and middle-aged people	Primarily older people
	Symptoms	Very few symptoms	Many symptoms late
	Course without treatment	• Long course • Rarely fatal	• Short course • Almost always fatal
	Metastases	Absent	Frequently
	Relapsing	Seldom	Frequently

Semimalignant Tumors

Although semimalignant tumors behave like malignant tumors in that they also grow invasively and destructively, the difference is that they do not metastasize.

Semimalignant tumors grow invasively and destructively but they do not metastasize.

Tumor Nomenclature

The naming of benign and malignant tumors depends on the cell of origin. The distinction is whether a neoplasm originates in epithelial or non-epithelial tissue (**Table 2.10**).

Epithelial Tumors

Epithelial tissue is a covering. It lines exterior and interior body surfaces as well as efferent glandular ducts.
- Benign epithelial tumors are called papillomas or adenomas. The latter originate in glandular epithelium.
- Malignant epithelial tumors are called carcinomas. In adults, they constitute up to 90% of all cancerous diseases.

Carcinomas are malignant tumors that originate in epithelial tissue.

Nonepithelial Tumors

Nonepithelial tumors originate, for instance, in connective tissue, muscle tissue, or nervous tissue.
- In benign nonepithelial tumors, the name of the cell of origin is followed by the suffix -*oma* (from Greek for "mass" or "lump").
- Malignant nonepithelial tumors are called sarcomas. Only about 1% of all malignant neoplasms are sarcomas.

Sarcomas are malignant nonepithelial tumors.

General Oncology

"Onkos" is the Greek word for a tumor. Oncology is the medical discipline that studies the diagnosis and therapy of *malignant* tumors.

Frequency

Adults

According to National Cancer Institute projections, there were 1 529 560 new cases of cancer in 2010,

Table 2.10 Systematics of epithelial and nonepithelial tumors (selection)

	Original cell		Benign tumor	Malignant tumor
Epithelial tumors	Squamous epithelium		Papilloma	Squamous epithelium carcinoma
	Glandular epithelium		Adenoma	Adenocarcinoma
Nonepithelial tumors	Connective and supporting tissue	Fibrocyte	Fibroma	Fibrosarcoma
		Fat cell	Lipoma	Liposarcoma
		Chondrocyte	Chondroma	Chondrosarcoma
		Osteocyte	Osteoma	Osteosarcoma
	Muscle tissue	Transversely striated muscle cell	Rhabdomyoma	Rhabdomyosarcoma
		Smooth muscle cell	Leiomyoma	Leiomyosarcoma
	Nervous tissue	Autonomic nerve cell	Gangliocytoma	(Ganglio-) neuroblastoma
		Schwann cell	Neurinoma	Neurogenic sarcoma
	Other	Vessels	Hemangioma Lymphangioma	Angiosarcoma
		Melanocytes	Melanocyte nevus	Malignant melanoma

Table 2.11 The most frequent cancer types in men (estimates of the Robert Koch Institute, 2006)

Rank	Cancer type	New cases per year	Page
1	Prostate carcinoma	60 100	–
2	Colon carcinoma	36 300	185
3	Bronchial carcinoma	32 500	157
4	Urinary bladder carcinoma	19 300	–
5	Stomach carcinoma	10 600	181
6	Kidney carcinoma	9000	213
7	Carcinoma in oral cavity and throat	7900	–
8	Lymphomas	7500	250
9	Malignant melanoma	7400	–
10	Pancreas carcinoma	6400	200
11	Leukemia	5100	247
12	Testicular tumors	5000	–
Total		approx. 229 000	

and 569 490 deaths were estimated for 2010. Tumor statistics are different for men and for women. The most frequent diseases in adults are presented in **Table 2.11** and **Table 2.12**.

▊ *Cancer is the second most frequent cause of death.*

Table 2.12 The most frequent cancer types in women (estimates of the Robert Koch Institute, 2006)

Rank	Cancer type	New cases per year	Page
1	Breast cancer	58 000	–
2	Colon carcinoma	32 400	185
3	Bronchial carcinoma	14 600	157
4	Endometrial carcinoma	11 100	–
5	Ovarian tumors	9700	–
6	Malignant melanoma	8500	–
7	Urinary bladder carcinoma	8100	–
8	Lymphomas	7200	250
9	Stomach carcinoma	7200	181
10	Pancreas carcinoma	7000	200
11	Kidney carcinoma	5800	213
12	Leukemia	4200	247
Total		approx. 198 000	

Children

After accidents, cancer is the second most frequent cause of death in children. According to the National Cancers Institute's most recent published figures (2007) approximately 10 400 children under age 15 were diagnosed in 2007 with cancer. In this age group, cancer is the most frequent cause of death after accidents.

The spectrum of malignant diseases in children is markedly different from the spectrum in adults, in whom carcinomas predominate with a frequency up to 90%. In children, carcinomas, originating in the skin or the mucosa, constitute only a bare 10% of all types of cancer. Children are much more likely to develop:

- Leukemia (about 35%, p. 247)
- Brain tumors (about 25%)
- Lymphomas (about 10%, p. 250)
- Neuroblastomas, originating in the sympathetic nervous system
- Nephroblastomas, originating in kidney tissue and also called Wilms tumors
- Bone tumors

Causes

Cells integrate themselves structurally and functionally into tissue and then into organs and entire organisms. For these purposes, each cell possesses numerous genes with control functions:

- Control of its own genome
- Control of cell growth
- Control of differentiation
- Control of the relationship with neighboring cells
- Control of programmed cell death

When several such genes in a cell are changed without being repaired, the cell changes step by step into a tumor cell. In simple terms, all factors that shift the balance between mutation rate and capacity for repair toward an increased mutation rate lead to the appearance of a tumor.

Age

Many malignant tumors predominantly manifest themselves in the elderly. The appearance of a tumor is based on the sum of genetic defects that exceeds a certain threshold value only in later years.

Nutrition

It is difficult to determine to what extent nutritional habits play a role in the development of cancer since they cannot be observed in isolation from other

Table 2.13 Important currently known carcinogens and their effects

Carcinogens	Occurrence	Resulting tumors
Polycyclic aromatic hydrocarbons, e.g.: • Benzopyrene • Benzanthracene	Substances contained in tar, soot, and smoke fumes	Tumors in numerous organs, e.g., bronchial carcinoma (p. 157)
Halogenated hydrocarbons, e.g., vinyl chloride	PVC-processing industry	• Angiosarcoma of the liver • Glioblastoma
Nitrosamines formed from nitrates and nitrite in pickling salt	• Meat and sausage • Fertilizer residue	Tumors of the gastrointestinal tract: • Stomach carcinoma (p. 181) • Colon carcinoma (p. 185)
Aromatic amines, e.g., aniline	Dye industry	Urinary bladder cancer
Mycotoxins, especially aflatoxin, the poison of the mold *Aspergillus flavus*	• Wheat • Spices • Nuts	Liver cell carcinoma (p. 196)
Arsenic	Previously used in: • Viticulture as herbicides • Psoriasis therapy	Skin tumors

causal factors. So far, it has been confirmed through countless laboratory studies and population studies that the following nutritional factors promote the development of various cancers:
• Overeating and overweight
• An excess of alcohol
• Lack of fiber, proteins, vitamins, minerals, and natural plant colorants and aroma compounds
• Natural harmful substances such as aflatoxin, the poison of the fungus *Aspergillus flavus*, and harmful substances that are introduced into food purposely or enter it inadvertently during growing and processing: e.g., environmental poisons such as lead and cadmium, fertilizer residues (nitrate), and such food additives as nitrite pickling salt, which can form nitrosamines (**Table 2.13**)

Chemical Factors

Chemical substances that promote development of cancer are called *carcinogens* (**Table 2.13**).
• Some carcinogens are harmful to the cell's genetic information and thus act as mutagens.
• Other carcinogens impair the DNA repair mechanisms of the cell.

Physical Factors

Radiation is the chief physical agent that acts as a mutagen and can thus contribute to tumor development:
• Ionizing radiation such as X-radiation and radiation used in oncological therapy (p. 67)

• Ultraviolet (UV) radiation, which triggers skin tumors because of its shallow depth of penetration

Genetic Factors

It is assumed today that about 5% of all tumor disease is genetically determined. Whereas in earlier years it was only possible to suspect that frequent occurrence in a family was genetically caused, it has recently been possible to identify some cancer-causing genes.

Examples
• *Breast cancer:* 5% of all cases can be traced to a defective *BRCA1* or *BRCA2* gene. Women with this gene defect develop breast cancer with a probability of 85%.
• *Colon cancer:* In patients with familial adenomatous polyposis (FAP), the colon is scattered with polyps. FAP is inherited by autosomal dominant transmission and is an obligate precancerosis; that is, affected individuals will definitely develop colorectal carcinoma (p. 185).

Viruses

Certain viruses can trigger the development of tumors by building their genome into that of the host cell and thus have a mutagenic effect or lead to immunosuppression.

Examples

- The large group of human papilloma viruses (HPV) leads to warts. HPV types 16 and 18 cause benign warts in the area of the genitalia (**Fig. 2.24**) and also cause cervical carcinoma.
- Hepatitis B viruses play an important role in the development of liver cell carcinoma (p. 192 and p. 196).
- The Epstein–Barr virus, a member of the group of herpes viruses, causes both mononucleosis and B cell lymphoma in immunocompromised patients, e.g., Burkitt lymphomas, which occur mainly in Central Africa, as well as carcinomas of the nose and throat found mainly in Asia (p. 275).
- Other herpes viruses trigger Kaposi sarcoma in AIDS patients (p. 283).

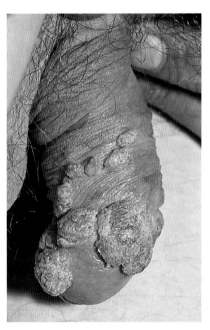

Fig. 2.24 Genital warts on male genitalia. (Jung 1998.)

Immune Deficiency

Congenital and acquired immune deficiency (p. 30) promote not only infectious diseases but also the development of tumors because neoplastic cells are not sufficiently recognized and eliminated.

Stages of Tumor Development

Cancerous diseases do not originate directly in a healthy cell but develop through a number of steps (**Fig. 2.25a–d**).

Precancerous Conditions

Precancerous conditions are tissue changes with a statistically elevated risk of becoming neoplastic. A distinction is made between:
- Facultative precancerous conditions, which turn into a malignancy only occasionally and after a long time
- Obligate precancerous conditions, which always turn into a malignant tumor and in a relatively short time

Metaplasia–Dysplasia–Carcinoma Sequence

- *Metaplasia:* Under continual stress, the cells of labile tissues change reversibly into more resistant cells. For instance, in chronic bronchitis the goblet cells proliferate in the respiratory tract, which is now protected by a thicker mucosal layer.
- *Dysplasia:* Dysplasia occurs when a tissue deviates from the norm as the result of disturbed differentiation. It is based on cell proliferation that is still controlled and that regresses if the stimulus is removed. Since a malignant tumor can develop under a continual stimulus, dysplasia is a precancerous condition.
- *Carcinoma in situ:* A carcinoma in situ (c.i.s.) is a severe cellular alteration in the epithelium that has not yet penetrated the basal membrane, i.e., is not yet growing invasively.

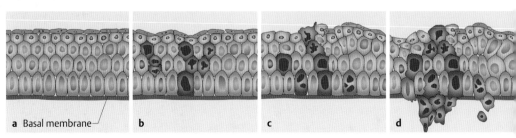

a Basal membrane   b   c   d

Fig. 2.25a–d Stages of tumor development. **a** Normal squamous epithelium. **b** Dysplasia: cellular and nuclear anomalies with cell layering retained. **c** Carcinoma in situ (c.i.s.): cellular layering destroyed with basal membrane preserved. **d** Invasive carcinoma: tumor cells have penetrated the basal membrane.

- *Carcinoma:* Carcinoma is characterized by invasive growth. Penetration into the lymphatic or blood vessels can result in metastasis.

Metastasis

Malignant tumors can form secondary lumps called metastases. In addition to local spread, in which the tumor attacks neighboring organs by increasing in size, a tumor can undergo lymphatic spread, i.e., through the lymph vessels, or hematogenous spread, i.e., through the blood vessels.

Lymphatic Metastasis

In lymphatic metastasis, tumor cells that have become detached from the periphery of a tumor break into the lymph vessels and are carried away via the lymphatic system. Penetration of the lymphatics does not even take 24 hours, since the anatomical structure of the vessel wall does not present a significant barrier. Usually the tumor cells are caught by the next lymph node and continue their autonomous growth there. From the first *lymph node metastasis*, neoplastic cells can travel through the lymphatics to distant lymph nodes and finally reach the blood system.

▪ *Lymphatic metastasis leads to lymph node metastases.*

Sometimes the cancer cells can start multiplying in the lymphatics because of favorable flow conditions, and grow along the vessel and occlude it. This process is called *lymphangitic carcinomatosis.*

Hematogenous Metastasis

Tumor cells penetrate into the smallest veins directly or via the lymphatics. In the bloodstream, most cancer cells are destroyed within 24 hours. The cells that are not destroyed reach other parts of the body and remain caught in the fine capillaries; they penetrate the organ tissue and can grow into daughter tumors.

▪ *Hematogenous metastasis leads to distant metastases.*

The distribution of the neoplastic cells depends on the localization of the primary tumor (**Fig. 2.26a–d**).
- In the *lung type,* the hematogenous metastasis originates from a primary lung tumor. Via the pulmonary veins and the left heart, the tumor cells reach the organs supplied by the systemic circulation, particularly the liver, bones, brain, and adrenal glands.
- In the *hepatic type,* a tumor travels from the liver via the veins of the systemic circulation and the right heart into the pulmonary circulation. Thus liver tumors lead first to lung metastases.
- The metastatic pathways of the *caval type* correspond to those of the liver type. Consequently, with primary tumors in the area of inflow into the vena cava, e.g., kidney and bone tumors, the first area of metastasis is the lungs.

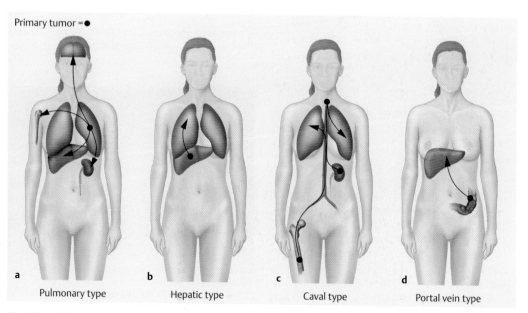

Primary tumor = ●

a Pulmonary type   b Hepatic type   c Caval type   d Portal vein type

Fig. 2.26a–d Hematogenous metastasis

- All intestinal tumors are of the *portal vein type.* Just as the portal vein normally carries nutrient-rich blood from the intestine to the liver, tumor cells are also brought from the intestine to the liver, which is the first location for metastases.

Tumor Classification

Therapy and prognosis are determined first of all on the basis of tumor spread (staging) and its differentiation grade (grading).

Staging

Solid tumors are classified internationally according to the TNM system.
- T_{0-4}: Size and extent of the primary tumor; the tumor stages are defined separately for each tumor type, e.g., bronchial carcinoma (p. 157) and colorectal carcinoma (p. 185).
- N_{0-4}: Extent of the lymph node invasion, which has been defined for each tumor type
- M_{0-1}: Absence or presence of distant metastases

To define the local and systemic extent of a tumor (staging), use is made chiefly of imaging techniques such as sonography, radiography, CT, and MRI.

Grading

The tumor tissue is histologically prepared in order to determine the degree of differentiation. This is identified as G_1 to G_4. Highly differentiated tumors are very similar to the tissue of origin and the malignity grade is usually low (G_1), whereas undifferentiated tumors have nothing in common with the tissue of origin and are usually highly malignant (G_4).

Complications of Tumors

The local and systemic effects of the primary tumor and its metastases determine the clinical picture.

Local Complications

Some important complications are:
- Functional disturbance of the affected organ by invasive, destructive tumor growth and tumor-caused circulatory disruption that causes necrosis
- Compression of neighboring structures resulting in venous stasis, e.g., in blood vessels, gastrointestinal tract, kidneys, and efferent urinary tract as well as infections in the stasis area
- Invasion in neighboring structures that can lead, for example, to bleeding, effusions, perforation of

hollow organs and fistulas. Fistulas are connections between two hollow organs or between a hollow organ and the body surface.

Paraneoplastic Syndromes

About 15% of all patients develop pathological general symptoms related to their cancerous disease. The cause of these paraneoplasias is unclear in many respects. They can become clinically observable before, during, or after a tumor disease.
- *Endocrine paraneoplasia:* Particular tumors that originate in endocrine-producing tissue can produce hormones or hormone-like substances. For instance, some bronchial carcinomas (p. 157) produce adrenocorticotropic hormone (ACTH), which stimulates cortisone production by the adrenal glands and thus leads to Cushing syndrome (p. 239).
- *Neuromuscular paraneoplasia:* The destruction of nerve cells or muscle fibers is probably caused by the fact that the tumor activates a latent viral disease or an autoimmune process, e.g., dermatomyositis (p. 264) that can occur as a paraneoplasm in bronchial, renal, or genital carcinomas.
- *Hematological paraneoplasia:* In a tumor disease, suppression of the bone marrow or destruction of erythrocytes can lead to anemia. On the other hand, activation of the bone marrow can result in polyglobulia with an elevated number of blood cells. Sometimes active clotting agents entering the bloodstream can lead to a thrombosis (p. 131).

> *Tumor patients must be considered at risk for thrombosis.*

- *Cutaneous paraneoplasia:* Certain skin changes can be a warning of tumors in the internal organs (**Fig. 2.27**).

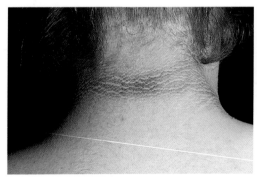

Fig. 2.27 Acanthosis nigricans maligna as an example of cutaneous paraneoplasm. The dermatologist saw the dirty-brown hyperkeratosis on the patient's neck as a signal and called for further diagnostic tests, which revealed a stomach carcinoma. (Jung 1998.)

Tumor Cachexia and Reduced Quality of Life

The general depletion and weakness of cancer patients is called tumor cachexia. This may be caused by the fact that the tumor directly inhibits sufficient dietary intake or the absorption of nutrients. In addition, mediators lower the appetite, increase energy consumption, and promote the breakdown of body proteins (catabolism).

The quality of life and autonomy of the oncological patient can be assessed and evaluated in the course of the disease by means of various scales. Table 2.14 summarizes the Zubrod scale and the Karnofsky index.

Diagnostic Aspects

Histology

> In spite of great advances in imaging procedures, the exact diagnosis of a tumor is only possible by means of histological examination of the tumor tissue.

Tumor Markers

Tumor markers are proteins produced in tumor cells that can often be detected in the blood. Since they can also occur in small amounts in healthy individuals, they are not suitable for tumor diagnosis. Rather, they serve to monitor the course of the disease. After a malignoma has been diagnosed, the specific tumor marker is determined. Elevated values will become normal again after successful therapy. During after-care, the tumor marker is determined regularly and rising values suggest the need to look for a relapse of the tumor or for metastases.

> Tumor markers are used to monitor the course of the disease.

Therapy

Curative therapy has the objective of healing the patient, whereas in palliative therapy, only mitigating measures are applied, for example pain therapy. Both curative and palliative approaches can be achieved in the following ways:

- Surgery
- Chemotherapy
- Radiation therapy
- Hormone therapy
- Immunotherapy

The individual measures are presented in detail in chapter 5 and together with the corresponding diseases in part 2 of this book.

Prognosis

The prognosis of patients with a particular cancer is given as the 5-year survival rate, indicating what percentage of patients will be alive in 5 years.

> The 5-year survival rate is a statistically calculated value that gives no information about the prognosis of the individual patient.

Table 2.14 Evaluation of the quality of life and the autonomy of a tumor patient

Zubrod scale		Karnofsky index	
	Patient carries out normal activity	100%	Patient is free of complaints
		90%	Patient is capable of normal activity, exhibits few symptoms
	Patient is living at home with tolerable tumor symptoms	80%	With some effort, normal activity is possible; moderate symptoms
		70%	Patient can take care of his/her self, but is unable to pursue normal activities
	Patient's tumor manifestations are an impediment but the patient only stays in bed half the day	60%	Patient occasionally needs help from others
		50%	Patient needs considerable help and often requires medical care
	Patient is severely handicapped and stays in bed more than half the day, but can get up	40%	Patient is handicapped and needs care
		30%	Patient is severely handicapped; admission to hospital is indicated
	Patient is seriously ill and completely bedridden	20%	The patient is severely ill and admission to hospital is essential
		10%	Patient is moribund; the life-threatening illness is progressing rapidly

Early Detection

Cancer is basically curable if it is detected early enough. For this reason, in Germany the statutory health insurance companies allow their members early cancer detection examinations. In the United States, insurance coverage of cancer screening procedures varies widely from state to state and from private insurance to Medicare. It also varies for different types of cancer. For instance, 26 states and the District of Columbia have laws requiring insurance coverage for a full range of colorectal cancer screening tests. A few other states require coverage of only certain tests. In all other states, either there are no laws requiring coverage or the law requires insurers to offer (not necessarily provide) coverage. There are various provisions for free or insurance-covered screening for breast cancer. Legislation for insurance coverage of screening for other types of cancer is under study in state legislatures.

3 Cardinal Symptoms

Changed Skin Color

■ Pallor

Skin color is determined chiefly by circulation and pigmentation. Pallor can be caused by physiological and pathological factors (**Table 3.1**, **Fig. 3.1**).

■ Reddening

Reddening of the skin is caused by dilation of the vessels and increased circulation. Physiological and pathological causes can lead to reddening (**Table 3.2**).

Important Concepts

- *Erythema:* Patches of redness, e.g.:
  - Palmar erythema in liver cirrhosis (p. 192)
  - Butterfly erythema in systemic lupus erythematosis (p. 261)
  - Erythema migrans in borreliosis (p. 279)
- *Erythroderma:* The entire skin is reddened.

■ Cyanosis

Definition and Pathomechanism

The bluish-red tint of skin and mucosa resulting from reduced oxygen in the blood is called cyanosis. It appears when more than ⅓ of the hemoglobin molecules in the blood are not saturated with oxygen (**Fig. 3.2**). Cyanosis is most pronounced at the chin, tip of the nose, fingers and toes (acrocyanosis; **Fig. 3.3**) or at the mucosa of the lips, tongue and oral cavity.

In case of anemia (p. 246), the cyanosis threshold is lowered, so that in spite of a decreased oxygen concentration, the blue tint does not necessarily appear.

Forms and Causes

In central cyanosis, the oxygen saturation in the lungs is decreased, whereas peripheral cyanosis

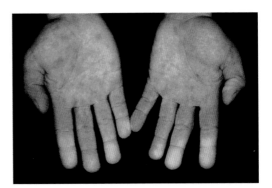

Fig. 3.1 Raynaud syndrome. Vascular spasms lead to transient insufficient perfusion of the fingers. At first the fingers become cold and pale, then cyanotic and later, as a result of reactive hyperemia, red. Raynaud syndrome can be the expression of collagenosis (p. 262). (Füeßl, Middeke 2005.)

Table 3.1 Differential diagnosis of pale skin

Causes	Important examples	Page
Physiological	• Predisposition • Cold • Fear	
Pathological	• Anemia • Arterial hypotension • Shock • Arterial perfusion disorder • Vascular spasms as in Raynaud syndrome (**Fig. 3.1**)	246 119 54 113 262

Table 3.2 Differential diagnosis of reddened skin

Causes	Important examples	Page
Physiological	• Exertion, e.g., in sports • Agitation • Heat	
Pathological	• Fever • Inflammation • Arterial hypertension	52 5 117

reflects an abnormally great extraction of oxygen from normally saturated arterial blood in the tissues (**Table 3.3**).

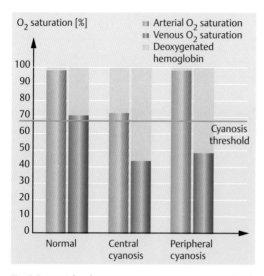

Fig. 3.2 Arterial and venous oxygen saturation in central and peripheral cyanosis.

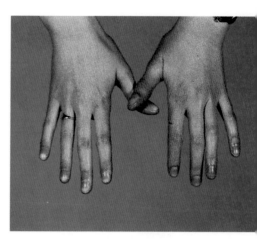

Fig. 3.3 Cyanosis and clubbed fingers in a girl with a congenital heart disease (p. 115). (Epstein 1994.)

Table 3.3 Types and causes of cyanosis

Cyanosis	Definition	Clinical differentiation	Causes	Page
Central	Decreased arterial O_2 saturation	Cyanosis of skin and mucosa	• Pulmonary disease • Congenital heart defects with right–left shunt	137 115
Peripheral	Increased arteriovenous O_2 difference	Cyanosis of skin	• Diseases with reduced blood circulation, e.g., heart failure • Elevated O_2 requirement in tissues, e.g., hypothermia	87

■ Icterus

Definition and Clinical Picture

Elevated bilirubin concentration causes the yellow tint of tissues and body fluids known as icterus.

- Starting at a serum bilirubin concentration of 1.5–2 mg/dL, a yellow tint can be seen in the connective tissue (**Fig. 3.4**). The term "icteric sclera" is used although the icterus is not in the sclera but in the conjunctiva.
- Starting at a bilirubin concentration of 3 mg/dL, the skin and all body fluids are also tinted yellow.

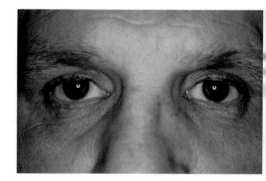

Fig. 3.4 Icterus. (Füeßl, Middeke 2005.)

Physiological Basis

Bilirubin is a breakdown product of hemoglobin at the end of red cell life. When hemoglobin is broken down, the globin components and iron are split off first and water-insoluble, toxic bilirubin (indirect bilirubin) is formed over a number of intermediate steps.

In the blood, it is reversibly bound to albumin and so reaches the liver. In the liver, it is transformed by conjugation with gluconic acid into the water soluble form (direct bilirubin) and is excreted with the bile into the intestine. In the intestine, the bilirubin is reduced to urobilinogen; 80% of it is excreted with the feces and 20% returns to the liver after resorption; a small portion is excreted by the kidneys (**Fig. 3.5**).

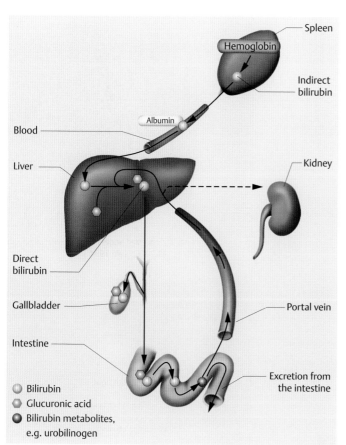

Fig. 3.5 Simplified diagram of bilirubin metabolism.

Table 3.4 Types and causes of icterus

Types	Important examples	Page	Laboratory values
Prehepatic icterus (hemolytic icterus)	Elevated hemolysis, e.g.: • Sickle cell anemia • (Auto-) Antibodies • Infectious diseases such as malaria	246	Indirect bilirubin ↑
(Intra-) Hepatic icterus	Liver damage, e.g.: • Viral hepatitis • Cirrhosis of the liver • Acute liver failure	192 192 195	• Indirect bilirubin ↑ • Possibly direct bilirubin ↑
Posthepatic icterus (cholestatic icterus)	Disturbed outflow of bile (cholestasis), e.g.: • Gallstones • Bile duct carcinoma • Cancer of the pancreas head • Defects in bile duct	197 198 200	Direct bilirubin ↑

Forms and Causes

After localization of the cause, a distinction is made between prehepatic, intrahepatic, and posthepatic icterus (**Table 3.4**).

Bleeding Tendency

When a blood vessel is injured, hemostasis occurs through a complex interplay of:
- Vessel wall
- Platelets
- Coagulation factors (p. 242)

Disorders in one or more of these systems result in a pathologically elevated tendency to bleed that is referred to as hemorrhagic diathesis (**Table 3.5**).

> *Hemorrhagic diathesis must also be taken into account in physical therapy treatment. Joints must be subjected to stress cautiously. Passive measures such as friction rubs should only be taken with restraint and the utmost care.*

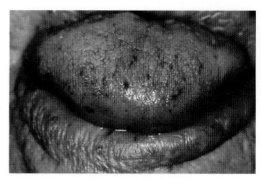

Fig. 3.6 Telangiectases (vascular dilatation) of the tongue in Osler disease. In Osler disease there are usually chronically bleeding telangiectases in the entire gastrointestinal tract. (Füeßl, Middeke 2005.)

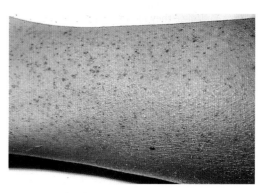

Fig. 3.7 Petechial bleeding in thrombocytopenia. (Füeßl, Middeke 2005.)

Table 3.5 Differential diagnosis of hemorrhagic diathesis

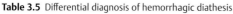

Localization of cause	External clinical appearance	Important examples	Page
Blood vessels	Punctiform petechial bleeding (Purpura; **Fig. 3.6**)	Vasculopathy, e.g.: • Vasculitis • Osler disease (**Fig. 3.6**) • Vitamin C deficiency (scurvy)	265

Platelets (clotting)	Punctiform petechial bleeding (Purpura; **Fig. 3.7**)	• Depressed platelet count (thrombocytopenia), e.g.:
		  – Damage to bone marrow
		  – Autoimmune processes (**Fig. 3.7**)
		  – Enlarged spleen (hypersplenism)
			252

		• Disorder of platelet function (thrombocytopathy) e.g.: – Rare congenital disorders	253
		– Inhibitor of platelet aggregation such as acetyl salicylic acid	73
		– Plasmocytoma	251
		– Chronic renal failure	209
Coagulation system	Extensive bleeding (ecchymoses; **Fig. 3.8**)	Coagulopathies, e.g.: • Hemophilia (**Fig. 3.8**) • Von Willebrand syndrome	253 254
		• Consumption coagulopathy	255

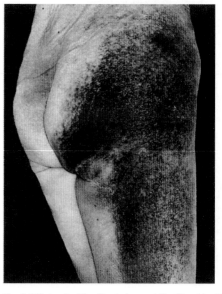

Fig. 3.8 Extensive bleeding in hemophilia. (Baenkler 1999.)

Accumulation of Fluid

$$P_{hydrostatic} > P_{oncotic} \rightarrow Filtration$$
$$P_{oncotic} > P_{hydrostatic} \rightarrow Resorption$$
$$Filtration = Resorption + Lymphatic\ flow$$

■ Edema

Definition

Edema is a painless swelling that is not reddened. It is caused by abnormal accumulation of fluid in the extracellular spaces of tissues. In skin edemas, pressure leaves a depression (**Fig. 3.9a, b**).

Pathomechanism

Edema results when more fluid is pressed into the tissue than is returned to the venous system by resorption and lymphatic flow (**Fig. 3.10a, b**).

▌ *Filtration > Resorption + Lymphatic flow → Edema*

Physiological Basis

Tissues are supplied by blood capillaries. Substances dissolved in the plasma and water pass through the approximately 8 nm sized pores of the capillaries. Blood cells and proteins do not pass through because they are too large; they remain in the vessel. The filtration is driven by the *difference in hydrostatic pressure* between the inside of the capillary and the tissue. At the arterial end of the capillaries, the average pressure is about 30 mmHg; at the venous end it falls to about 15 mmHg.

Only 90% of the filtered fluid returns to the capillaries by resorption. The remaining 10% returns to the venous system through the lymphatic circulation. The filtrate is brought back into the blood circulation by proteins that build up a so-called *oncotic pressure*, which is the driving force of the resorption.

The following factors disturb the balance and contribute to the formation of edema (**Table 3.6**):

- With increasing blood pressure at the venous end of the capillaries, filtration increases and resorption decreases.
- Decreased lymphatic flow also promotes edema. Primary lymphedema results from malformation of the lymph vessels and secondary lymphedema results from tumors, inflammation, trauma, or iatrogenic causes, e.g., after surgery, oncological therapy with removal of lymph nodes, or radiation therapy (p. 136).
- Protein deficiency in the blood (hypoproteinemia) causes low oncotic pressure and thus a decrease in resorption.
- Inflammation increases the permeability of the capillaries to both fluid and proteins.

Table 3.6 Factors promoting edema

Factors	Important examples	Page
Venous stasis	• CVI	129
	• Thrombosis	129
	• Heart failure	87
Lymph stasis	• Malformation of lymph vessels	
	• Tumor infiltration	34
	• Infections, e.g. erysipela	274
	• Trauma and surgery	
	• Lymph node excision	
	• Radiation	67
Hypoproteinemia	• Reduced protein synthesis, e.g.:	
	– Cirrhosis of the liver	195
	– Malabsorption	173
	• Protein loss, e.g.:	
	– Nephrotic syndrome	205
	– Burns	
Elevated capillary permeability	• Inflammation	5

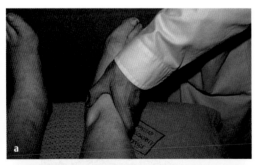

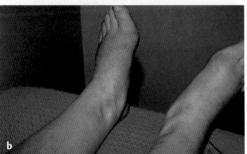

Fig. 3.9a, b Ankle edema (Epstein 1994).

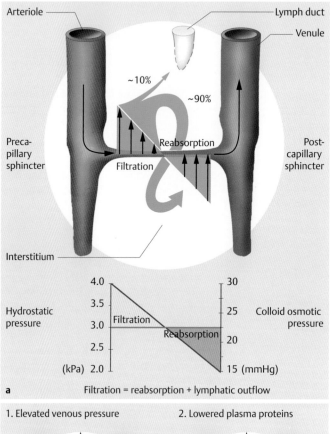

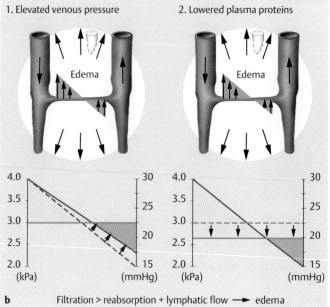

Fig. 3.10a, b Pathological mechanism of edema. **a** Fluid exchange at the capillaries. **b** Formation of edema.

Effusion

Definition

An accumulation of fluid in an anatomically defined body cavity is called effusion, e.g.: joint effusion, pericardial effusion (p. 115), pleural effusion (p. 167), ascites (ascites, p. 192)

Causes

Like edema, effusion can be caused by:
- Venous stasis, i.e. engorgement due to slow or impaired blood flow
- Inflammation
- Protein deficiency

> Any appearance of effusion must raise the question of malignancy.

Transudate and Exudate

Analysis of puncture fluid provides diagnostic information:
- Inflammatory and malignant processes make the vessels become so porous that large protein molecules and blood cells can escape the circulation (**Table 3.7**).
- In addition, the fluid is checked for blood, microorganisms, and tumor cells.

Dyspnea

Dyspnea is an abnormally uncomfortable awareness of breathing and presents one of the principle symptoms of pulmonary and cardiac disease. This can be an expression of decreased oxygen in the blood (hypoxemia), although there are numerous causes for dyspnea (**Table 3.8**).

Patients with chronic hypoxemia often show clubbing of the digits (**Fig. 3.3**, **Fig. 3.11**).

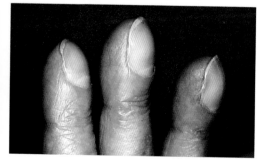

Fig. 3.11 Clubbed fingers in a patient with bronchial carcinoma (p. 157). (Füeßl, Middeke 2005.)

Table 3.7 Differentiation between transudate and exudate

Fluid	Protein and cell content	Causes
Transudate	Low	• Congestion • Protein deficiency
Exudate	High	• Inflammation • Malignancy

Table 3.8 Differential diagnosis of dyspnea

Localization	Important examples	Page
CNS	• Encephalitis • Cerebral bleeding • Cerebral space-consuming lesion	
Upper respiratory tract	• Malformations • Rhinitis • Tonsillitis • Foreign bodies	
Larynx	• Epiglottitis • Laryngitis • Laryngospasm • Spasm of recurrent laryngeal nerve • Trauma	
Trachea	• Malformations • Foreign bodies	
Bronchi	• Acute bronchitis • Chronic bronchitis • Mucoviscidosis • Bronchiectases • Foreign bodies	148 148 161 143
Lung	• Malformations • Lack of surfactants • Pneumonia • Emphysema • Bronchial carcinoma • Pulmonary fibrosis • Atelectasis • Pneumothorax • Pleural effusion	155 148 157 160 142 166 167
Heart	• Coronary artery disease • Myocardial infarction • Cardiac arrhythmias • Valvular heart disease • Myocarditis • Cardiomyopathies • Pericardial effusion • Congenital heart disease	98 101 104 111 113 113 115 115
Blood	• Anemia • Acidosis • Intoxication	246
Nerve and muscle	• Poliomyelitis • Neuropathies • Myopathies	
Other	• Psychiatric • Psychosomatic	

Nausea and Vomiting

Vomiting is triggered by a stimulus to the vomiting center at the floor of the fourth ventricle in the brain, situated close to various vegetative centers and the center of balance. A stimulus to any of these centers can stimulate the vomiting center (**Table 3.9**).

Table 3.9 Differential diagnosis of vomiting

Localization, cause	Important examples	Page
Gastrointestinal tract	• Inflammation, e.g.:	
	– Acute gastroenteritis	272
	– Appendicitis	185
	– Pancreatitis	198
	– Ulcerative disease	180
	– Peritonitis	197
	• Pain, e.g., biliary colic	
	• Obstruction, e.g.:	
	– Ileus	187
	– Diabetes mellitus with autonomous neuropathy	215
	• Postoperative intestinal atonia	
Severe pain	• Myocardial infarction	101
	• Renal colic	212
	• Migraine	
	• Glaucoma	
	• Testicular torsion	
Metabolic decompensations	• Uremia in renal failure	209
	• Diabetic ketoacidosis	215
Intoxication	• Alcohol	
	• Drugs	
	• Food	
	• Medication	
CNS	• Elevated cerebral pressure, e.g.:	
	– Meningitis	
	– Encephalitis	
	– Tumors	
	– Bleeding	
Other	• Vestibular vertigo	57
	• Pregnancy	
	• Exposure to ionizing radiation	
	• Eating disorders like:	
	– Anorexia nervosa	
	– Bulimia	

Pain

■ Physiological Basis

Pain is a vital alarm signal.

The main pain receptors are free nerve endings that occur everywhere in the skin, the internal organs, the muscles, and the joints; they are called *nociceptors*. These react to signal substances that are released in case of cell and tissue injury or inflammatory reactions (p. 5).

Pain receptors do not accommodate, as a sustaining risk could otherwise be ignored.

The pain signal travels first to the spinal cord over peripheral nerves and crosses to the opposite side in the same segment. The stimulus travels along the spinothalamic tract in the anterolateral strand of the spinal cord, via the brainstem to the thalamus, the "gate of consciousness." Here the stimulus is transferred to the third neuron, running to the sensory portion of the cerebral cortex, the postcentral gyrus.

The Feeling of Pain

- The subjective feeling of pain is influenced by various factors, e.g., social and cultural origin as well as upbringing.
- There is no direct relationship between the intensity of the experienced pain and the severity of the disease. For instance, a patient with functional heart problems can have the most severe retrosternal pain (p. 120), while a patient with advanced stomach cancer can be free of pain (p. 181).

■ Chest Pain

Pain in the area of the thorax can be of both thoracic and extrathoracic origin (**Table 3.10**).

■ Abdominal Pain

Overview

Localization

Principal suspected diagnoses depending on the localization of abdominal pain are shown in **Fig. 3.12**.

Extra-abdominal illness can cause abdominal pain (myocardial infarction, pneumonia, and spinal disease).

Table 3.10 Differential diagnosis of chest pain

Localization of cause	Important examples	Page
Cardiac	• Coronary artery disease • Myocardial infarction • Pericarditis • Hypertensive crisis	98 10 115 117
Pulmonary or pleural	• Pulmonary embolism • Pneumothorax • Pleuritis	163 166 167
Mediastinal	• Aortic dissection • Esophagitis • Mediastinitis	127 177
Abdominal	• Pancreatitis • Gallbladder colic	198 197
Other	• Orthopedic causes • Functional heart problems	 120

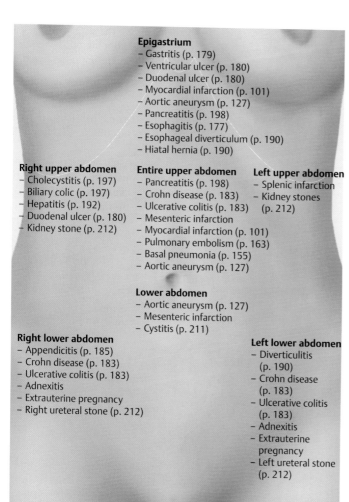

Epigastrium
– Gastritis (p. 179)
– Ventricular ulcer (p. 180)
– Duodenal ulcer (p. 180)
– Myocardial infarction (p. 101)
– Aortic aneurysm (p. 127)
– Pancreatitis (p. 198)
– Esophagitis (p. 177)
– Esophageal diverticulum (p. 190)
– Hiatal hernia (p. 190)

Right upper abdomen
– Cholecystitis (p. 197)
– Biliary colic (p. 197)
– Hepatitis (p. 192)
– Duodenal ulcer (p. 180)
– Kidney stone (p. 212)

Entire upper abdomen
– Pancreatitis (p. 198)
– Crohn disease (p. 183)
– Ulcerative colitis (p. 183)
– Mesenteric infarction
– Myocardial infarction (p. 101)
– Pulmonary embolism (p. 163)
– Basal pneumonia (p. 155)
– Aortic aneurysm (p. 127)

Left upper abdomen
– Splenic infarction
– Kidney stones
  (p. 212)

Lower abdomen
– Aortic aneurysm (p. 127)
– Mesenteric infarction
– Cystitis (p. 211)

Right lower abdomen
– Appendicitis (p. 185)
– Crohn disease (p. 183)
– Ulcerative colitis (p. 183)
– Adnexitis
– Extrauterine pregnancy
– Right ureteral stone (p. 212)

Left lower abdomen
– Diverticulitis
  (p. 190)
– Crohn disease
  (p. 183)
– Ulcerative colitis
  (p. 183)
– Adnexitis
– Extrauterine
  pregnancy
– Left ureteral stone
  (p. 212)

Fig. 3.12 Localization of abdominal pain and possible diagnoses.

Character

Visceral Pain

Visceral pain is mainly caused by:
- Distension of hollow organs
- Smooth-muscle spasms
- Circulatory disorders
- Inflammation

It is conveyed via visceral nervous pathways whose nociceptors are located in the region of the organs. Such visceral pain is described as dull, hard to localize, and of varying intensity. The patient can obtain relief through movement.

Somatic Pain

Somatic pain is carried by nociceptors in the peritoneum and neighboring tissues. It begins as acute pain that is intense, sharp, burning, and easy to localize. Since somatic pain is intensified by movement, a person with somatic pain often adopts a protective posture.

Course

Abdominal pain can be expressed as continuous pain or as colics in the form of periodically recurring pain.

Acute Abdomen

Cardinal Symptoms

In addition to abdominal pain with sudden onset, a patient with an acute abdomen has the following symptoms:
- Reduced general condition
- Guarding tension ("boardlike" abdomen) as an indication of peritonitis (inflammation of the peritoneum)
- Changed intestinal sounds
- Possible fever, nausea, vomiting, diarrhea, or constipation

Causes

Numerous causes can lead to the clinical picture of an acute abdomen (**Table 3.11**).

> Since an acute abdomen is often caused by a life-threatening condition, it requires immediate diagnosis and therapy.

Table 3.11 Causes of an acute abdomen

Localization	Important examples	Page
Gastrointestinal tract	• Inflammation, e.g.:	
	– Appendicitis	185
	– Pancreatitis	198
	• Occlusion of a hollow organ, e.g.:	
	– Ileus	187
	– Choledocholithiasis	197
	• Perforation of a hollow organ, e.g.:	
	– Ventricular or duodenal ulcer	180
	– Trauma	
	• Gastrointestinal bleeding, e.g.:	172
	– Ventricular or duodenal ulcer	180
	– Trauma	
	• Perfusion disorders, e.g.:	
	– Mesenteric infarction	
	– Incarcerated hernia	190
Heart and aorta	• Myocardial infarction	101
	• Ruptured abdominal aneurysm	127
Lung and pleura	• Pneumonia	155
	• Pleuritis	167
Urogenital tract	• Nephro- and urolithiasis	212
	• Adnexitis	
	• Extrauterine pregnancy	
	• Testicular torsion	
Spinal column	• Vertebral fractures	
	• Herniated intervertebral disks	

Fever

Physiological Principles

Body temperature is kept stable within a physiological range by the temperature regulation center of the hypothalamus. Characteristically, there are physiological variations throughout the day, with the lowest temperature in the morning and the highest in the afternoon. Values vary depending on the method of measurement (**Table 3.12**).

After physical exertion, there is a physiologically normal rise in body temperature. There is also a rise in temperature of about 0.5 °C in the second half of the menstrual cycle after ovulation.

Definition

We speak of fever when the body temperature exceeds the physiological limits or when rectal or auricular temperature is increased above 38 °C.

Table 3.12 Normal range of various methods for measuring body temperature

Location of measurement	Temperature
Axillary (armpit)	34.7–37.3 °C
Oral (mouth)	35.5–37.5 °C
Auricular (ear)	35.8–38.0 °C
Rectal (rectum)	36.5–38.0 °C

- Temperatures up to 38.5 °C are considered to be subfebrile.
- Temperatures above 38.5 °C are considered to be febrile.

Three courses of fever can be distinguished, depending on the range of temperature variation:
- Continuous, with the temperature fluctuating through the day by no more than 1 °C
- Remittent fever with fluctuations of 1–2 °C
- Intermittent fever with broader temperature fluctuations

Causes

In fever, the target temperature value in the temperature regulation center of the hypothalamus is shifted upward. In comparison to this target temperature, the body temperature is at first too low, causing shivering and sometimes rigor, to generate heat. Later the body becomes too hot and the fever is combated by sweating as the result of vasodilatation. Causes of temperature regulation disorders include:
- Central cerebral processes
- Pyrogenic (fever-causing) substances such as mediators from inflammation-activated leukocytes (p. 5), breakdown or metabolic products from damaged cells, bacteria and other pathogens

There can be many different underlying diseases and triggers for fever:
- Infectious diseases caused by bacteria, viruses, fungi, and other pathogens (p. 19)
- Inflammatory diseases of the rheumatic spectrum, such as rheumatoid arthritis, collagenoses, and vasculitis (p. 256)
- Other autoimmune processes (p. 29)
- Leukemia (p. 247) and lymphoma (p. 250)
- Other tumors (p. 33)
- Hyperthyroidism (p. 235)
- Medications ("drug fever")
- Dehydration

Enlarged Lymph Nodes

Swollen lymph nodes occur very frequently; they can be localized or generalized and are confirmed by inspection and palpation (**Fig. 3.13**). Any lymph node that can be palpated is considered to be enlarged.

The following lymph node locations are accessible for examination:
- In front of and behind the ears
- In front of and behind the sternocleidomastoid muscle
- At the angle of the jaw
- In the neck
- Above and below the clavicle
- In the axilla
- Inside the elbow
- In the groin

Causes

Localized Lymph Node Enlargement

- In case of acute inflammation of the drainage area of the lymph node, e.g., tonsillitis, erysipelas (p. 274) or injury, the enlarged lymph nodes are tender to the touch. Lymphangitis with visible red stripes may be present.
- Lymph node metastases of malignant tumors are usually not tender to the touch and can grow together or form adhesions with surrounding tissue (p. 34).

Generalized Lymph Node Enlargement

In case of generalized swelling of the lymph nodes, the spleen and liver are usually also enlarged. Causes may include:

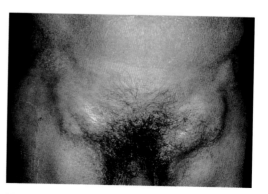

Fig. 3.13 Enlarged inguinal lymph nodes in a patient with non–Hodgkin lymphoma (p. 251). (Füeßl, Middeke 2005.)

- Systemic lymphatic disease caused by infection, e.g, HIV lymphadenopathy (p. 283) or infectious mononucleosis (p. 277)
- Systemic lymphatic disease caused by malignancy, e.g., lymphoma (p. 250)

Shock

Shock is the greatest threat to life in emergency and intensive care patients. Various factors can contribute to critically reduced microcirculation, which causes tissue hypoxia.

> Definition: Critical decrease of microcirculation with tissue hypoxia.

Pathophysiology

Figure 3.14 shows the pathophysiological vicious circle, which may begin at various points, e.g., decreased blood volume in hypovolemic (lack of volume) shock.

As a result of the hypovolemia, the cardiac output decreases. Mechanisms for regulation of the circulation, such as the pressor receptor reflex and the renin–angiotensin–aldosterone system (RAAS, p. 85), maintain the blood pressure first of all by creating vasoconstriction in the gastrointestinal tract, in the kidneys, and in the skin and muscles. The circulating blood volume is redistributed to the heart and brain, which, thanks to centralization, at first still receive sufficient blood.

However, in the tissue with lower blood supply, increasing hypoxia and acidosis lead to autoregulatory vascular atonia. The capillaries become more permeable, so that more fluid escapes into the extravascular space and the lack of volume increases.

Once this vicious circle closes, events progress independently of the cause.

Types and Causes of Shock

Figure 3.14 also shows the four important types of shock that initiate the vicious circle at different locations.

- *Hypovolemic shock* can be the result of extensive bleeding (hemorrhagic shock) or of fluid loss through the kidneys or the gastrointestinal tract or in the case of extensive burns.
- Primary pump failure of the heart is associated with *cardiogenic shock*, which can be caused by any disease that leads to acute heart failure (p. 87). The most frequent cause is myocardial infarction (p. 101).
- *Allergic shock* is due to an allergic type I reaction in which histamine causes vasodilatation and increased vascular permeability (p. 27).
- In *septic shock*, vasodilatation and increased vascular permeability are mediated by bacterial toxins or other inflammatory mediators.

Symptoms

The symptoms can be explained by falling blood pressure, centralization, and the mechanisms for circulatory regulation (p. 85):
- Restlessness, anxiety, and confusion
- Clouding of consciousness
- Paleness in hypovolemic shock and cardiogenic shock
- Cold sweat
- Vital parameters
  - Tachypnea
  - Tachycardia
  - Arterial hypotension
- Decreased diuresis

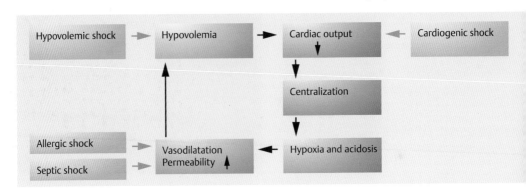

Fig. 3.14 Shock spiral and forms of shock.

Shock Index

The shock index is the quotient of heart rate and systolic blood pressure. At values larger than 1, there is a danger of shock.

▮ *Shock index ≥ 1 → danger of shock*

Complications

The chief complications are:
- Acute kidney failure (shock kidney, p. 209)
- Acute pulmonary failure (shock lung, p. 163)
- Myocardial ischemia (p. 98)
- Acute liver failure (shock liver, p. 195)
- Disseminated intravasal clotting and consumption coagulopathy (p. 255)

Altered States of Consciousness

A distinction is made between:
- Quantitatively altered states of consciousness in which the degree of alertness diminishes and
- Qualitatively altered states of consciousness with altered conscious content

Quantitatively Altered States of Consciousness

Stages

In quantitatively altered states of consciousness or disruption of alertness, the increasing clouding of consciousness can be subdivided into several stages.
- *Somnolence:* The patient is abnormally sleepy, apathetic, and dazed, presenting psychomotor retardation but can be awakened, to the point of being completely oriented.
- *Sopor:* The patient is in a sleeplike state and can only be brought to consciousness by strong stimuli such as loud calling or application of pain stimuli.
- *Stupor:* The patient can no longer be awakened, but still reacts to intense pain stimuli.
- *Coma:* In coma, there are no longer any reactions to environmental stimuli, the native and foreign reflexes are extinguished, vegetative functions are disturbed, and vital functions such as breathing and circulation can be adversely affected.

Glasgow Coma Scale

The Glasgow Coma Scale permits a more detailed classification of consciousness status and is used, among other purposes, for emergency medicine (**Table 3.13**). The point count is at least 3 and at most 15. Coma is present when the score is 8 points or fewer.

Causes

- Primary cerebral traumatic and nontraumatic damage, e.g., skull–brain injuries, tumors, bleeding, cerebral seizure disease, or stroke
- Secondary cerebral damage, e.g., by:
  - Hypoglycemia (p. 215)
  - Other metabolic disorders such as thyrotoxic crises (p. 235), myxedemic coma (p. 236) and hypophyseal coma (p. 232)
  - Shock (p. 54)
  - Intoxication
  - Hypoxemia

Scope

In contrast to syncope (p. 56), the alertness disorders discussed here are not usually spontaneously reversible. It is also always important to determine whether there are signs of death (p. 9) and whether resuscitation measures are indicated (p. 108).

Table 3.13 Glasgow Coma Scale

Function	Best patient reaction	Points
Opening eyes	• Spontaneous	4
	• On being addressed	3
	• On pain stimulus	2
	• No opening	1
Verbal reaction	• Orientated	5
	• Confused, disorientated	4
	• Unconnected words	3
	• Meaningless sounds	2
	• No verbal reaction	1
Motor reaction (to standard commands and pain stimuli)	• Obeys commands	6
	• Specific defense against pain	5
	• Unspecific defense against pain	4
	• Kinematic synergy	3
	• Stretch synergy	2
	• No motor reaction	1

Qualitatively Altered States of Consciousness

Clarity of consciousness is characterized by normal orientation and realistic perception of one's own person and the environment, as well as by appropriate mental activity. Disorders can be manifested, for instance, by:

- Hallucinations
- Difficulties in perception
- Orientation disorders
- Poor recognition of persons and situations
- Decreased accountability

Qualitative consciousness disorders often occur in endogenous and organic psychoses.

- Schizophrenia is the classical example of an endogenous psychosis.
- Examples of acute organic psychoses are delirium, e.g., alcohol withdrawal delirium and postsurgery psychosis that can occur after anesthesia.
- Dementia is a chronic organic psychosis.

Syncope

Definition and Significance

Syncope is defined as a sudden transient loss of consciousness with loss of muscle tone and spontaneous complete recovery.

- Up to 5% of all referrals to emergency departments take place with this diagnosis.
- At least 3% of all individuals suffer a syncope in their lifetimes.
- The prevalence of isolated incidents of syncope is age-dependent; at ages 35–44 years, the incidence is 0.8% and rises to 4% in individuals over the age of 75 years. Approximately 80% of all syncope patients are over 65 years old.
- 35% of patients have a relapse within 3 years.

Causes

Although many and sometimes very costly research methods are used, a cause is found in a bare 60% of patients (**Table 3.14**).

Prognosis

- Cardiac syncope is associated with a 1-year mortality of 18%–33%.
- The prognosis of noncardiac syncope at a 1-year mortality of 0%–12% is more favorable.

Table 3.14 Differential diagnosis of syncope

Causes (frequency)	Important examples	Page
Reflex-mediated decrease in vascular resistance (about 25%)	• Orthostatic hypotension • Autonomic dysfunction, e.g., in diabetes mellitus • Neurocardiac syncope • Cough syncope • Micturition syncope	119 215

Cardiac (about 20%)	• Cardiac arrhythmias:
	  – Bradyarrhythmias
	  – Tachyarrhythmias
	• Ischemia
	• Obstruction of flow, e.g., in:
	  – Aortic valve stenosis
	  – Hypertrophic cardiomyopathy
	  – Pulmonary embolism
		104
		
		98
		111
		113

Cerebrovascular (about 10%)	• Vertebral insufficiency • Transient ischemic attack (TIA) • Stroke • Seizures	
Other (about 5%)	• Medication • Psychiatric causes	
Unknown (about 40%)		

Vertigo

Definition

Vertigo is a disturbance of the body's spatial orientation in which affected individuals experience the perception of movement of their body or the environment when no such movement actually takes place. Vertigo can be associated with vegetative symptoms such as nausea and vomiting.

Forms and Causes

Systemic Vertigo

In systemic or vestibular vertigo, the direction of movement experienced is constant. It is expressed as spinning, disequilibrium, or lightheadedness and can be present at rest as well as during motion. Systemic vertigo is caused by disorders of the vestibular apparatus, e.g.:

- Peripheral-vestibular or labyrinthine in diseases of the inner ear
- Central-vestibular in diseases of the CNS

Vestibular vertigo is often associated with ringing in the ears, so-called tinnitus, and with unintentional eye movements (nystagmus).

Nonsystemic Vertigo

In nonsystemic vertigo, patients feel groggy or dazed. The perceived direction of movement is not constant. The causes are varied and can be more closely defined by a detailed history and physical examination:

- Cardiovascular vertigo typically occurs after standing up or during exertion. Affected individuals see blackness or flickering and become groggy to the point of collapse (syncope, p. 56). Anyone who straightens up abruptly after bending down is familiar with this form of vertigo. It can be caused by arterial hypotension, e.g., in orthostatic dysregulation (p. 119) or heart failure (p. 87).
- Cerebral vertigo is often associated with neurological symptoms and is caused by insufficient cerebrovascular perfusion or brain damage, e.g., in cases of stroke, tumor, encephalitis, or multiple sclerosis.
- Other causes are eye diseases, cervical spine diseases, and psychosomatic diseases.

4 Diagnostic Procedures

For a disease to be identified, a large amount of data must be collected, documented and evaluated. The initial important information comes from the medical history and the physical examination.

On this basis, the physician decides whether additional examinations are necessary, such as:

- Laboratory studies
- Imaging
- Functional studies
- Invasive or endoscopic procedures

The process of information gathering usually leads the physician to a *diagnosis* (Greek: the distinguishing), which forms the basis of therapeutic planning.

Medical History

The starting point for diagnosis is the medical history or anamnesis (Greek: memory). If this is obtained by conversation with the patient, it is called a self-reported history; otherwise, it is a third-party history.

> The "yield" of the medical history depends decisively on the physician's skill at questioning and on the patient's ability to remember.

Self-Reported History

A self-reported history is preferable if at all possible. The physician questions the patient systematically and specifically on the following points:

- Current complaints
- Autonomic history
- Previous illnesses
- Medications and addictive drugs
- Social history
- Family history (**Table 4.1**)

Third-Party History

In the third-party history, other persons—for example, parents, work colleagues or eye witnesses—give information about the patient. While only a third-party history is possible for infants, small children, and the unconscious, it can also be a useful supplement to a self-reported history, especially for psychiatric patients.

Physical Examination

In the physical examination of the patient, the physician uses all his or her senses and also, where applicable, technical resources. **Table 4.2** summarizes the evaluation criteria of the five basic examination steps:

- Inspection, in which the patient is observed
- Palpation, in which palpatory findings are collected
- Auscultation, in which auditory phenomena of the heart, blood vessels, lung, and intestine are assessed by using a stethoscope
- Percussion, in which the surface of the patient's body is percussed so as to draw conclusions about the underlying organs from the different sounds
- Clinical functional tests

Table 4.1 Contents of the self-reported medical history

Current complaints	Autonomic history	Previous illnesses	Social history	Family history
The "7 Ws" • What is the problem? • Where do you notice the problems? • When do the complaints arise? • What do the complaints feel like? • What triggers, intensifies, or weakens the complaints? • When did these complaints begin? • What has been done about them so far?	• Weight changes • Sweating • Fever • Stool habits • Urination • Sleep	• Hospital stays • Serious illness • Start of chronic disease • Surgeries • Accidents and injuries • Pregnancies and deliveries • Medications and addictive drugs	• Family status • Lifestyle • Occupation • Sports and hobbies	• Hereditary diseases • Cardiovascular diseases • Malignancies • Metabolic diseases, e.g., diabetes mellitus • Serious infectious illnesses

Laboratory Studies

In principle, all the patient's bodily fluids can be examined for their components. The chief substances to be examined are:
- Blood
- Urine
- Stool
- Cerebrospinal fluid
- Pathological bodily fluids (**Table 4.3**, **Fig. 4.1**)

Imaging

Wilhelm Conrad Röntgen was a pioneer of diagnostic imaging. In 1895 he discovered high-energy electromagnetic radiation (X-radiation) that is able to penetrate various bodily tissues to different degrees. Since the discovery of X-radiation, diagnostic imaging has undergone continuous and rapid development and today is a vital part of medicine.

■ Radiographic Procedures

Basic Principles

X-radiation is invisible to the eye but it darkens photographic plates. This radiation has shorter wave-

Table 4.2 Summary of physical examination

Inspection	Palpation	Auscultation	Percussion	Clinical functional testing
• Demeanor • Movement • Malposition • Skin color • Swelling • etc.	• Skin temperature • Pulses (p. 121) • Lymph nodes • Size and consistency of organs • Surface sensation • etc.	• Heart (p. 90) • Vessels (p. 121) • Lung (p. 144) • Intestinal peristalsis	• Pulmonary borders in respiration • Hepatic borders • Intestinal air content	• Joint mobility • Muscle status • Blood pressure measurement (p. 90); • Walking distance (p. 123) • Ratschow position test (p. 123) • Reflex status • etc.

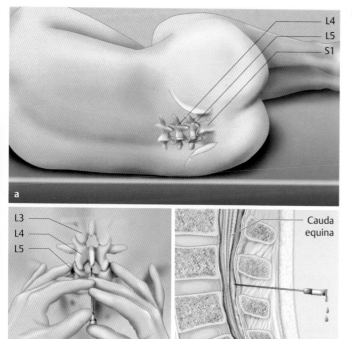

Fig. 4.1a–c Lumbar puncture

Table 4.3 Overview of the most important laboratory tests

Test medium	Sampling	Important test or issue

Blood	• Venipuncture	• Hematologic tests
		  – Blood count (p. 245)
		  – Sedimentation rate
		• Clinical chemistry
		  – Electrolytes
		  – Enzymes
		  – Blood proteins
		  – Blood sugar (p. 214)
		  – Blood lipids (p. 220)
		  – Coapulation parameters (p. 245)
		  – Kidney retention values (p. 205)
		  – Hormones
		• Serological–immunological studies
		  – Blood groups
		  – Proof of infection (p. 19)
		  – Allergy diagnosis (p. 26)
		• Blood culture to detect bacteria and bacterial count

	• Arterial puncture	• Blood gas analysis (p. 147)

Urine	• Midstream urine
	• One-time catheterization
	• Suprapubic bladder puncture (rare)
		• Urine status or orienting test strip to examine for:
		  – Erythrocytes
		  – Leukocytes
		  – Bacteria
		  – Protein
		  – Glucose
		• Urine sediment to examine solid components
		• Urine culture to detect bacteria and bacterial count

Stool	Stool sample	• Detection of occult blood • Stool culture to detect bacteria and bacterial count • Determination of lipids on suspicion of malassimilation (p. 173) • Chymotrypsin determination on suspicion of exocrine pancreatic insufficiency (p. 171)

Cerebrospinal fluid	Lumbar puncture
	(**Fig. 4.1a–c**)
		• Findings on inspection
		  – Opacity
		  – Blood in cerebrospinal fluid
		• Clinical chemistry
		  – Protein content
		  – Sugar content
		• Microscopic examination
		  – Cell count
		  – Bacteria
		• Cerebrospinal fluid culture to detect bacteria and bacterial count
		• Serological-immunological studies

Pathological body fluids, e.g.: • Sputum • Wound secretions • Effusion	• Smear • Puncture	Conclusions regarding causes of disease, e.g., by • Detection of microorganisms • Detection of tumor cells

lengths than visible light and has high penetration ability for most materials and high ionization capacity.

X-radiation is damaging to embryos (teratogenic; p. 16) and is carcinogenic (p. 34).

The radiation is generated in X-ray tubes and directed toward the patient. The patient is situated between the X-ray tube and a film that records the transmitted radiation (**Fig. 4.2**). The patient's different tissues absorb the radiation to different degrees.

- Thus X-ray-dense tissues like bone have a high absorption fraction, i.e., they pass only a small amount of radiation and the film is barely blackened. Thus, in the negative, bone appears light.
- The air-filled lung is transparent to radiation and the film is blackened.

A distinction is made between conventional and digital radiographic procedures; both can be conducted with and without contrast agents.

Conventional Radiographic Procedures

In conventional radiographic procedures, the resulting image is visualized directly on an X-ray film or is examined on a monitor, for example, for a radiographic image of the thorax.

In some cases, the natural differences in tissue density are not sufficient to provide reliable differentiation among the different anatomical structures. In such cases, radiographic contrast agents yield better imaging (**Table 4.4**).

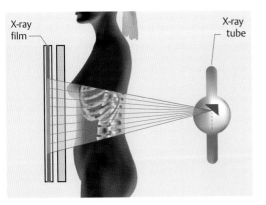

X-ray film

X-ray tube

Fig. 4.2 Image creation in conventional radiography.

Digital Radiographic Procedures

Computed tomography (CT) is a digital radiographic procedure. The absorption differences of the tissues are measured with specialized instruments and further processed by a computer before computer-constructed cross-sectional images of the body appear

Table 4.4 Overview of the most important radiographic images with contrast agent

Organ system	Test	Administration of contrast agent	Important examples of indications	Page
Respiratory tract	Bronchography	Inhalation	• Malformations • Bronchiectases	 143
Digestive tract	Esophagography	Barium swallow	• Esophageal carcinoma • Esophageal diverticuli	178 190
	Stomach–intestine passage	Barium swallow	• Tumors • Gastroduodenal ulcer disease	181 180
	Colon contrast imaging	Enema	• Polyps • Colon carcinoma • Colon diverticuli	189 185 190
	Cholangiopancreatography	Endoscopy (ERCP, p. 176)	• Gallstones • Bile duct tumors • Pancreas tumors	197 198 200
Kidney and urinary tract	Urography	Intravenous injection	• Malformations • Urinary stones • Tumors	 212 213
Vessels	Angiography	Intra-arterial injection	• Peripheral arterial disease • Acute arterial occlusion	123 123
	Coronary angiography	Left heart catheter (p. 95)	• Coronary artery disease • Myocardial infarction	98 98
	Phlebography	Intravenous injection	Thrombosis	131

on a monitor (**Fig. 4.3a–c**). For certain issues, administration of a radiographic contrast agent is necessary here as well.

◼ Sonography

The mechanical vibrations of ultrasound have frequencies above the threshold of human hearing.

Ultrasound diagnosis or sonography makes use of the fact that tissues reflect the sound waves to some extent and absorb them to some extent. During the examination, a transducer emits ultrasound waves, captures the reflected "echoes" and transforms them by the same principles as echo sounding (sonar) into image information.

Examples:
- Abdominal sonography permits external evaluation of organs such as liver, gallbladder, pancreas, spleen, kidneys, abdominal aorta, and urogenital organs. Pathological fluid accumulations in the abdominal cavity can also be visualized.
- For certain investigations, the transducer can even be introduced into hollow organs. For instance, this so-called endosonography can be used to determine how deep a tumor extends.
- Echocardiography is an important component of noninvasive cardiological diagnosis (p. 93).

- By means of Doppler and color-coded duplex sonography, the movement of the blood can be imaged. Vascular diagnosis is mainly established with these techniques (p. 121).
- Sonography functions without radiation exposure, so it can be used without hesitation in pregnancy to observe the development of the fetus (**Fig. 4.4**).

◼ *Sonography does not entail exposure to radiation.*

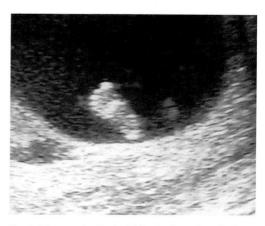

Fig. 4.4 Sonography. Tamina's* foot in the 13th week of pregnancy.

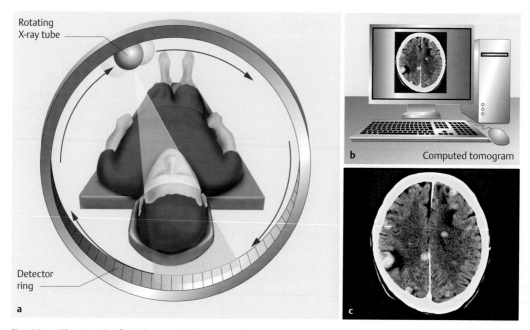

Rotating X-ray tube

Detector ring

a

b   Computed tomogram

c

Fig. 4.3a–c The principle of CT. The example shows cranial CT in a patient with brain metastases.

*the auther's niece.

Magnetic Resonance Imaging

Utilizing the phenomenon of nuclear magnetic resonance, the tomographic technique of magnetic resonance imaging (MRI) is a sectional imaging procedure that, in contrast to computed tomography, does not make use of ionizing radiation.

MRI does not entail exposure to ionizing radiation.

The patient is subjected to a strong magnetic field in which the magnetic moments of atomic nuclei (usually those of hydrogen, i.e., protons) of the tissues line up. This alignment is disrupted by short high-frequency pulses. As they return to their starting (random) alignments, the atomic nuclei emit electromagnetic waves that are captured by specialized sensors and transformed into image information.

Healthy and pathologically changed tissues have different proton densities and thus pathological processes such as brain tumors can be detected by MRI.

Scintigraphy

In nuclear medicine, scintigraphy is an examination technique in which radionuclides are administered to the patient. These are unstable radioactive isotopes of a chemical element that accumulates in the organ or tissue being examined. There they decay to stable isotopes of the element while emitting radiation that can be measured with the appropriate instruments. This makes it possible to draw conclusions regarding the metabolic activity of the region of interest.

Examples:
- Thyroid scintigraphy (p. 234, **Fig. 4.5**)
- Skeletal scintigraphy; e.g., to visualize bone metastases

Functional Studies

It is occasionally necessary to monitor the specific functioning of an organ or an organ system. In addition to clinical function tests (p. 58), the following procedures may be used:
- Measurement of electrical phenomena (**Fig. 4.6**)
- Pulmonary function tests (p. 144)
- Stress testing, as in bicycle ergometry, treadmill test, stress echocardiography (pp. 92, 93)

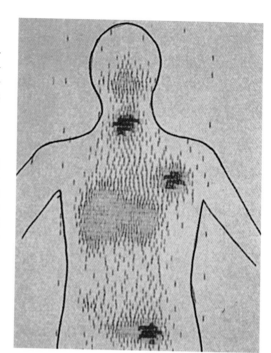

Fig. 4.5 Whole-body scintigram with iodine-131 in a patient with metastasized thyroid carcinoma. Radionuclide accumulation is seen in remnants of surgically removed thyroid gland as well as in metastases in the lungs and the pelvic bones. (Gerlach 2000.)

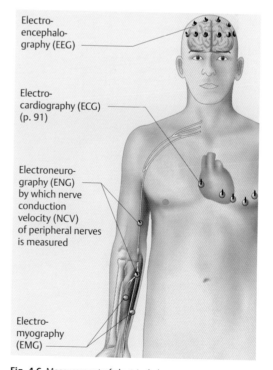

Electro-encephalo-graphy (EEG)

Electro-cardiography (ECG) (p. 91)

Electroneuro-graphy (ENG) by which nerve conduction velocity (NCV) of peripheral nerves is measured

Electro-myography (EMG)

Fig. 4.6 Measurement of electrical phenomena.

- Functional diagnosis by means of imaging procedures, e.g., thyroid scintigraphy, myocardial perfusion imaging (MRI or scintigraphy), PET imaging
- Functional diagnosis by means of laboratory tests, e.g., of hormone levels

Table 4.5 Overview of the most important endoscopic procedures

Organ system	Test	Organ examined
Respiratory tract	Bronchoscopy (p. 147)	Respiratory tract
	Mediastinoscopy	Mediastinum
	Thoracoscopy	Lung and pleura
Digestive tract	Esophagoscopy	Esophagus
	Gastroscopy	Stomach
	Duodenoscopy	Duodenum
	Colonoscopy	Large intestine
	Sigmoidoscopy	Sigmoid portion of the large intestine
	Rectoscopy	Rectum
	Proctoscopy	Section of the intestine close to the anus
Urogenital tract	Cystoscopy	Urinary bladder
	Ureteroscopy	Ureters
	Pyeloscopy	Renal pelvis
	Hysteroscopy	Uterus
Joints	Arthroscopy	Joint cavity

Endoscopic Procedures

In endoscopy particular instruments are introduced into hollow organs or body cavities. These endoscopes comprise optical systems with light sources that permit direct observation of different organs (**Table 4.5**). If the findings are suspicious, tissue samples are taken with biopsy forceps and worked up histologically as, for instance, in tumor diagnosis.

For certain situations, endoscopic and imaging techniques are combined, e.g., endoscopic retrograde cholangiopancreatography (ERCP, p. 175), in which duodenoscopy and contrast radiography are combined. Sometimes a diagnostic endoscopy becomes a therapeutic intervention when, for instance, colon polyps are removed during a colonoscopy (p. 189).

Laparoscopy

Laparoscopy is a special form of endoscopic observation. Under anesthesia, gas is introduced into the abdominal cavity through a cannula. After the abdomen has been "pumped up," a light source, a video camera and, where needed, instruments, are introduced through several small abdominal incisions (**Fig. 4.7a, b**).

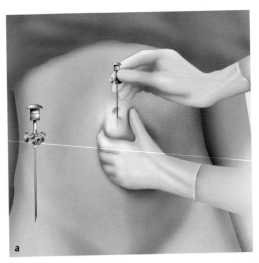
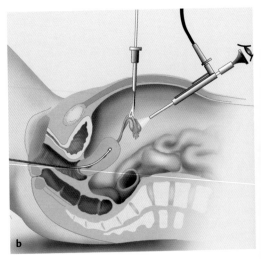

a   **b**

Fig. 4.7a, b Example of therapeutic laparoscopy. **a** Insertion of cannula through which gas is introduced into the abdominal cavity. **b** Surgical sectioning of the fallopian tubes.

Diagnostic Laparoscopy

Diagnostic (exploratory) laparoscopy is indicated for oncological issues and to elucidate unclear abdominal complaints, for example:

- To obtain histological samples
- For tumor staging
- For therapy monitoring

Therapeutic Laparoscopy

In minimally invasive surgery (MIS), numerous operations can be performed endoscopically, for example:

- Endoscopic appendectomy (removal of the vermiform appendix)
- Endoscopic cholecystectomy (removal of the gallbladder)

5 Principles of Therapy

Overview

Requirements

> A requirement for any useful therapy is a firm diagnosis or at least a justifiable suspected diagnosis. This is true both for the physician and the physical therapist.

Procedure

Indication

First of all a decision has to be made whether there is an *indication* for treatment, i.e., whether therapeutic measures are necessary.
- If there is an *absolute indication*, treatment is absolutely necessary; e.g., therapy for a myocardial infarction (p. 101). A *vital indication* is a special case when the patient's life is in danger and therapeutic measures must be taken even without the patient's consent, e.g., if the patient is unconscious.
- There is a *relative indication* when the patient is endangered only to a limited extent or when the success of the treatment is not certain.

Objective

Curative Therapy

The objective of any treatment is to cure disease.

Palliative Therapy

There are still today diseases whose course cannot be significantly influenced. In these cases palliative therapy is intended to:
- Relieve the patient's complaints
- Improve the quality of life
- Extend the remaining lifespan

Palliative measures are an important component of oncological therapy (p. 66).

Selection of Measures

Contraindications

In selecting the appropriate form of therapy, possible secondary effects, treatment duration and resulting limitations in the patient's life must be taken into account. These considerations may reveal contraindications for certain measures.
- If there are *absolute contraindications,* the therapy may not be applied.
- Where there is a *relative contraindication,* particular care must be taken.

Causal and Symptomatic Treatment

- Ideally, a *causal* treatment eliminates the causes of illness.
- In contrast, *symptomatic* measures such as pain medication only eliminate the signs of the illness and should, if possible, be employed as useful supplements to causal treatment.

Conservative and Surgical Therapy

- In *noninvasive or conservative therapy,* the patient's body remains intact.
- *Invasive or surgical therapy* must be distinguished from this. **Figure 5.1** shows the approaches for various operative interventions.

Oncological Therapy

Therapy for malignant diseases can be curative or palliative:
- *Curative therapy* pursues the objective of healing the patient. A requirement is that the tumor must be diagnosed at an early stage.
- *Palliative therapy* is introduced when there is no prospect of a cure. Palliative treatment is intended to alleviate the suffering and improve the patient's quality of life, e.g., through pain relief.

Both approaches are possible, either alone or in combination, using the following systemic or local measures:

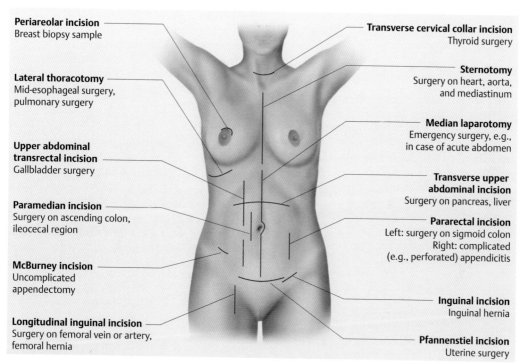

Periareolar incision
Breast biopsy sample

Transverse cervical collar incision
Thyroid surgery

Lateral thoracotomy
Mid-esophageal surgery,
pulmonary surgery

Sternotomy
Surgery on heart, aorta,
and mediastinum

Upper abdominal
transrectal incision
Gallbladder surgery

Median laparotomy
Emergency surgery, e.g.,
in case of acute abdomen

Transverse upper
abdominal incision
Surgery on pancreas, liver

Paramedian incision
Surgery on ascending colon,
ileocecal region

Pararectal incision
Left: surgery on sigmoid colon
Right: complicated
(e.g., perforated) appendicitis

McBurney incision
Uncomplicated
appendectomy

Inguinal incision
Inguinal hernia

Longitudinal inguinal incision
Surgery on femoral vein or artery,
femoral hernia

Pfannenstiel incision
Uterine surgery

Fig. 5.1 Surgical approaches

- Local measures:
  - Surgery
  - Radiation
- Systemic measures:
  - Chemotherapy
  - Hormone therapy
  - Immunotherapy

■ Surgery

In surgical therapy, the primary tumor with an adequate margin of neighboring tissue and the regional lymph nodes are removed. Surgical treatment can sometimes be considered for a solitary metastasis, for example, in the liver or lung.

■ Radiation

Radiation therapy is an important mainstay of oncology. Radiation therapy is a relatively young field as an autonomous discipline, which has been recognized as a specialty since the 1980s.

Ionizing Radiation

Ionizing radiations are used in radiation therapy with such high energy that electrons become detached from atoms or molecules. In reaction to irradiation tissues may suffer:
- DNA damage
- Disruption of cell function
- Cell death

The effect of ionizing radiation is used to kill radiation-sensitive tumor cells. However, it also triggers a number of adverse side-effects in healthy tissues.

Radiation Techniques

In contrast to systemic chemotherapy, use of radiation is a local measure that affects only the irradiated field.

Percutaneous Radiation Therapy

In percutaneous radiation therapy, the tumor is irradiated from outside, through the intact skin. To protect healthy tissue, the radiation dose required to destroy the tumor is administered in numerous small doses and at intervals. The healthy tissue recovers better than the tumor tissue and is less severely damaged. This effect can also be achieved if the tumor is irradiated from several directions in one session.

Contact Irradiation

In this form of radiation therapy, the radiation source and tumor are brought into direct contact. Radioactive substances can be directly inserted into body cavities or tissues. In both cases, the range of the radiation is small, so that healthy tissue is spared.

Side-effects

A distinction is made between acute side-effects that set in during the period of radiation therapy, and late reactions that can emerge months or years after the radiation treatment.

Acute Side-effects

- A "radiation hangover" with general symptoms such as nausea or exhaustion occurs mainly when large areas in the abdominal region are irradiated.
- Irritation of the skin and mucosa are possible as well as hair loss when the skull is irradiated. Care of the skin (see below) and good irradiation techniques make "burns" a rarity.
- Irradiation of bone tissue can suppress blood formation.

Late Reactions

The chief possible late reactions are:
- Infertility when ovaries or testicles are irradiated
- Fibrosis, i.e., proliferation of connective tissue in irradiated tissues; e.g., pulmonary fibrosis after irradiation for breast cancer (p. 160)
- Secondary neoplasia: the probability that a new tumor will develop 10–30 years later as a consequence of radiation lies in the "per thousand" range.

Skin Care

> Some consequences of radiation may be of significance for physical therapists.

In the case of percutaneous irradiation, the skin area marked out with waterproof pen for irradiation requires special care.
- Whether and how intensely the skin may be washed must be discussed with the patient by the treating physician.

- Since the skin is very sensitive, it must not be subjected to mechanical stress from time of the first radiation treatment to 3 weeks after the end of treatment. For instance, brushing, rubbing, massaging, heat and cold treatments, or local application of alcohol (e.g., in deodorants and the like) should be avoided.

■ Chemotherapy

Chemotherapy involves the use of cell poisons. These are called cytostatics, which primarily attack dividing cells at various developmental stages. Tumor cells multiply unimpeded and usually faster than healthy cells; in the ideal case, they are more severely damaged. The medications are often combined in polychemotherapy.

Objectives

- Curative or palliative (see above)
- Neoadjuvant chemotherapy: preoperative chemotherapy to reduce the size of the tumor, achieving *downstaging* and thus improving operability
- Adjuvant chemotherapy: chemotherapy, for instance after surgical local therapy, to prevent relapses or metastases in a patient clinically free of tumors. Adjuvant chemotherapy is used for a curative approach.

Phases

The phases of therapy comprise:
- Induction therapy, intended to achieve complete remission and thus freedom from symptoms
- Consolidation therapy, to stabilize remission
- Maintenance therapy, which is intended to achieve freedom from relapse and thus, a cure

Side-effects

Cytostatics attack not only the tumor cells but the healthy cells as well. The most vulnerable tissues are those with rapid cell growth. These include in particular:
- Blood-generating bone marrow
- Lymphatic tissue
- Intestinal and oral mucosa
- The sperm-producing tissue of the testicles

The effects on the bone marrow are particularly serious, since the consequences for patients under chemotherapy can be life-threatening. Serious infections, anemia, and bleeding occur as a result of the decreased leukocytopoiesis, erythrocytopoiesis, and thrombocytopoiesis. Patients must be protected from infections by isolation from microorganisms and careful hygienic measures (protective isolation). In case of fever, patients must be immediately examined and treated with antibiotics.

Frequent general side-effects of cytostatics are:
- Nausea and vomiting, which can be prevented with medication
- Inflammation of oral and intestinal mucosa leading to diarrhea
- Reversible hair loss

Long-term side-effects are:
- Toxic effect on the gonads
- Carcinogenic effects

Certain medications have organ-specific side-effects and can damage the heart, lungs, kidneys, liver, CNS, and peripheral nerves among others.

Hormone Therapy

Hormones are messenger substances that can promote the growth of healthy tissue but also of tumor tissue. Clinically relevant examples of tumors that may exhibit hormone receptors are:
- Carcinoma of the breast, whose growth may depend on estrogen or gestagen
- Endometrial carcinoma, originating in the uterus mucosa, which can also be influenced by estrogen and gestagen
- Prostate carcinoma, which may grow under the influence of androgens

In testing the tissue of these tumors, the pathologist will look for hormone receptors. The presence of hormone receptors is a positive factor in the prognosis because hormone therapy, among other measures, can be employed.
- Hormone receptors of the tumor cells are blocked with an anti-hormone so that the body's own hormones can no longer bind to them (**Fig. 5.2**). Isolated tumor cells can no longer divide and are eliminated by the immune system before metastases can form. An example is the anti-estrogen treatment of breast cancer.
- In addition, hormone synthesis can be blocked, e.g., by aromatase inhibitors in breast cancer.

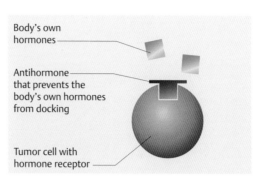

Body's own hormones

Antihormone that prevents the body's own hormones from docking

Tumor cell with hormone receptor

Fig. 5.2 The mechanism of action of hormone therapy.

- Ablative hormone therapy, in which the hormone-synthesizing gland is removed (e.g., removal of the ovaries in breast cancer), is not used very frequently today.

Hormone therapy does not entail as many side-effects as chemotherapy. However, the examples mentioned here do bring about early menopause in female patients.

Immunotherapy

There is great hope for immunotherapy, which is in part still in the experimental stage.
- It is hoped that immunity-stimulating therapy with interleukins I and II and alpha-interferon can activate the body's defense system to eliminate individual tumor cells.
- Genetically engineered antibodies can mark tumor cells quite specifically to be destroyed by the immune system. This procedure is equivalent to passive inoculation.

Organ Transplantation

Transplantation (Latin: transplantare, to remove and plant in another place; Tx) is the transfer of cells, tissues, or organs to another individual or another site in the body for therapeutic purposes. This usually requires a surgical intervention performed by specially trained surgeons. Exceptions are transfers such as blood or bone marrow transfusions that can be carried out intravenously (p. 247). Determination of the indication for transplantation as well as preparation and aftercare of patients are usually within the specialty of internists.

Table 5.1 Organ transplantations in the US in the year 2008

Organ	Kidney	Kidney and pancreas	Pancreas	Liver	Heart	Heart and lung	Lung	Intestine
Number of transplants in 2008	16 520	873	436	6 319	2 163	27	1 478	185
Number of patients on the waiting list of November 2009	82 364	2 220	1 488	15 915	2 884	83	1 863	229

In the United States, regulation of organ donation is left to states, within the limitations of various federal laws. The distribution of organs is governed by the United Network for Organ Sharing (UNOS). Allocation and matching of organs is carried out on a national scale. See **Table 5.1** for an overview of transplantations carried out and patients on the waiting list in the United States in the year 2008.

Historical Overview

Organ transplantation was attempted early, but it was not until the beginning of the twentieth century that advances in vascular surgery and operative techniques created the conditions for successful transplantation.
- In Vienna in 1902 the surgeon Emmeric Ullmann performed the first successful kidney transplantation in a dog.
- In 1933, the Ukrainian surgeon Yurii Voronoy risked the first kidney transplantation in a human patient; it failed on account of tissue incompatibility, which could not be managed at that time.
- In Boston in 1954, Joseph Murray performed the first successful kidney transplantation between two identical twin brothers.
- Beginning in 1962, great progress was made in the pharmacology of immunosuppression. In 1980, ciclosporin (cyclosporine A, CSA) was developed, contributing to a breakthrough in transplantation medicine.
- In 1967 in Cape Town, Christiaan Barnard performed the first successful heart transplantation. In the same year, Thomas Starzel performed the first successful liver transplantation.
- A lung was first transplanted in 1985 in the United States.
- In 1988, in Hanover, Germany, Rudolf Pichelmayr succeeded in performing the first partial liver transplantation; that is, he divided a donor liver between two recipients.

Procedure

Today, the following organs are regularly transplanted:
- Cornea
- Heart (p. 97)
- Lung
- Kidney (p. 209)
- Liver
- Vessels
- Intestine
- Endocrine organs such as pancreas and adrenal gland
- Bone marrow and stem cells (p. 247)

Table 5.2 summarizes the usual concepts in transplantation medicine.

Recipient

Indications and contraindications have been determined for each organ, for example, heart transplantation (HTX; p. 97). Acute infections and malignancies are usually contraindications, since they would "explode" under immunosuppression therapy.

Moreover, a potential recipient is required to exhibit a high level of cooperation and an understanding of the need for lifelong aftercare and immunosuppression.

Donor

There are two possibilities of organ donation:
- Living donation
- Cadaver donation

Living Donation

A living donation can be considered in the case of:
- Kidney transplantation
- Partial transplantation of the liver
- Bone marrow or stem cell transplantation

In the case of a living donation by a relative, a suitable donor is sought among relatives of the first and

Table 5.2 Overview of concepts in transplantation (TX) medicine

Characteristic	Terminology	Definitions	Examples
Degree of genetic compatibility of donor and recipient	• Autogenous TX • Autologous TX	Donor and recipient are identical	Skin transplantation
	• Syngenic TX • Isologous TX	Donor and recipient are genetically identical	Transplantation between identical twins
	• Allogenic TX • Homologous TX	Donor and recipient belong to the same species	Usual transplantation procedure, from human to human
	• Xenogenic TX • Heterologous TX	Donor and recipient belong to different species	Pig to human, limited to only a few indications, e.g., heart valve replacement
Correspondence of explantation and transplantation site	Isotopic TX	Correspondence of site and of tissue	(A rather theoretical concept)
	Orthotopic TX	Correspondence of site	Heart transplantation
	Heterotopic TX	No correspondence of site	Kidney transplantation

second degrees with similar tissue characteristics. The tissue characteristics are called histocompatibility antigens (see below). In the United States, state and federal statutes govern living donations of organs to both related persons and nonrelated persons.

A prerequisite for a living donation is that no significant harm to the donor will result from organ removal. This prerequisite is only met if the remaining organ functions perfectly. Moreover, there must be no risk factors present that make later organ damage probable, such as arterial hypertension (p. 117) or diabetes mellitus (p. 215).

Cadaver Donation

Prerequisites for organ removal from a cadaver are:
- Brain death must be confirmed according to specific criteria by two physicians independently of each other and playing no role in the transplantation (p. 9).
- There must exist written permission expressed by the donor before his or her death, for instance in the form of an organ donor ID. Since in practice such a document is often absent, permission or refusal must be given by a close relative.

Contraindications

Those who cannot be considered as organ donors are:
- Patients with infectious diseases such as tuberculosis or HIV
- Patients with malignancies
- Patients with known preexisting diseases of the organs to be transplanted

Risks of Transplantation

Overview

- Transplantation is a serious surgical intervention with the usual risks related to surgery and anesthesia, e.g., danger of bleeding and infection.
- In spite of extensive organ testing, there is a residual risk that pathogens such as cytomegalovirus, human immunodeficiency viruses or hepatitis viruses and tumor cells could be transferred together with the transplanted organ.
- The transplant recipient has the possibility of tissue rejection.
- The necessary immunosuppression leads to a permanently elevated susceptibility to infection and increases the long-term risk of malignancy. In addition, immunosuppressive medications have specific side-effects.
- Physical and psychological problems require complex interdisciplinary care for the transplant patient.

Transplant Rejection

The success of a transplantation is determined to a significant extent by the immune response of the recipient.
- In *autogenous* transplantation, e.g., transfer of skin from one site on the body to another site in the same individual, as well as in *syngenic* transplantation, there is no rejection reaction.
- Immune reactions against the transplant arise when donor and recipient tissues exhibit different antigen patterns, that is, in *allogenic* and *xenogenic* transplants.

Histocompatibility Antigens

Histocompatibility antigens are genetically determined tissue characteristics.

Histocompatibility antigens of the donor tissue do not occur in the recipient and are recognized as foreign. The result is an immune reaction with formation of specifically sensitized T lymphocytes that attack the transplant. The cellular immune response corresponds to the type IV allergic reaction (p. 27). Moreover, B lymphocytes create specific antibodies that attack the foreign tissue.

To avoid the rejection reaction or keep it at a minimum, the tissue compatibility of donor and recipient is tested before a transplantation for optimal compatibility. In addition, the immune reaction after transplantation of a foreign tissue is inhibited by lifelong immunosuppressive therapy. Only corneal transplantation is barely subject to rejection reactions because there are very few blood and lymph vessels in the anterior chamber of the eye.

Medications Relevant to Physical Therapists

■   Forms of Administration

The manner in which a medication is administered depends on:
- The properties of the medication, e.g., capacity to be absorbed
- When and how long the medication is expected to act
- Whether the medication is intended to act systemically or locally
- The patient's condition

Forms of Local Administration

For local use, medication is applied to the skin or the mucosa, e.g., oral mucosa, auditory canal, connective tissue of the eye, nasal mucosa, and vaginal mucosa. An active substance is also applied locally in inhalation therapy.

Depending on the active agent, a portion of it can be absorbed and thus function systemically as well.

Forms of Systemic Administration

Enteral Administration

In enteral administration, a medication enters the organism through the mucosa of the gastrointestinal tract. There are several possibilities for enteral administration:
- In *oral* administration, the patient swallows the medication.
- In *sublingual* administration, a medication is placed under the tongue and absorbed through the oral mucosa.
- In *rectal* administration, a suppository is introduced into the rectum and absorbed through the intestinal mucosa.

Parenteral Administration

In parenteral administration, a medication is administered by means other than the alimentary tract. Various types of injection fall into this category (**Fig. 5.3**):
- Intradermal (ID), i.e., into the epidermis
- Subcutaneous (SC), i.e., into the subcutaneous tissue
- Intramuscular (IM), i.e., into a muscle
- Intravenous (IV), i.e., into a vein
- Intra-arterial (IA), i.e., into an artery
- Intra-articular, i.e., into a joint
- Intrathecal, i.e., into the spinal canal

Infusion

In infusion, large quantities of fluid, usually containing medications, are administered, usually drop by drop, via one of the following venous approaches:
- Peripheral venous approach, especially with an indwelling venous catheter (e.g., the Venflon).
- A central venous catheter (CVC) inserted into the superior vena cava via the internal jugular vein or the subclavian vein, particularly for long-term infusions, infusion of medications that irritate the vessel walls, and for measurement of central venous pressure.

To ensure an exact inflow rate, infusion pumps such as syringe drivers (**Fig. 5.4**) or syringe pumps (**Fig. 5.5**) are used.

> *If infusion systems are in the way during physical therapy treatment, they may only be removed by the nursing staff or the physician.*

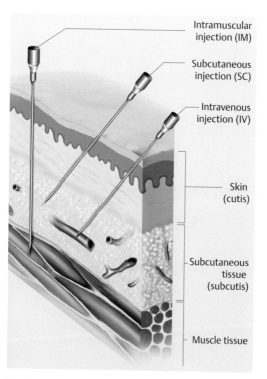

Intramuscular injection (IM)

Subcutaneous injection (SC)

Intravenous injection (IV)

Skin (cutis)

Subcutaneous tissue (subcutis)

Muscle tissue

Fig. 5.3 Various modes of injection.

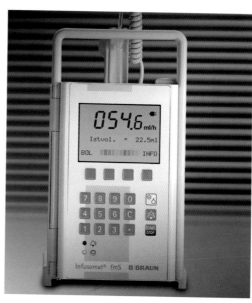

Fig. 5.4 Electrical infusion pump (Braun, Germany) (Kellnhauser 2004).

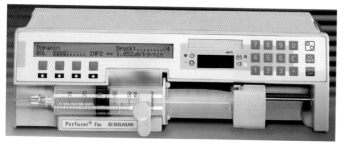

Fig. 5.5 Electrical syringe pump (Braun, Germany) (Kellnhauser 2004).

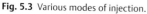

■ Medications That Affect Hemostasis

Physiological Basis

The physiological basis of hemostasis, coagulation, and fibrinolysis is described in detail on page 242.

Mechanism of Action and Typical Indications

The following groups of active agents influence hemostasis:

- *Platelet aggregation inhibitors:* Active agents in this group, such as acetylsalicylic acid or clopidogrel produce changes in platelets that decrease aggregation. This avoids thrombi, particularly in the arteries.

- *Heparins:* Heparins inhibit clotting by activating antithrombin III (AT III). AT III is a natural inhibitor that blocks the next to last step in the coagulation cascade. Since heparins are unstable in gastric acid, they must be administered subcutaneously or intravenously (**Fig. 5.6**).

- *Direct inhibitors of coagulation factors*: Newer substances are capable of inhibiting certain coagulation factors directly, e.g., Factor II or Factor X. They can be administered orally.

- *Coumarins:* Coumarins (such as Coumadin) inhibit the synthesis of coagulation factors in the liver, where they are formed with the help of vitamin K (Factors II, VII, IX and X). In contrast to heparins, coumarins can be administered orally.

Overdose and the resulting risk of bleeding can be countered by giving vitamin K (**Fig. 5.6**).

• *Fibrinolytics:* Fibrinolytics can dissolve blood clots in part or entirely through the activation of plasminogen (**Fig. 5.7**).

Important members of this group, together with their indications, are summarized in **Table 5.3**.

Side-effects

Medications that affect hemostasis and coagulation must be taken into account in physiotherapeutic treatment because of the increased risk of bleeding. Joints may only be stressed with care. Passive measures such as friction are to be used with restraint.

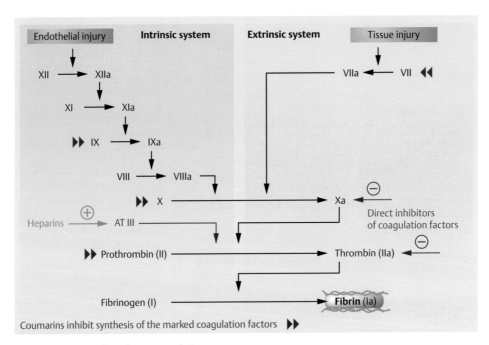

Fig. 5.6 Medications that influence coagulation.

Table 5.3 Medications that affect hemostasis and their indications

Active agents	Typical indications
Platelet aggregation inhibitors such as: • Acetylsalicylic acid • Clopidogrel	Prophylaxis and therapy of arterial thrombi, e.g., in: • Coronary artery disease (CAD, p. 98) • Myocardial infarction (p. 101) • Stent implantation (vessel support) • Ischemic cerebral infarction
Heparins	Prophylaxis and therapy of venous thrombi in: • Thrombosis (p. 131) • Pulmonary emboli (p. 163)
Coumarins such as • Coumadin • Phenprocoumon	• Prophylaxis of venous thromboses • Embolism prophylaxis in atrial fibrillation (p. 107) • Embolism prophylaxis for artificial heart valves (p. 111)
Fibrinolytics such as: • Urokinase • Streptokinase • Tissue plasminogen activators	Acute vascular occlusion by thrombus or embolus, e.g.: • Myocardial infarction (p. 101) • Thrombosis (p. 131) • Pulmonary embolism (p. 163) • Embolic cerebral infarction

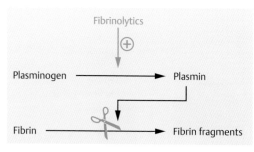

Fig. 5.7 Fibrinolytics

■ **Medications That Affect the Autonomic Nervous System**

Physiological basis

The autonomic nervous system (ANS), together with the endocrine system, controls the internal environment of the body. Its two branches adjust the functioning of the different organ systems to the various needs of the organism.
- The *sympathetic* branch is the component of the ANS that prepares the organism for "fight or flight" (**Fig. 5.8**).
- The *parasympathetic* branch regulates the energy uptake and storage of the body at rest (**Fig. 5.9**).

Mechanism of Action and Typical Indications

In illness, an attempt is often made to control and normalize organ functions with the help of medications that affect the function of the ANS.
- *Sympathomimetics* and *parasympathomimetics* imitate the functions of the respective branches of the autonomic nervous system.
- *Sympatholytics* and *parasympatholytics* inhibit the functions of the respective branches of the autonomic nervous system.

Sympathomimetics

- Sympathomimetics or catecholamines such as epinephrine (adrenaline) and norepinephrine (noradrenaline) are used in intensive and emergency medicine because of their effect on the circulation, e.g., in arterial hypotension (p. 119), in shock (p. 54), and in resuscitation (p. 108).
- Sympathomimetics administered by inhalation are bronchodilators and are therefore a component of therapy for obstructive respiratory diseases such as COPD (p. 148) and bronchial asthma (p. 153).

- In obstetrics, sympathomimetics are used to inhibit labor (tocolysis) since they relax smooth muscles such as the uterus.

Sympatholytics

The sympathetic nervous system acts on various receptors that can be blocked by sympatholytics.
- Alpha receptor blockers (alpha blockers) act to dilate blood vessels and thus lower blood pressure.
- Beta receptor blockers (beta blockers) suppress the action of the sympathetic nervous system, especially on the heart. Heart rate, excitability, contractility and oxygen requirement of the myocardium decrease. Important indications for beta blockers are:
  - Arterial hypertension (p. 117)
  - Coronary artery disease (p. 98)
  - Chronic heart failure (p. 96)
  - Various cardiac arrhythmias (p. 104)

Adverse effects of beta blockers are caused by increased tonus of the smooth muscles, for example, bronchoconstriction, peripheral vasoconstriction with circulatory disturbances, and uterine contractions with premature labor.

> In physiotherapeutic treatment, it must be kept in mind that under exertion the acceleration in heart rate is lower in a patient treated with a beta blocker. Heart rate is not an appropriate indicator for stress in these patients.

Parasympathomimetics

- Systemic administration of parasympathomimetics is used to treat intestinal atonia (paralytic ileus, p. 187).
- Eye drops containing parasympathomimetically active agents can decrease the internal pressure of the eye in glaucoma.

Parasympatholytics

Parasympatholytics such as atropine suppress the action of the parasympathetic system. They are used as:
- Spasmolytics
- Bronchodilators
- Mydriatics, i.e., to dilate the pupils before an ophthalmological examination

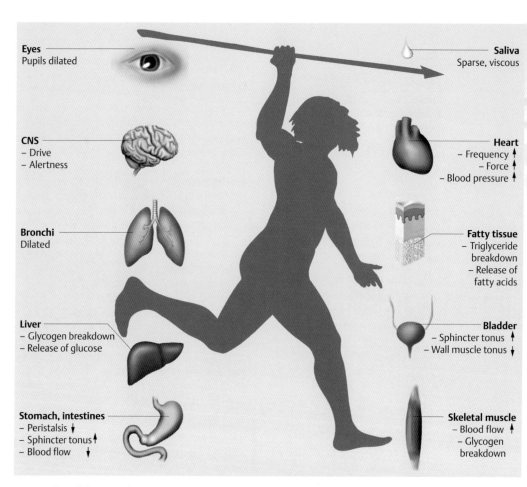

Eyes
Pupils dilated

Saliva
Sparse, viscous

CNS
– Drive
– Alertness

Heart
– Frequency ↑
– Force ↑
– Blood pressure ↑

Bronchi
Dilated

Fatty tissue
– Triglyceride
  breakdown
– Release of
  fatty acids

Liver
– Glycogen breakdown
– Release of glucose

Bladder
– Sphincter tonus ↑
– Wall muscle tonus ↓

Stomach, intestines
– Peristalsis ↓
– Sphincter tonus ↑
– Blood flow ↓

Skeletal muscle
– Blood flow ↑
– Glycogen
  breakdown

Fig. 5.8 Effect of the sympathetic nervous system (adopted from Heinz Lüllmann, Klaus Mohr, and Albrecht Ziegler).

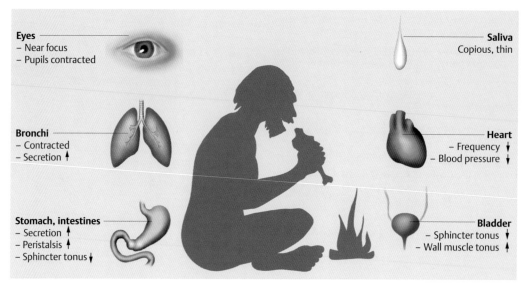

Eyes
– Near focus
– Pupils contracted

Saliva
Copious, thin

Bronchi
– Contracted
– Secretion ↑

Heart
– Frequency ↓
– Blood pressure ↓

Stomach, intestines
– Secretion ↑
– Peristalsis ↑
– Sphincter tonus ↓

Bladder
– Sphincter tonus ↓
– Wall muscle tonus ↑

Fig. 5.9 Effect of the parasympathetic nervous system (adopted from Heinz Lüllmann, Klaus Mohr, and Albrecht Ziegler).

■ Glucocorticosteroids

Physiological Basis

Naturally occurring glucocorticosteroids are hormones of the adrenal cortex, named after their effect on carbohydrate metabolism. Their main role is to make glucose and fatty acids available as energy sources, so that they are released in greater quantities in stress situations (**Table 5.4**). The most important member of this group is cortisol.

Mechanism of Action and Typical Indications

The main pharmacological application of glucocorticosteroids is based on their effect on the immune system. Their action is:
- Anti-inflammatory
- Antiallergic
- Immunosuppressive
- Antiproliferative (**Table 5.4**)

Typical indications for glucocorticosteroids are, for example:
- Autoimmune diseases (p. 29) such as the rheumatic diseases (p. 256)
- Allergic reactions (p. 26)
- Bronchial asthma (p. 153)

- Organ transplantation
- Substitution therapy in adrenocortical insufficiency (p. 241)

Side-effects

In long-term therapy with glucocorticosteroids, the dose may be such as to trigger exogenous Cushing syndrome. Most side-effects can be traced to their effect on metabolism:
- Steroid diabetes as a result of glucose availability (p. 215)
- Consequences of protein breakdown:
  - Parchment skin
  - Hemorrhaging as a result of capillary fragility
  - Connective tissue weakness and tears in the dermis, leading to the typical red stripes
  - Disturbance of wound healing
  - Muscle atrophy
  - Osteoporosis, which is also promoted by decreased calcium absorption in the intestine and increased calcium excretion by the kidneys (p. 225)
  - Rarely, aseptic bone necrosis
- Redistribution of deposited fat with full moon face, bull neck, and central obesity (p. 239)

Table 5.4 Effect of glucocorticosteroids

Site of action	Effect	Mechanisms
Carbohydrate, lipid and amino acid metabolism (alarm reaction)	Glucose availability	• Gluconeogenesis through catabolic action, i.e., protein breakdown in: – Muscles – Bones – Skin – Lymphatic tissue • Redistribution of fat
Coronary circulation (alarm reaction)	Elevated blood pressure	• Enhancement of epinephrine action • Vasoconstriction • Sodium and water retention by the kidneys
Kidneys	Decrease in diuresis	At higher doses, it acts like aldosterone, i.e., causes retention of sodium and water
Immune system	• Anti-inflammatory • Antiallergic • Immunosuppressive	At high doses it inhibits: • Lymphocyte formation • Antibody formation (proteins) • Phagocytosis • Histamine release
Stomach	Increase in production of gastric juice	
Brain	At high doses it: • Acts on the hypothalamus • Causes psychological alterations	

Further consequences of hypercortisolism include:
- Secondary arterial hypertension (p. 117)
- Tendency to edema
- Susceptibility to infection
- Gastric ulcers (ulcus ventriculi, p. 180)
- Psychological changes, such as depression
- Loss of libido and impotence in men; menstrual disturbances in women

> *In physiotherapeutic treatment, the most important problems to watch for are risk of osteoporosis, parchment skin, fragile vessels, and arterial hypertension.*

Cushing Threshold Dose

The adverse effects mentioned only occur after long-term therapy with unphysiologically high doses. Synthetic glucocorticosteroids, which are more active than cortisol, induce side-effects even at low doses (**Table 5.5**).

Table 5.5 Cushing threshold dose for different glucocorticosteroids

Active agent	Potency	Threshold dose
Cortisol	1	30 mg/day
Prednisolone	4	7.5 mg/day
Methylprednisolone	5	6 mg/day
Triamcinolone	5	6 mg/day
Paramethasone	10	3 mg/day
Betamethasone	30	1 mg/day
Dexamethasone	30	1 mg/day

Study Questions on General Pathology

Review the text and increase your understanding of it to prepare for the examination. (The page numbers in parentheses indicate where the answers can be found.)

1. What are the factors that can provoke an inflammatory reaction? (p. 5)

2. Name the signs of local and systemic inflammation. (p. 6)

3. What are the laboratory parameters that indicate the presence of inflammation? (p. 7)

4. What causes an aberration in the number of chromosomes? (p. 11)

5. Explain autosomal dominant inheritance. (p. 14)

6. Explain autosomal recessive inheritance. (p. 14)

7. Explain gonosomal recessive inheritance. (p. 15)

8. What characterizes multifactorially determined diseases? (p. 16)

9. What is the difference between embryopathies and fetopathies (p. 17–18)

10. What is the structure of bacteria? (p. 21)

11. What is the structure of viruses? (p. 23)

12. How do viruses reproduce? (p. 24)

13. Name some fungi that are human pathogens. (p. 24)

14. What is atopic diathesis? (p. 27)

15. Describe the type I allergic reaction. (p. 27)

16. What is the purpose of hyposensitization? (p. 28)

17. Describe the type IV allergic reaction. (p. 29)

18. What is an autoimmune disease? Give some important clinical examples. (p. 29)

19. Name the vascular risk factors. (p. 32)

20. What are the possible consequences of arteriosclerosis? (p. 32)

21. What is the difference between benign and malignant tumors? (p. 33)

22. What is a carcinoma? (p. 34)

23. What is a sarcoma? (p. 34)

24. Name the three most frequent forms of malignant tumors in men, women, and children, respectively. (p. 34–36)

25. What are the factors that can affect the growth of malignant tumors? (p. 36)

26. What is a precancerous condition? (p. 38)

27. What is a carcinoma in situ? (p. 38)

28. Name some pathways of metastasis. (p. 39)

29. Name some paraneoplastic syndromes. (p. 40)

30. What are tumor markers? (p. 41)

31. What is the difference between central and peripheral cyanosis. Give some important examples. (p. 43)

32. What causes icterus? (p. 44)

33. What are the factors that promote a tendency to bleed? (p. 46)

34. What causes edema? (p. 47)

35. What is an effusion? What is the difference between exudate and transudate? (p. 49)

36. Which differential diagnoses must be considered for a patient with dyspnea? (p. 49)

37. What are the differential diagnoses for thoracic pain? (p. 51)

38. Name some causes of an acute abdomen. (p. 52)

39. What can cause fever? (p. 52)

40. What is the shock spiral and what are the chief forms of shock? (p. 54)

41. Describe the signs and symptoms of shock. (p. 54)

42. What are the stages of quantitatively altered states of consciousness? (p. 55)

43. What can cause a syncope? (p. 56)

44. Which differential diagnoses must be considered in a patient with vertigo? (p. 57)

45. What must be included in a self-reported medical history? (p. 58)

46. What are the most important imaging techniques? (p. 59–63)

47. Which organs can be evaluated endoscopically? (p. 64)

48. What is the difference between curative and palliative therapy, between causal and symptomatic treatment, and between conservative and operative therapy? (p. 66)

49. What measures are applied in oncological therapy? (p. 67)

50. What are the risks of an organ transplantation? (p. 71)

51. Which medications affect hemostasis and clotting? What are the consequences for physiotherapeutic treatment? (p. 73–74)

52. How do sympathomimetics and sympatholytics work? (p. 75)

53. How do parasympathomimetics and parasympatholytics work? (p. 75)

54. When are glucocorticosteroids indicated? (p. 77)

55. What are the signs and symptoms of Cushing syndrome? What consequences of physiotherapeutic treatment must be taken into account? (p. 78)

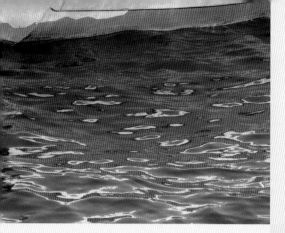

Part 2
Internal Medicine

This section of the book discusses all areas of internal medicine:

- Cardiology
- Vascular Medicine
- Pneumology
- Gastroenterology
- Nephrology
- Metabolism and Endocrinology
- Hematology
- Rheumatology
- Infectiology

Each chapter begins with a summary of the anatomical and physiological basis of each organ system. Then the causes, symptoms, diagnoses and therapy of the most important disease pictures are developed and physiotherapeutic aspects are pointed out.

6 Cardiology

Physiological Basis

◼ Excitation and Conduction

Specialized myocardial cells are responsible for excitation and conduction in the heart (**Fig. 6.1**). The sinus rhythm is the basic physiological rhythm. The cells of the sinus node can produce an action potential independently, i.e., without a nerve impulse. This potential spreads over the myocardial cells of the atria and to the atrioventricular node (AV node). Finally, the ventricular myocardium is excited by the His–Tawara bundle and the Purkinje fibers.

Each of these structures can evoke action potentials (**Table 6.1**). Since the sinus node, at 60–80 beats/min has the highest intrinsic frequency, it is at the head of the hierarchy and determines the heart rate. But if it fails, in a disease condition, the myocardium is stimulated by the next intact pacemaker at a correspondingly lower frequency.

The autonomic nervous system influences the sinus node to adjust the heart rate to the requirements of the organism.
- The heart rate increases under the influence of the sympathetic nervous system and under physical stress.
- The vagus nerve exercises parasympathetic control and lowers the heart rate. This occurs, among other things, during sleep or in athletes at rest.

◼ Mechanical Performance of the Heart

After an electrical impulse, the myocardium contracts. The cardiac cycle (**Fig. 6.2a, b**) is basically a temporal sequence of the following mechanical events:
- Systole, consisting of myocardial contraction and ejection phase
- Diastole, consisting of myocardial relaxation and filling phase

These concepts apply to the action of the ventricles.

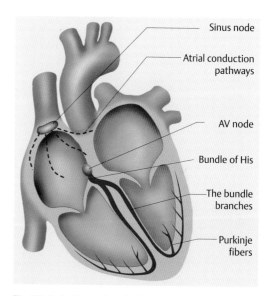

Fig. 6.1 Excitation and conduction system.

Table 6.1 Physiological cardiac pacemakers

Pacemaker	Anatomical structures	Essential frequency
Primary	Sinus node	60–80/min
Secondary	AV node	40–60/min
Tertiary	• Bundle of His • Tawara bundle • Purkinje fibers • Ventricular myocardium	20–40/min

Systole

At the start of systole (Greek: contraction), all heart valves are closed. Ventricular pressure starts to build up in the early contraction phase and exceeds that in the atria. As soon as the ventricular pressure is higher than the pressure in the aorta and pulmonary trunk, the semilunar valves open and the ejection phase begins (**Fig. 6.2a, b**). Of the 120 mL of blood in each chamber at the start of systole, about 80 mL is ejected. The *ejection fraction* (EF) is the ratio of stroke volume and the end-diastolic filling volume.

◼ *Normal EF value: 60%–75%.*

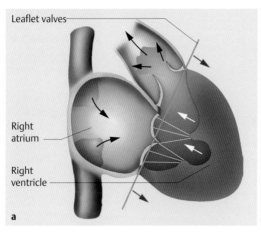
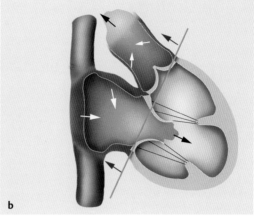

Leaflet valves

Right
atrium

Right
ventricle

a

b

Fig. 6.2a, b The heart as pressure-suction pump. **a** Systole. **b** Diastole.

At the end of the ejection phase, the ventricular pressure decreases below the pressure in the aorta and the pulmonary trunk, and the semilunar valves return to the closed position. This is the end of the systole.

When the end-systolic volume is less than the equilibrium volume, recoil forces are generated due to shortened muscle fibers in the ventricles acting as a compressed spring. The resulting suction and pressure decrease in the atria permits filling of the atria and venous blood return to the heart.

Diastole

The ventricular myocardium relaxes and the recoil forces occur in early diastolic phase (Greek: diastole, derived from the two words *to send* and *apart*). The ventricular pressure drops, while the atrial pressure rises above the pressure of the ventricles. Then the valve leaflets open and the relaxation phase is followed by the filling phase. End-diastolic contraction of the atria helps to complete diastole and contributes to about 20% of ventricular filling.

Cardiac Output

The cardiac output is calculated from the stroke volume times the heart rate and at rest amounts to about 5 L/min. Generally, three mechanisms cause it to rise to 25–30 L/min under physical stress:
- The Frank–Starling mechanism
- The autonomic nervous system (ANS) via the sympathetic nervous system
- Myocardial hypertrophy

Frank–Starling Mechanism

To a certain extent the heart, which consists of striated muscles, functions as a self-regulating pump. When the venous backflow, and thus the final diastolic filling, increases, the actin and myosin filaments overlap optimally, the subsequent contraction is stronger, and the stroke volume increases as needed.

In the case of pathological dilatation, actin and myosin filaments are pushed so far apart that there are scarcely any cross-bridges between them, and the contraction force decreases.

Sympathetic Nervous System

The sympathetic nervous system is the component of the ANS that prepares the organism for "fight or flight." It increases the cardiac output by:
- Increasing the heart rate; the so-called positive chronotropic effect
- Shortening the conduction time of the AV node; the so-called positive bathmotropic effect
- Increasing the contractility; the so-called positive inotropic effect

However, an increase in heart rate is not an unlimited advantage, since it is only possible at the expense of the diastole (**Table 6.2**).
- This gives the ventricles less time to fill and, as a result, stroke volume is decreased.
- In systole, the blood vessels embedded in the myocardium are compressed, so that the myocardium is supplied with blood mainly during diastole. Consequently, the blood supply to the myocardium is diminished if diastole is shortened.

� *Rule of thumb: Maximal heart rate = 220 – age.*

Table 6.2 Duration of systole and diastole with increase in heart rate

Heart rate	Duration of systole	Duration of diastole
70/min	0.28s	0.58s
150/min	0.25s	0.15s

Myocardial Hypertrophy

Both the Frank–Starling mechanism and the sympathetic nervous system can increase cardiac output for a brief time. When the myocardium is continuously stressed, as in athletes, it reacts, like any muscle, with hypertrophy.

If a critical heart weight of 500g is exceeded as a result of myocardial hypertrophy, there is a risk of decreased blood circulation and disorders of heart rhythm.

■ Circulation

Anatomically, the circulation can be divided into systemic circulation and pulmonary circulation (or the large and small circulation), or according to the prevailing pressure into a high-pressure and a low-pressure system (**Fig. 6.3, Table 6.3**).

Low-Pressure System and Venous Blood Return to the Heart

The veins of the systemic circulation are part of the low-pressure system. In spite of the low pressure, the following factors guarantee an adequate circulation speed and thus venous return (**Fig. 6.4a, b**):

- Venous valves direct the flow of blood toward the heart and prevent the blood from flowing back into the periphery.
- Veins are compressed when neighboring muscles contract. This is the so-called muscle pump (**Fig. 6.4a**).
- Veins are compressed by the pulse wave of neighboring arteries, the so-called arteriovenous pump (**Fig. 6.4b**).
- Through the suction mechanism of the heart, pressure in the atria falls during systole and, in this way, the blood is "sucked" out of the veins (**Fig. 6.2a,b**).
- In breathing, there is continual alternation between intra-abdominal or intrathoracic pressure increase and decrease, and these states are transmitted to the veins.

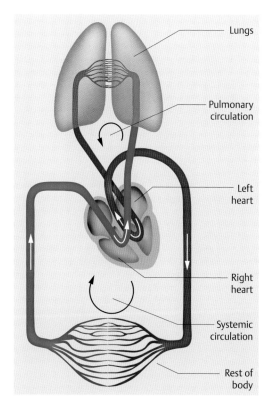

Fig. 6.3 Systemic and pulmonary circulation.

Lungs

Pulmonary circulation

Left heart

Right heart

Systemic circulation

Rest of body

Table 6.3 Division of the circulation into high- and low-pressure systems

System and related structures	Pressure
High-pressure system: • Left ventricle • Arteries of the large circulation	80–120 mmHg
Low-pressure system: • Veins of the large circulation • Right heart • Pulmonary circulation • Left atrium	5–20 mmHg

High-Pressure System and Blood Pressure Regulation

The pressure prevailing in the arteries of the systemic circulation is termed *blood pressure* (BP). **Figure 6.5** shows the course of blood pressure in the aorta as a function of heart action.

- The maximal pressure is about 120 mmHg. Since this is the prevailing pressure when the heart is in systole, it is called the *systolic blood pressure* (SBP).

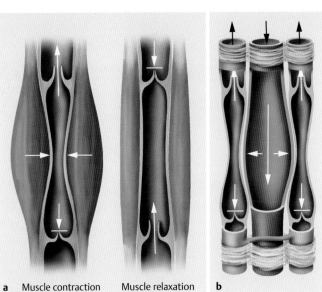

Fig. 6.4a,b Venous blood return.
a Muscle pump. **b** Arteriovenous coupling.

a   Muscle contraction   Muscle relaxation   **b**

Fig. 6.5 Time relationship between ECG and mechanical heart action.

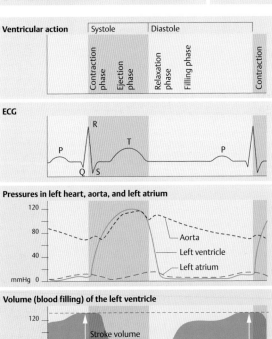

- The minimal pressure is about 80 mmHg. Since this is the prevailing pressure when the heart is in diastole, it is called the *diastolic blood pressure* (DBP).

The indirect, bloodless method of measuring blood pressure by means of an upper-arm cuff is documented in the form:

▌ *BP 120/80 mmHg.*

Various mechanisms maintain blood pressure and thus circulation to the organs. Of these mechanisms, we will explain here the pressor receptor reflex and the renin–angiotensin–aldosterone system.

Pressor Receptor Reflex

In the aortic arch and the carotid artery there are receptors that measure the blood pressure. These pressor receptors transmit the result of their measurement to the circulation control center in the medulla oblongata. This reacts to a drop in blood pressure by activating the sympathetic system and inhibiting the parasympathetic system. The blood pressure rises again. In contrast, when the pressure rises, the parasympathetic system is activated and the sympathetic system is inhibited, causing blood pressure to fall again.

▌ *Pressor receptors adapt—i.e., they accept a steady high pressure as the new normal value.*

Renin–Angiotensin–Aldosterone System

A specific pressure of the blood reaching the kidneys is important for their function. The kidneys (Latin *renes*, cf. "renal") react to a fall in blood pressure by releasing renin, which transforms angiotensinogen to angiotensin I. Angiotensin I is converted to the active agent angiotensin II by *angiotensin-converting enzyme* (ACE), which causes vasoconstriction and release of aldosterone from the adrenal glands.

Aldosterone causes a sensation of thirst and decreases diuresis by increasing resorption of sodium and water in the kidneys. Increased fluid uptake and decreased fluid excretion increases blood volume and this, together with vasoconstriction, raises blood pressure. The renin–angiotensin–aldosterone system (RAAS) is outlined in **Fig. 6.6.**

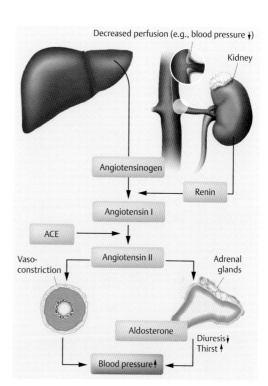

Fig. 6.6 The renin–angiotensin–aldosterone system.

Cardinal Cardiological Symptoms

▪ Overview

Some important cardinal cardiological symptoms are:
- Signs of heart failure
- Chest pain, especially retrosternal pain
- Syncope
- Racing pulse, palpitation, pounding heartbeat

While in Part 1 of the book we discussed the differential diagnosis of chest pain and syncope, in this second part we will explain symptoms that can occur in patients with heart failure.

▪ Cardinal Syndrome Heart Failure

Definition and Significance

All heart diseases can reduce cardiac function to such an extent that the heart is no longer able to provide tissues with sufficient blood and oxygen to ensure metabolism under exertion or even at rest in advanced diseases. The resulting signs are combined under the term *heart failure*.

Heart failure is one of the most frequent syndromes in internal medicine and affects 1–2% of the population. The frequency of occurrence, like that of underlying diseases, increases with age. Prevalence rises from under 1% in persons aged from 45 to 55 years to about 10% in persons aged 80 years.

Classification and Causes

The underlying heart diseases can be divided into four groups according to their immediate effects (**Table 6.4**):
- In most diseases, the left ventricle is too weak to increase the stroke volume in response to demand. In that case, we are dealing with a *systolic functional disorder.*
- More rarely it is an *isolated diastolic functional disorder,* in which ventricular relaxation and ventricular filling are impaired. The blood backs up in the veins on its return to the heart, which leads to congestion.
- Some diseases produce increased resistance in the systemic and pulmonary circulation that the left or the right ventricle must overcome and thus lead to increased afterload.
- Increased preload is equivalent to the increased volume that must be pumped by the heart.

Acute and chronic heart failure are distinguished by their time course.
- *Acute heart failure* appears within minutes to hours with symptoms of cardiogenic shock as a result of abrupt decrease in cardiac output, e.g., in an extensive myocardial infarction or in the form of cardiogenic pulmonary edema by backward failure of the left ventricle.
- *Chronic heart failure* occurs when the underlying disease and the signs persist over a period of at least 6 months. The main causes of chronic heart failure are arterial hypertension and coronary artery disease (CAD).

Symptoms and Compensation Mechanisms

For a better understanding of symptoms, a distinction is often made between the signs of left-sided and right-sided heart failure. Often there is only a slight connection between complaints and the degree of ventricular dysfunction.

Symptoms of Left-Sided Heart Failure

A weak left ventricle is not able to supply sufficient blood flow to meet the body's need (so-called for-

Table 6.4 Causes of heart failure

Underlying diseases	Immediate effects
• Coronary artery disease (CAD) • Myocardial infarction • Cardiac arrhythmias • Myocarditis • Dilated cardiomyopathies	Systolic dysfunction
• Left ventricular hypertrophy, as in arterial hypertension • Hypertrophic and restrictive cardiomyopathy • Pericarditis and pericardial tamponade	Diastolic dysfunction
• Stenoses of the semilunar valves • Arterial hypertension • Pulmonary hypertension	Increased afterload
• Valve regurgitation • Stenoses of the AV valves • Congenital heart diseases with left-to-right shunt • Volume overload	Elevated preload

ward failure). At the same time, backward failure causes congestion in the pulmonary circulation. The following symptoms result from *forward failure:*
- Physical capacity is decreased. Weakness, exhaustion, and tiredness are frequent first symptoms.
- Sleep disorders, confusion, and syncope occur as a result of insufficient circulation to the brain.
- Arterial hypotension and shock (p. 54) are the expression of a severe output failure.

In *backward failure* of the left ventricle, the blood congests in the pulmonary circulation and pulmonary edema develops (p. 91, see **Fig. 6.15**). Possible consequences include:
- Dyspnea that first occurs only on exertion and in severe cases even at rest
- Orthopnea, that is, position-dependent air hunger, especially when lying in supine position
- Cough caused by irritation or fluid congestion; can be dry or associated with foaming sputum, possibly flecked with blood
- Paroxysmal nocturnal dyspnea, that is, air hunger and attacks of coughing that awaken the patient abruptly
- Central cyanosis, since the blood is insufficiently oxygenated (p. 43)

Symptoms of Right-Sided Heart Failure

Figure 6.7 shows edema, with the associated weight gain and engorged neck veins as visible signs of right heart failure. They are caused by fluid congestion due to right ventricular backward failure.

At first, edemas form symmetrically around the feet, around the ankles, and pretibially; later they can be generalized as so-called anasarca. Since fluid collects primarily in lower levels of the body, in response to gravity, edema in bed-bound patients tend to be found in the sacrum, flanks, thighs, and genitals. Collections of fluid increase during the day; at night they are washed out.

Venous congestion also impairs the function of many organs, resulting in:

- Pleural effusions
- Congested liver, even cirrhosis of the liver
- Congestive gastritis with a feeling of fullness and loss of appetite
- Renal congestion with nocturia (urinating at night) and proteinuria

Global Heart Failure

Isolated right-sided heart failure rarely occurs. Usually it is the result of left-sided heart failure with accumulation of fluid in the lungs that applies secondary stress to the right ventricle. This is also called global or biventricular heart failure.

"Compensatory Vicious Spiral"

Initially, the cardiac output can still be increased by the physiological compensatory mechanisms that were described on page 85, ensuring sufficient circulation to the organs. But in the long term, they contribute to worsening of heart failure (**Fig. 6.8**).

- The activated sympathetic system increases the heart rate and the contractility of the myocardium, and leads to vasoconstriction. But the increased myocardial oxygen demand and shortened diastole, as well as the increased afterload, have a negative long-term effect.
- Since cardiac output decreases, and with it the renal perfusion, the RAAS is activated. Angiotensin narrows the vessels, elevating the afterload, while aldosterone increases the available volume and the preload.

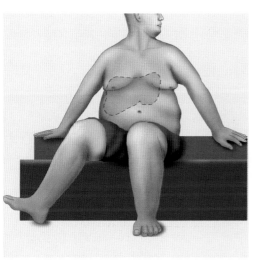

Fig. 6.7 Patient with right heart failure. Congested jugular veins, peripheral edema and acrocyanosis are remarkable.

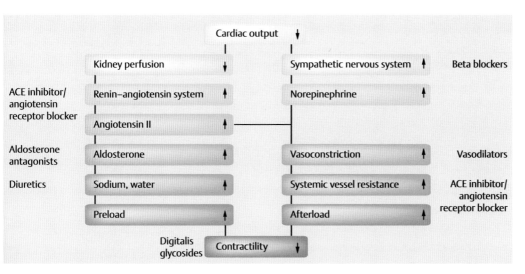

Fig. 6.8 Compensatory vicious spiral and drug therapy in chronic heart failure.

Degrees of Clinical Severity

Heart failure is classified into stages I–IV, according to the classification of the New York Heart Association (NYHA) (**Table 6.5**).

Course of the Disease and Prognosis

Heart failure is usually progressive, even when no new or additional myocardial damage occurs. The clinical picture can suddenly become worse, i.e., decompensate acutely and lead to complications such as acute pulmonary edema or cardiogenic shock (p. 54). In addition, patients are more susceptible to life-threatening cardiac arrhythmias and thrombotic and thromboembolic events.

The prognosis becomes worse with increasing NYHA stage. About 10% of patients in NYHA stage I die within 2 years. In the same period of time, about 40% of all NYHA stage IV patients die. Very rarely, heart failure can improve, for instance after myocarditis or after elimination of a clearly identifiable cause such as an arrhythmia by antiarrhythmic treatment or a defective heart valve by means of a valve replacement.

Table 6.5 Degrees of clinical severity of chronic heart failure according to the revised NYHA classification

Stage	Functional classification
I	Heart disease without physical limitation
II	Heart disease with slight limitation of physical capacity under everyday activity
III	Heart disease with marked limitation of physical capacity under everyday activity
IV	Heart disease with complaints during all activities and at rest

Cardiological Diagnosis

■ **Patient History and Physical Examination**

Patient history and physical examination findings usually lead to a correct initial diagnosis. Inspection, palpation of the heart region and pulses, and percussion and auscultation with the stethoscope provide important information about the condition of the heart and circulatory system.

A significant part of examining a heart patient is taking the blood pressure. Additional technical examinations help to confirm the diagnosis, determine the degree of severity of the heart disease, and arrive at the right program of therapy.

Auscultation

The first and the second heart sound is produced by the mechanical action of the heart (**Fig. 6.9**).
- The first heart sound is heard at the beginning of ventricular contraction. It is an acoustic signal of the start of systole.
- The second heart sound is produced when the semilunar valves close. It identifies the end of systole and the onset of diastole.

Pathological heart murmurs are mainly an indicator of valvular defects. Depending on the time of appearance, a distinction is made between:
- Systolic murmurs, occurring in systole, beginning with or after the first heart sound
- Diastolic murmurs, occurring in diastole, beginning with or after the second heart sound

Examples
- In mitral regurgitation, the mitral valve does not close correctly and during systole blood rushes

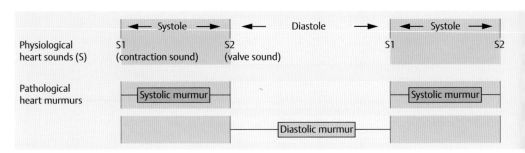

Fig. 6.9 Schematic representation of heart sounds and heart murmurs.

back through the leaking valve into the atrium. This creates a systolic murmur.

• In mitral stenosis, the mitral valve does not open correctly, so that filling is impeded. As a result of turbulent flow, a diastolic murmur is heard.

Blood Pressure Measurement

• The pressure in the arteries of the systemic circulation can be measured directly and indirectly. The direct, bloody method for blood pressure measurement is only indicated in exceptional cases, such as in intensive care treatments. The bloodless method (p. 85) has become generally used. In this method, arterial pressure is determined by means of a sphygmomanometer.

• A rubber sleeve (cuff) is connected to a scale with a column of mercury, allowing the examiner to take a reading. The cuff is wrapped around the upper arm and inflated to a pressure of about 30 mmHg above the expected systolic blood pressure. Since the cuff is compressing the artery, no radial pulse can be detected and no sounds can be heard when the stethoscope is placed over the brachial artery. The pressure in the cuff is slowly released while listening to the pulse and reading on the scale. When the pressure falls below the systolic blood pressure, blood flows through the artery synchronously with the pulse. This flow can be heard as the so-called Korotkoff sounds. When the pressure in the cuff falls below the diastolic blood pressure, blood can flow through the artery continuously and the Korotkoff sounds disappear. The corresponding values can be read on the manometer scale.

The best picture of the actual blood pressure situation can be obtained by using ambulatory blood pressure monitoring over 24 hours. An upper arm cuff measures the blood pressure at defined intervals. A portable storage medium registers the measured data, which are evaluated by a computer.

Normal values:
• Daytime average below 135/85 mmHg
• Nighttime average below 120/75 mmHg
• The frequency of values above 140/90 mmHg is less than 25% during the day and less than 20% at night.
• The nighttime decrease in systolic and diastolic blood pressure is greater than 10 mmHg.

■ Electrocardiogram

For many cardiological problems, it is useful to record an electrocardiogram (ECG). This procedure gives a graphic representation of the electrical behavior of the heart. **Figure 6.10** shows the basic arrangement of electrodes for the ECG and **Table 6.6** shows how the ECG is read.

There are various recording modes for an ECG: Standard 12-lead ECG at rest, ECG in exercise stress testing, long-term ECG recording, ECG monitoring.

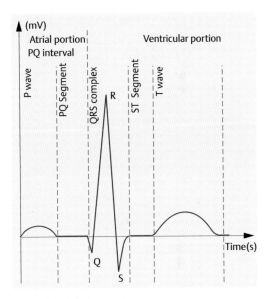

Fig. 6.10 ECG: basic recording

Table 6.6 Basic principles of the ECG

ECG	Significance and comments
P wave	Atrial depolarization
PQ segment	• Conduction time, i.e., the time required by the AV node to conduct excitation from the atria to the ventricles • Isoelectric, i.e., no voltage registered because all atrial cells are at the same level of excitation
QRS complex	Ventricular depolarization
ST segment	Isoelectric, i.e., no voltage registered because all ventricular cells are at the same level of excitation
T wave	Ventricular repolarization

Standard 12-lead ECG at Rest

The standard ECG is recorded at rest using 12 leads (**Fig. 6.11a, b**) in order to collect as much information as possible:

- Standard limb leads according to Einthoven (I, II, III)
- Limb leads according to Goldberger (aVR: right arm, aVL: left arm, aVF: foot)
- Precordial leads according to Wilson (V_1–V_6)

The resting ECG serves chiefly to determine heart rhythm and conduction disorders as well as to recognize a myocardial infarction and evaluate its course. In addition, ECG changes arise in myocardial hypertrophy, CAD, myocarditis, electrolyte disorders, and many other clinical conditions.

ECG in Exercise Stress Testing

The examination takes place with continuous recording of the ECG and closely spaced blood pressure measurements in the presence of a physician. The patient is subjected to incremental stress increases, under standard conditions, until he or she reaches at least 85% of the age-dependent maximal heart rate. Exercise protocols involve bicycle ergometry, treadmill protocols, arm ergometry, or step stairs to apply dynamic exercise. The procedure serves to determine the general performance capacity and, in particular, to identify myocardial ischemia. If a relevant coronary stenosis is present, the capacity to increase coronary blood flow in response to increased oxygen demand, is abolished. This can result in chest pain (angina pectoris) or dyspnea as well as changes in the ECG. Possible indications for exercise testing are:

- Preventive examination of patients with cardiac risk factors
- Clinical suspicion of coronary artery disease
- Determination of performance capacity after myocardial infarction
- Determination of the blood pressure response to exertion. At a level of 100 watts, the blood pressure should not exceed 200/100 mmHg; higher values indicate stress hypertension while resting values are normal.

Long-term ECG Recording

In a long-term or Holter ECG, an ECG is registered continuously over a period of 24–48 hours. The electrical signals are conducted and recorded by

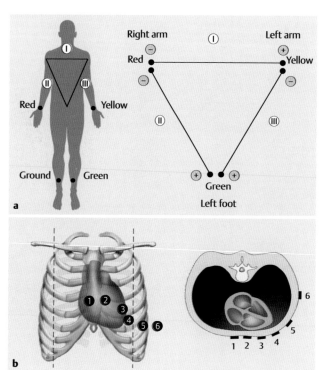

Fig. 6.11a, b ECG: position of the electrodes.

electrodes applied to the chest and recorded on a portable storage medium. This examination makes it possible to record occasional disturbances of heart rhythm. The recording can be extended over several weeks or months by means of special instruments called event recorders.

ECG Monitoring

The patient is attached to a monitor, for instance for continuous monitoring of the heart rhythm in an intensive care unit or an ambulance.

◼ Noninvasive Imaging

Echocardiography

Echocardiography is an ultrasound examination that can produce moving images of the heart's structure and function (**Fig. 6.12**). Blood flow and blood flow direction can be evaluated by means of Doppler and color Doppler echocardiography.

Transthoracic Echocardiography (TTE)

In this standard examination, the transducer is applied to the chest in order to obtain the following information:
- Size and function of atria and ventricles
- Morphology and function of the heart valves
- Thickness of the myocardial walls

During Stress Test Echocardiography

This is a special procedure for the diagnosis of coronary artery disease and myocardial ischemia. Contraction of the myocardium is observed during dynamic stress testing, e.g., in the bicycle exercise test, or with pharmacological stress testing using infusion of the stress hormone dobutamine. In case of myocardial ischemia, the corresponding area of myocardium will show wall motion abnormalities.

Transesophageal Echocardiography (TEE)

Certain problems can be better studied by transesophageal echocardiography. In this procedure, an ultrasound probe is introduced into the esophagus behind the heart. This provides a more exact image of the left atrium, the heart valves, and the ascending aorta and permits a more certain diagnosis of:
- Atrial thrombi in atrial fibrillation (**Fig. 6.13**)
- Vegetations (growth of tissue) on the valves in endocarditis
- Aortic dissection

However, this procedure is less pleasant for the patient. Local spray anesthesia of the pharynx and sometimes even sedation is necessary so that the patient can swallow and tolerate the probe.

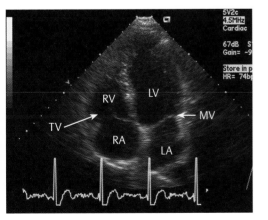

Fig. 6.12 Echocardiography: four-chamber view (MV, mitral valve; TV, tricuspid valve; RA, right atrium; LA, left atrium; RV, right ventricle; LV, left ventricle). (Flachskampf 2004.)

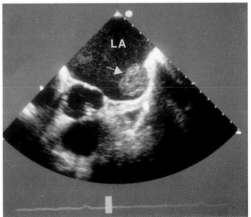

Fig. 6.13 Echocardiography: atrial thrombi in atrial fibrillation (LA, left atrium). (Baenkler 1999.)

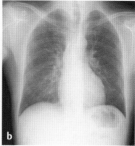

Fig. 6.14a, b Posterior–anterior view of the thorax: normal heart shape and position.

Aorta
Superior vena cava
Left atrium
Pulmonary trunk
Right atrium
Left ventricle
Right ventricle
a
b

Chest Radiography

Radiography of the chest is used for cardiac and pulmonary diagnosis, both in acute cases and to follow the course of a disease. Preferably images are made in two planes, with posteroanterior and lateral irradiation (**Fig. 6.14a, b**). In cardiological diagnosis, the radiographs provide the following information:

- The outline and size of the heart are changed when individual sections of the heart are enlarged or subject to stress.
- Increased prominence of the pulmonary vessels occurs when blood backs up into the vessels of the pulmonary circulation in the presence of left heart failure.
- Pulmonary edema is characterized by diffuse, spotty structures over the entire lung (**Fig. 6.15**).
- In a standing patient, a pleural effusion can be seen first in the angle of the diaphragm.

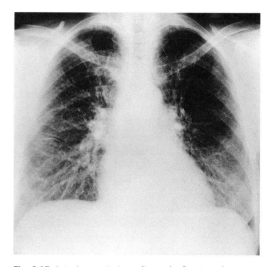

Fig. 6.15 Anterior–posterior radiograph of acute pulmonary edema. (Baenkler 1999.)

Procedures in Nuclear Medicine

In nuclear medical diagnosis, radioactive substances are injected and their diffusion throughout the body is followed by a specialized camera. Scintigraphy of the myocardium, for instance, is used in diagnosing ischemia where there is known or suspected stable coronary disease. It provides information as to the vitality and perfusion of the heart muscle. As in stress echocardiography, the examination is carried out at rest and during stress testing.

Sectional Imaging Procedures

Cardiac magnetic resonance imaging (MRI) uses magnetic fields to generate images in planes that can be selected at will. In this way, the morphology and function of the heart can be presented in three dimensions and without the stress of irradiation. The method is used, for instance, in the diagnosis of myocardial diseases and congenital heart disease. Cardiac MRI is also being used increasingly to study function. For instance, it is used to determine whether myocardial sections are still vital or have already been transformed to scar tissue and whether they are being perfused at rest and under stress.

Computed tomographic (CT) scanning is being used for the detection of the amount of calcification in the coronary arteries to evaluate cardiovascular risk in selected asymptomatic patients. A current research question is whether the coronary calcification has any prognostic value. In a CT scan, the patient is exposed to X-rays, as in a left heart catheterization.

■ **Heart Catheterization**

Left Heart Catheterization

Figure 6.16 shows the principle of left heart catheterization. After administration of local analgesia, a guide catheter is inserted into an easily accessible, large artery, usually the femoral artery in the groin or the brachial artery in the crook of the elbow or the radial artery. Through this, under radiographic control, a probe is advanced via the aorta to the heart and on into the ostium of the coronary artery to be examined. The aorta and the coronary arteries can be visualized by using radiographic contrast agents. The respective examinations are called:

- Aortography
- Coronary angiography

If there is narrowing of vessels or even occlusion, the vessel is slow to fill with the contrast agent or does not fill at all. Any stenoses present can be located and possibly even dilated in the same session (p. 98).

In ventriculography, the catheter is advanced into the left ventricle through the aortic valve and, after administration of contrast agent, the wall movement of the myocardium and the pumping function can be evaluated.

In addition, in a left heart catheterization, pressure in the aorta or the left ventricle is measured. Thus, for example, the extent of an aortic valve stenosis can be evaluated because the pressure difference between ventricle and aorta increases with increasing degree of stenosis.

Aftercare

After the femoral artery has been punctured, there is a danger of bleeding. To avoid this, a pressure bandage is applied. The following precautions are advised:

- *The leg should remain extended.*
- *The patient should remain in bed for at least 4 hours (observe individual physician's orders).*
- *The patient should avoid heavy physical activity for 7 days.*

Right Heart Catheterization

To permit one to reach the right heart with a catheter, a large, easily accessible vein is punctured, for example, the femoral vein in the groin or the jugular vein in the neck or the subclavian vein near the collar bone. The catheter is advanced toward the heart with the bloodstream. Depending on the problem to be investigated, it can be placed in the right atrium, the right ventricle or the pulmonary artery. The catheter is used to measure pressures and the cardiac output.

- A right heart catheter is inserted to evaluate the effects on the circulation of certain congenital or acquired heart and valvular diseases.

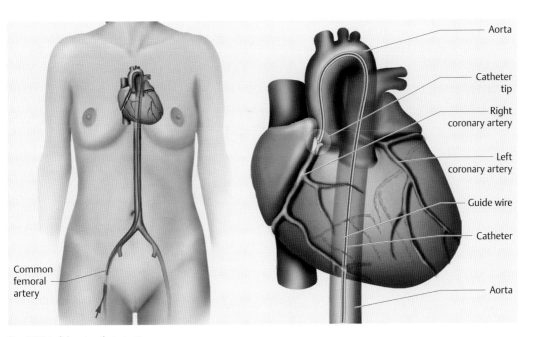

Aorta

Catheter tip

Right coronary artery

Left coronary artery

Guide wire

Catheter

Common femoral artery

Aorta

Fig. 6.16 Left heart catheterization

- In intensive-care medicine, the right heart catheter is used to monitor the circulation of unstable patients and to control therapy.
- It is also possible to obtain a biopsy specimen of the myocardium in the right ventricle for histological study. This can be useful in unexplained diseases of the heart muscle and in patients with a heart transplant, in order to recognize organ rejection.

> After a vein has been punctured, it is usually sufficient to apply a pressure bandage and maintain reduced activity for about 3 hours.

Electrophysiological Study

In an electrophysiological (EP) study, electrode catheters are inserted into the right heart via the femoral vein and electrical signals are recorded. Usually one catheter is placed in the right atrium near the bundle of His and one is placed in the right ventricle, under radiographic control. In this way, the excitation and conduction events taking place in the heart can be observed.

The heart can also be electrically stimulated by the catheter, which is connected to a computer, in order to trigger certain disorders of heart rhythm and localize their origin and their course in the heart. Various cardiac arrhythmias can be eliminated through this procedure by using current or very low temperatures to destroy the structures that cause them. This is called high-frequency ablation or cryoablation.

Therapeutic Principles

■ Therapy of Chronic Heart Failure

Causal Treatment

First of all, the underlying diseases must be treated. The therapeutic options are discussed for each clinical picture.

Symptomatic Therapy

Symptomatic therapy, summarized in **Table 6.7**, includes general measures as well as drug therapy.

General Measures
- Normalizing the patient's weight helps to avoid additional strain on the patient during physical activity.

Table 6.7 Symptomatic therapy of chronic heart failure

General measures	Drug therapy
• Normalization of weight	• ACE inhibitors or angiotensin-receptor blockers
• Limited fluid intake	• Beta blockers
• Limited salt intake	• Diuretics
• Cessation of smoking	• Spironolactone
• Cessation of alcohol use	• Cardiac glycosides
• Regular physical activity	
• Bed rest only in NYHA stage IV	
• Daily weight check	

- Fluid intake should be restricted to 1.5–2 L per day.
- Limitation of salt consumption can delay or decrease fluid retention.
- Abstinence from cigarette smoking and drinking alcohol prevents additional damage to the myocardium.
- In chronic, stable heart failure, regular exercise improves physical capacity and wellbeing. Dynamic forms of exercise, such as walking and cycling are useful in this respect.
- Strict limitation of activity and bed rest are required only in NYHA stage IV chronic heart failure.
- Daily weight monitoring helps timely recognition of fluid retention.

Medication
The primary purpose of drug treatment is to interrupt the compensation mechanisms described above, which would aggravate heart failure in the long term (**Fig. 6.8**).
- ACE inhibitors and angiotensin-receptor-blockers interrupt the renin–angiotensin–aldosterone system.
- Beta blockers inhibit the effects of the sympathetic system and thus measurably increase life expectancy.
- Diuretics promote the production of urine, excretion of fluid, and decrease of the preload.
- Spironolactone reduces the secretion and effect of aldosterone and thus supplements the ACE inhibitors or angiotensin-receptor-blockers.
- Cardiac glycosides act to increase myocardial contractility and decrease the heart rate.

Therapy of Acute Heart Failure

Therapy of acute heart failure or acutely decompensated chronic heart failure consists, first of all, in treating the underlying disease and eliminating triggering factors.

In cardiac pulmonary edema or cardiogenic shock, the compensation mechanisms described above, which become damaging over the long term, are necessary for life because they maintain or stabilize important circulatory functions in the acute situation. Patients with pulmonary edema struggle for air; they should receive oxygen through a face mask as a primary measure and be placed in an upright position with the legs hanging down. **Figure 6.17** shows the cardiac bed position that produces "blood pooling" thus reducing venous blood return to the heart and decreasing the preload.

Initial therapeutic measures in pulmonary edema:
- *Administer oxygen.*
- *Place the patient in the cardiac bed position, i.e., in an upright sitting position.*

Further therapy of acute heart failure is provided by the emergency physician or by an intensive care unit with constant monitoring of the circulatory parameters—heart rhythm, blood pressure, respiration, oxygen saturation—as well as the patient's general condition and alertness. Medications such as nitroglycerin and rapidly acting diuretics like furosemide enhance the preload lowering. Morphine can eliminate the patient's anxiety and lowers the volume overload in the pulmonary circulation.

In cardiogenic shock—i.e., unstable circulatory conditions with decline in blood pressure, cardiac arrhythmias, or other worsening of the condition with insufficient oxygen saturation—mechanical ventilation and pharmacological support with catecholamines are usually required.

Heart Transplantation

History

In 1967, Christiaan Barnard performed the first heart transplantation (HTX) in the Groote-Schuur Hospital in Cape Town. A sober mood soon followed the first euphoria, because most of the patients died within a year after this major intervention.

In 1980, ciclosporin (cyclosporine A; CSA) was developed. This immunosuppressive drug created a breakthrough in transplantation medicine. Since that time, more than 50 000 hearts have been transplanted worldwide and, on average, patients enjoy a 10-year increase of life expectancy.

Indications and Contraindications

HTX must be considered in terminal NYHA stage IV heart failure that can no longer be treated conservatively. Most of these patients are suffering from cardiomyopathies (p. 113) or CAD (p. 98).

In adding a patient to the waiting list for HTX, a factor in the decision is whether a successful transplantation can be expected in light of the patient's overall medical condition. The contraindications listed in **Table 6.8** apply.

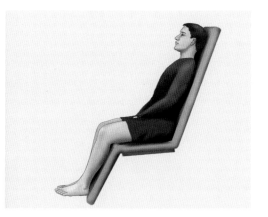

Fig. 6.17 Cardiac bed position

Table 6.8 Contraindications or heart transplantation

Absolute contraindications	Relative contraindications
• Severe pulmonary hypertension	• Age > 65 years
• Active infectious diseases	• Limited pulmonary function
• Malignancies	• Insulin-dependent diabetes mellitus
• Active ulcer	• Epilepsy
• Severe liver function disorders	• History of malignancy
• Significant peripheral arterial occlusive disease	
• Untreatable cerebral perfusion disorders	
• Psychiatric illness, poor medical compliance	

Bridging Procedures

Mechanical support systems, so-called *assist devices*, employed to bridge the waiting time until transplantation, include:
- Completely implantable left ventricular pump (left ventricular assist system or device)
- External blood pumps, used only in intensive care units

Consequences and Complications of Denervation

In transplantation, the autonomic innervation of the heart cannot be restored. Although the parasympathetic effect of the vagus nerve is totally absent, the sympathetic system can still affect the heart via the adrenal hormone epinephrine that reaches the heart in the bloodstream and binds to the beta receptors. Consequences of denervation and the predominantly sympathetic effect that are relevant to physical therapy are listed below:

- *High resting heart rate*
- *Slower rise in heart rate during physical activity*
- *Lack of pain mediation, therefore no complaints of angina pectoris*

In addition to surgical complications, there is the risk of organ rejection and the side-effects of immunosuppressive therapy. Rejection can be acute or chronic:
- Acute rejection primarily attacks the myocardium and can be well treated with high doses of glucocorticosteroids.
- Chronic rejection primarily attacks the grafted coronary vessels. Transplantation vasculopathy is the chief cause of death in the long-term course after HTX. As a result of surgical denervation, there are no complaints of angina pectoris.

Prognosis

Most patients return to NYHA stage I; 90% of patients experience no limitations of activity 1–2 years after surgery. Current survival rates are:
- 1-year survival rate > 80%
- 5-year survival rate 70%

The main causes of death vary over the postoperative course:
- Acute transplant rejection in the first month
- Infections in the first year
- Later, transplant vasculopathy as an expression of chronic rejection

Ischemic Heart Diseases

■ Coronary Artery Disease

Arteriosclerosis of the coronary arteries is called coronary artery disease (CAD). The pathological mechanism of arteriosclerosis is described on page 31. About 20% of men and up to 10% of women in middle age suffer from CAD, which is the most frequent cause of death in industrialized countries.

Classification

Depending on the number of coronary arteries affected, as given in **Fig. 6.18**, we speak of 1-, 2- or 3-vessel disease. Depending on the extent of stenosis, four degrees of severity are recognized (**Fig. 6.19**, **Table 6.9**).

Manifestation

The first manifestation of CAD is seen as:
- Angina pectoris in 40% of patients
- Myocardial infarction in 40% of patients
- Sudden cardiac death in 20% of patients

In addition to the signs of heart failure (p. 83) an *attack of angina pectoris* is a cardinal symptom of CAD. This is retrosternal pain, as a result of reversible myocardial ischemia, that can radiate to the following regions (**Fig. 6.20a, b**):
- Left arm, but also right arm
- Lower jaw
- Upper abdomen
- Between the shoulder blades

Table 6.9 Degree of severity of CAD

Grade	Severity of diameter reduction	Comment
I	25%–49%	Coronary sclerosis but no significant stenosis
II	50%–74%	Significant stenosis
III	75%–99%	Critical stenosis: If no collateral vessels are present, coronary reserve is exhausted and stress-related angina pectoris results
IV	100%	Occlusion

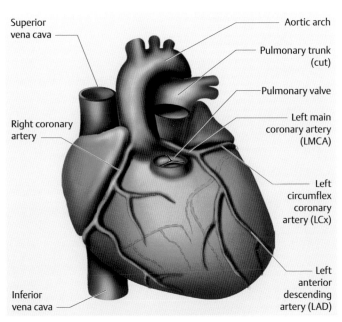

Fig. 6.18 Coronary arteries

Superior vena cava

Aortic arch

Pulmonary trunk (cut)

Pulmonary valve

Right coronary artery

Left main coronary artery (LMCA)

Left circumflex coronary artery (LCx)

Inferior vena cava

Left anterior descending artery (LAD)

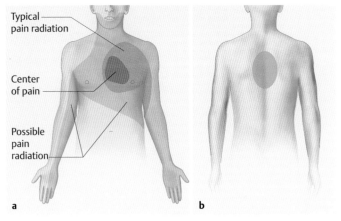

Fig. 6.19 Coronary angiography: stenosis in the left circumflex artery (arrow). (Baenkler 1999.)

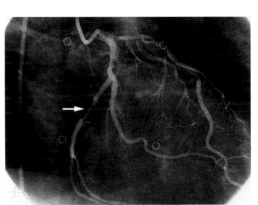

Fig. 6.20a, b Possible radiation of angina pectoris pain.

Typical pain radiation

Center of pain

Possible pain radiation

a

b

Course of Angina Pectoris

Stable Angina Pectoris

Stable angina pectoris is regularly triggered by specific stresses and responds well to glyceryl trinitrate preparations. Factors that lead to an imbalance between myocardial oxygen supply and demand and thus can trigger an angina pectoris attack are summarized in **Table 6.10**.

Unstable Angina Pectoris

When severity, duration and frequency of the pain attacks increase and respond less and less to glyceryl trinitrate preparations, the angina pectoris is unstable. Since the risk of infarction is 20%, this is also called *preinfarct syndrome.* Every first attack is treated like an unstable angina pectoris.

Prinzmetal Angina

This special form of angina pectoris is caused by coronary spasms.

Diagnosis

- Diagnostic indicators are provided by 12-lead ECGs at rest and during stress testing.
- Supplementary noninvasive procedures are stress echocardiography, myocardial scintigraphy, and cardiac MRI.
- The definitive diagnosis is provided by coronary angiography, an invasive procedure.

Therapy

Stable Angina Pectoris

Minimizing Vascular Risk Factors

The patient is advised to:
- Normalize body weight
- Eat a balanced diet
- Stop smoking
- Exercise regularly
- Learn and use relaxation techniques

A changed lifestyle has a positive effect on:
- Arterial hypertension
- Type 2 diabetes mellitus
- Disorders of lipid metabolism

Drug Therapy

- Acetylsalicylic acid (ASA) is a platelet inhibitor.
- Beta blockers lower myocardial oxygen demand.
- Nitrates and calcium antagonists are vasodilators.
- Statins reduce cholesterol synthesis and protect the vascular endothelium.

Measures for Revascularization

Catheterization techniques: During a cardiac catheterization, the stenosed vessel can be dilated by inflating a balloon catheter. Balloon dilation is called *percutaneous transluminal coronary angioplasty* (PTCA, **Fig. 6.21a**). During this procedure, usually a stent is inserted to support and maintain the dilation result. Stents reduce the rate of restenosis (**Fig. 6.21b**).

Surgical techniques: The chief indications for coronary bypass operations are left main stem stenosis, 3-vessel disease, and failed PTCA. In addition to

Table 6.10 Possible causes of an angina pectoris attack

Factors decreasing myocardial O_2 supply	Factors causing elevated O_2 demand
Intraluminal narrowing of coronaries, e.g., by: • Arteriosclerosis • Thrombus formation, for instance in plaque rupture • Coronary spasms	Increased heart activity, e.g., in: • Left heart failure • Physical activity • Fever • Hyperthyroidism
Extraluminal compression, e.g., due to rise in ventricular pressure	Myocardial hypertrophy, e.g., as a result of: • Arterial hypertension • Stenosis of the semilunar valves
Decreased perfusion pressure, e.g., due to drop in blood pressure	
Shortened diastole with increasing heart rate	
Extracardial causes, e.g.: • Respiratory insufficiency • Anemia	

opening the thorax with a sternotomy, in certain cases a minimally invasive procedure is possible. **Figure 6.22a, b** shows the usual procedures:

- In coronary artery bypass grafting (CABG), the stenosis is usually bridged with a surface leg vein, for example the saphenous vein.
- Better long-term results are obtained by using the internal mammary artery (IMA), in which the right or left internal thoracic artery is grafted into a coronary artery to go around the diseased part of the coronary vessel.

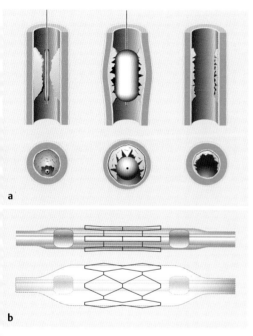

a

b

Fig. 6.21a, b **a** Principle of balloon dilatation. **b** Stent before and after unfolding in the vessel.

If causal treatment is no longer possible in terminal heart failure, i.e., in NYHA stage IV, and symptomatic measures have been exhausted, heart transplantation must also be considered for young patients.

Unstable Angina Pectoris

Therapy of unstable angina pectoris is the same as for myocardial infarction (p. 101) and is carried out under intensive care conditions. The following medication is administered:

- Heparins
- Platelet inhibitors such as ASA among others
- Glyceryl trinitrate
- Beta blockers

If the patient remains symptomatic, or troponin values are rising, coronary angiography should be performed within 48 hours.

Prognosis

The prognosis is first of all dependent on remaining vascular risk factors. Patients with appreciable main stem stenosis have the worst prognosis if they receive exclusively drug treatment. About 30% of patients with a main stem stenosis exceeding 70% die within 1 year.

■ Myocardial Infarction

In the United States, approximately 1.5 million persons a year suffer a myocardial infarction (heart attack). As many as 50000 of these persons die. It is the most frequent cause of death in the Western industrialized nations.

Fig. 6.22a, b Bypass types. **a** Aortocoronary venous bypass. **b** Mammary artery bypass.

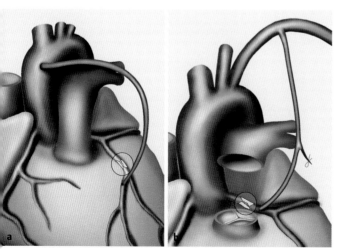

a   b

A myocardial infarction is a circumscribed area of necrosis in the heart muscle; the underlying cause is usually CAD. A vessel-occluding thrombus forms at the point where an arteriosclerotic plaque breaks up (plaque rupture, p. 31). As a result of the interrupted blood flow, the zone of myocardium supplied by that vessel loses its function and dies if reperfusion is not reestablished within a very short time. In 40% of patients, the infarction is the first sign of CAD.

Symptoms

Intense, long-lasting angina pectoris that is scarcely affected by glyceryl trinitrate is a cardinal symptom. Retrosternal pain, frequently radiating into the left arm, is typical. Atypical pain localization can make diagnosis difficult (**Fig. 6.20a, b**).

- Pain radiating to the right arm can be erroneously interpreted as "shoulder–arm syndrome."
- Pain in the lower jaw can be erroneously considered "tooth ache."
- Upper abdominal pain that may arise with infarction of the inferior wall can be erroneously ascribed to "stomach problems."
- Pain between the shoulder blades can be erroneously considered "back pain" or "muscular or skeletal problem."

Atypical radiation of pain can lead to erroneous diagnoses.

From 15% to 20% of all myocardial infarctions are not accompanied by pain. The tendency to "silent infarctions" is found especially in the elderly and in diabetics, as a result of autonomic neuropathy.

"Silent infarctions" are possible.

Additional symptoms are:
- Severe fear
- Attendant autonomic symptoms such as sweating, nausea and vomiting
- Symptoms caused by complications

Complications

The typical early complications, occurring within the first 48 hours, include cardiac arrhythmias (p. 104). These range from relatively rare atrial fibrillation to conduction blocks, ventricular extrasystoles, and ventricular tachycardia (VT) to ventricular fibrillation (VF). VT and VF are fatal without treatment and constitute the most frequent cause of death in patients with infarctions.

As a result of pumping failure, about 30% of patients develop left heart failure of varying severity; 10% of patients develop cardiogenic shock (p. 54).

Extensive tissue defects can result in:
- Rupture of the myocardial wall with pericardial tamponade
- Rupture of the ventricular septum
- Papillary muscle dysfunction with mitral valve regurgitation

Ventricular aneurysm is the most important late complication, developed by about 10% of patients with infarctions. The weakening and bulging of the infarcted heart muscle can promote left heart failure, arrhythmias, or thrombus formation. A thrombus can cause embolic complications.

Diagnosis

In addition to the typical symptoms, the first indicator of an infarction event is provided by the medical history with information about vascular risk factors and previously diagnosed CAD. In general, further diagnosis is based on:
- Changes in the ECG
- Laboratory parameters
- Coronary angiogram

A specific sign in the ECG of acute myocardial infarction is the ST elevation that appears in characteristic form in only 60% of patients within the first 24 hours. **Figure 6.23a–d** shows how the ECG typically changes with time.

When heart muscle cells die, their "contents" can be detected in the blood. Cardiac troponins and the enzyme creatine kinase (CK) or the myocardium-specific CK-MB are clinically significant (**Table 6.11**).

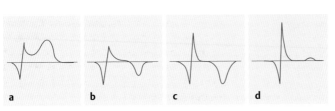

Fig. 6.23a–d ECG changes in myocardial infarction. **a** Initial stage (first minute to about sixth hour). **b** Acute infarction (first day to 10 days). **c** Intermediate stage (second week to 2 months). **d** End stage (fourth–sixth week to several years).

Table 6.11 Course of important laboratory parameters in myocardial infarction

Parameter	Increase (h)	Maximum (h)	Normalization (d)
Troponin	3	20	7–14
CK-MB	4–8	12–18	2–3

Stenoses and occlusions become visible in coronary angiography.

Therapy

To limit the extent of the infarction and thus the complications, treatment must be started as soon as possible. The emergency physician who accompanies the patient to the hospital initiates general measures. Reperfusion must take place as soon as possible after the start of symptoms.

General Measures

In the early phase, the patient is cared for in an intensive care unit, assigned to strict bed rest, and is psychologically sheltered and receives oxygen through a nasal tube. In order to recognize early complications, the circulatory functions of heart rhythm and blood pressure as well as breathing are continually monitored.

Drug Therapy

- Acetylsalicylic acid (ASA) among other platelet inhibitors and anticoagulants prevent the vascular thrombus from being enlarged.
- Beta blockers decrease the myocardial oxygen demand and reduce the frequency of threatening arrhythmias.
- Glyceryl trinitrate eases angina pectoris and decreases the load on the heart by dilating the coronary arteries as well as the afferent and efferent vessels.
- ACE inhibitors slow structural modification processes in the myocardium ("remodeling") and decrease the afterload.
- Morphine preparations reduce pain and have an anxiolytic effect.

Reperfusion Therapy

Ideally, the affected coronary artery is recanalized as soon as possible by means of immediate PTCA and stent-insertion (**Fig. 6.21a, b**). This procedure depends on personnel and instrumentation but produces better results than the alternative thrombolytic therapy.

If no heart catheterization laboratory is available or the time to intervention is more than 90 minutes, immediate systemic thrombolysis (fibrinolysis or lysis therapy) is indicated. Lysis therapy should be followed by coronary angiography and possibly PTCA within the next 24 hours.

Long-Term Therapy after Myocardial Infarction

Long-term therapy after a myocardial infarction is also called *secondary prevention*. Vascular risk factors must be minimized by means of the general measures described for CAD therapy (p. 98).

Standard medication includes:

- Lifelong ASA
- Clopidogrel or similar platelet inhibitor in addition to ASA, for a limited period
- Beta blocker for at least 2 years or lifelong in heart failure
- Long-term ACE inhibitors or angiotensin-receptor blockers if there is reduced ventricular function or heart failure
- Statins

Rehabilitation

Rehabilitation proceeds in three phases:

- Early mobilization
- Early rehabilitation
- Late rehabilitation and aftercare phase

For an acute myocardial infarction, intensive monitoring for at least 24–48 hours is necessary. If the course is without complications, physical therapy can begin on the second day of treatment with early mobilization. The objective of the early mobilization, individually adapted to the clinical course, is to avoid physical and psychological consequences of unnecessary immobilization. The capacity to perform light everyday activities can be achieved by low-risk patients within 1 week; most high-risk patients can reach this level within 3 weeks.

After the acute phase of the illness follow-up treatment is established, the so-called early rehabilitation, which takes place in rehabilitation clinics or in an outpatient setting and usually lasts for 3 weeks.

Ideally, this is followed by late rehabilitation and an aftercare phase with lifelong continual maintenance in local heart groups.

Exercise therapy is a low-risk therapeutic measure for coronary artery disease, accepted worldwide and delivered under a physician's supervision by trained exercise instructors. This therapy can increase physical and psychological capacity for daily life, professional life, and leisure time, decrease coronary risk factors, and improve cardiac function directly and indirectly.

Prognosis

About 50% of patients do not survive the infarction event; the chief cause of death is ventricular fibrillation:

- 30% of all patients die before they reach the hospital.
- 10%–20% of all patients die in the hospital.
- Within 2 years, an additional 5% suffer sudden cardiac death, that is, they die from malignant arrhythmias.

Case Study: Mr. M., 53 years old, wakes up in the early morning hours with violent retrosternal pain radiating to the left arm and lower jaw. His wife calls the emergency physician, who finds a pale patient in cold sweat with the following vital parameters:
- Heart rate 104/min
- Blood pressure 125/85 mmHg
- Respiration 24/min

Oxygen saturation, at 96%, is still within normal range. Inspection and auscultation give no indication of acute heart failure. While the ECG electrodes are being applied, the emergency physician takes the history. Mr. M. reports that he takes hypertension medication. He has been smoking 20 cigarettes a day for the last 30 years.

The ECG exhibits sinus tachycardia and ST elevations, which confirm the suspected diagnosis of acute myocardial infarction.

The patient is given oxygen through a nasal tube and ASA, heparin, a beta blocker, and morphine intravenously. The emergency physician accompanies the patient, who is being monitored in the ambulance, to the hospital. On the way, ventricular fibrillation sets in and the patient must be resuscitated. Defibrillation is successful.

In the hospital, the diagnosis of an acute anterior wall infarction is made on the basis of a standard 12-lead ECG. After blood samples are taken, the patient is immediately taken to the cardiac operation room. Coronary angiography shows an occlusion of the left anterior descendent artery (LAD) that can be reopened by PTCA and stenting. The patient, now free of complaints, is moved to the intensive care unit for further monitoring and therapy.

Cardiac Arrhythmias

■ Overview

As soon as the heart rhythm deviates from the normal sinus rhythm, cardiac arrhythmia is present. The clinical significance ranges from harmless variations of normal to sudden cardiac death, the cause of death in the United States of 300 000 to 400 000 persons annually.

Causes

The course of excitation described in on page 83 depends primarily on intact myocardium, sufficient oxygen supply, and physiological electrolyte concentrations, which makes it susceptible to disturbances. Important arrhythmogenic factors are:

- Lack of oxygen through cardiac causes such as CAD and extracardiac causes such as pulmonary disease and anemia
- Altered myocardial structure, e.g., hypertrophy, infarction scar, myocarditis and cardiomyopathy
- Disturbed electrolyte and water balance
- Medications that affect the electrolyte balance or ion channels, such as digitalis, diuretics, antiepileptics, psychopharmaceuticals, certain antibiotics and, paradoxically, even antiarrhythmics
- Congenital alterations in the myocardial ion channels, e.g., congenital long QT syndrome
- Stimulants such as tobacco, alcohol, and drugs that stimulate beta-1 and other receptors, e.g., caffeine, cocaine, amphetamines
- Fever
- Hyperthyroidism (excessive functioning of the thyroid gland)
- Physical and mental stress

Classification of Cardiac Arrhythmias

Cardiac arrhythmias are classified by heart rate as bradycardial and tachycardial arrhythmias:

- Bradycardia; i.e., fewer than 60 beats/min
- Tachycardia; i.e., more than 100 beats/min
- Arrhythmia; i.e., irregular heart beat
- Tachyarrhythmia; i.e., irregular, overly rapid heart beat
- Bradyarrhythmia; i.e., irregular, overly slow heart beat
- Extrasystole, in which heart beats appear outside the basic rhythm

Table 6.12 Classification of cardiac arrhythmias

Tachycardial arrhythmias	Bradycardial arrhythmias

• Supraventricular arrhythmias:
  – Sinus tachycardia
  – Supraventricular extrasystole
  – Atrial fibrillation and atrial flutter
  – Atrial tachycardia
  – Reentry tachycardia
• Ventricular arrhythmias:
  – Ventricular extrasystole
  – Ventricular tachycardia
  – Ventricular flutter and ventricular fibrillation
	• Sick sinus syndrome
	• AV block
	• Carotid sinus syndrome
	• Asystole

Tachycardia is classified, depending on origin, as supraventricular, i.e., emanating from the atrium, and ventricular tachycardia (**Table 6.12**).

Symptoms

The clinical expression of the disease depends mainly on the type of cardiac arrhythmia and the resulting ventricular frequency as well as on the possibilities for compensation—in other words, on the patient's underlying disease. Some patients are asymptomatic; others notice subjective complaints such as palpitations, racing heart, or fluttering heart.

A cardiac arrhythmia can also be noticed through noncardiac symptoms. Often, atrial fibrillation that was at first unrecognized (p. 107) is finally noticed because of a thromboembolic event such as a stroke. Moreover, arrhythmias are always threatening when the circulation is no longer supplied with blood and oxygen. Under those conditions, the following signs can arise:

- Vertigo
- Visual and speech disorders
- Sudden loss of consciousness, so-called syncopes
- Angina pectoris
- Signs of heart failure

Ventricular fibrillation and asystolic arrest are not compatible with life, since the heart is functionally at a standstill (p. 108).

Diagnosis

The first step is the taking of a detailed medical history with questions about the frequency and duration of the arrhythmia, symptoms, and possible triggers and previous diseases. For patients with stable circulation, the clinical examination includes count-

ing the pulse for at least 1 minute and blood pressure measurement, supplemented with additional instrumental diagnostic procedures:

- ECG at rest, to identify any current arrhythmia
- Stress ECG, if arrhythmias occur in stress situations
- Long-term ECG or event recorder, to identify rarely occurring arrhythmias
- If necessary, an invasive electrophysiological study for purposeful provocation of suspected arrhythmias
- Monitoring ECG, to supervise patients in doubtful or life-threatening situations

Therapeutic Principles

If a disorder of cardiac rhythm is clinically significant, it must be treated. As a first step, underlying diseases must be treated or their triggers must be eliminated. If causal treatment is insufficient or if immediate intervention is necessary in acute, life-threatening arrhythmias, a combination of drug and nondrug treatment measures is considered. This includes electrotherapeutic measures:

- Catheter ablation
- Pacemaker therapy
- Cardioversion and defibrillation

Drug Therapy

Simply stated, antiarrhythmics act by blocking various ion channels or beta receptors at the myocardium. By virtue of this action they are sometimes even proarrhythmic. Therefore, the indication must be very carefully determined. Examples for frequently used antiarrhythmic drugs are beta blockers and calcium antagonists of the verapamil type, as well as amiodarone, dronedarone and flecainide.

Catheter Ablation

During an electrophysiological study (p. 95), structures of the cardiac excitation and conduction system that trigger or maintain tachycardia can be located and then targeted and destroyed.

- High-frequency ablation; i.e., destruction by electric current
- Cryoablation; i.e., destruction by cold

Success rates depend on the underlying disease and exceed 90% in case of certain supraventricular tachycardias.

Pacemakers

A cardiac pacemaker can be indicated for bradycardial cardiac arrhythmia. It can be applied permanently or temporarily.

In an emergency, a pacemaker can be applied by means of:

- Transcutaneous stimulation with electrodes pasted to the skin
- Transvenous stimulation, in which electrodes are temporarily inserted into the cavities of the right heart via the internal jugular vein or the subclavian vein
- Epicardial stimulation, which is often used during cardiac surgery. Here, electrodes are inserted directly into the heart muscle from the outside and led to the exterior through the skin; they can be removed from this position after a few days.

If long-lasting pacing is necessary, a pacemaker is implanted permanently. This device consists of a module with a battery and a minicomputer and is usually implanted subcutaneously on the right side on the major pectoral muscle (**Fig. 6.24**). The patient's natural rhythm is registered via leads with electrodes inserted transvenously into the cavities of the right heart. The pacemaker delivers electric stimuli to the heart when necessary. The following configurations of leads and functions are possible:

- "One-chamber" systems with just one lead in the right atrium, indicated, for instance, in the sick sinus syndrome (p. 107)
- "One-chamber" systems with one lead in the right ventricle, indicated, for instance, in chronic atrial fibrillation and very slow conduction (p. 107)
- A "two-chamber" system with one lead in the right atrium and one lead in the right ventricle. These two leads can coordinate the activity of atrium and ventricle with each other and thus imitate physiological excitation, e.g., in high-grade AV block (p. 107).
- Complex systems with an additional lead that can also stimulate the left ventricle via the coronary sinus, so-called cardiac resynchronization therapy (CRT)

Defibrillation and Cardioversion

In external defibrillation or electrocardioversion, the patient receives a direct current impulse over two electrodes applied to the thorax in order to synchronize the electrical activity of the myocardium and restore the normal sinus rhythm.

- *Defibrillation* is an emergency measure used for patients who must be resuscitated after sudden heart death resulting from ventricular fibrillation. The electric current is delivered randomly during the already chaotic cardiac action.
- *Electrical cardioversion* is different from defibrillation because the current delivered is synchronized with the ECG and delivered at a specific moment in the cardiac cycle. It is required in order to restore sinus rhythm in a patient with atrial fibrillation or ventricular tachycardia. A random electrical impulse could lead to life-threatening ventricular fibrillation if there is orderly ventricular activity present. Electrocardioversion is performed with monitors under light anesthesia.

During external defibrillation or cardioversion, no one is allowed to touch the patient or the patient's bed.

Patients who have already survived a sudden cardiac death or who are in danger of death from ventricular arrhythmias receive an *implantable cardioverter defibrillator* (ICD) to protect them from sudden cardiac death. This device is constructed on the same principle as a pacemaker and is implanted in a similar way, but usually in the left pectoral site. The ICD is a "built-in emergency physician" with the task of continually monitoring the cardiac rhythm and intervening automatically in case of a hazardous arrhythmia. If the rhythm is too slow, the ICD can raise the pulse by the continually available pacemaker function. Persons in contact with the patient are not endangered by an ICD shock.

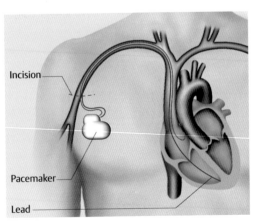

Fig. 6.24 Cardiac pacemaker implanted subcutaneously in the right side of the thorax with leads in the right ventricle and in the right atrium.

Incision

Pacemaker

Lead

Physical therapists should keep the following cautions in mind with wearers of pacemakers and ICDs:
- *No jerking or excessive abduction in the shoulder joint, so as not to displace the leads.*
- *No direct mechanical force applied to the units.*
- *Electrotherapy only after consultation with the treating physician.*
- *Wearers of ICDs usually suffer from severe heart disease, i.e., they are patients with heart failure.*

■ Selected Cardiac Arrhythmias

Figure 6.25a–f shows changes in the ECG for some cardiac arrhythmias that are discussed here in detail:
- Sick sinus syndrome
- AV blockages
- Atrial fibrillation
- Other supraventricular tachycardias
- Ventricular tachycardias and ventricular fibrillation

Sick Sinus Syndrome

The *sick sinus syndrome* includes persistent sinus bradycardia and sinoatrial block in which conduction of excitation from the sinus node to the muscles of the atria is delayed or absent, the so-called sinus arrest. A permanent pacemaker is implanted in symptomatic patients.

Atrioventricular Conduction Disorders

Three degrees of severity can be distinguished in AV block:
- In *first-degree* AV block, there is a delay in conduction of excitation from the atria to the ventricles. The finding is usually made by chance; the PQ interval in the ECG is prolonged.
- In *second-degree* AV block, conduction is delayed and sometimes completely missing. In 2:1 block, only one of two impulses from the sinus node reaches the ventricles. If a patient has symptoms such as vertigo or syncope, pacemaker therapy is indicated.
- In *third-degree* AV block, excitation of the atria is never conducted to the ventricles. The ventricles are excited at a lower frequency by secondary or tertiary pacemakers (**Table 6.1**). This can result in vertigo or syncope, designated as *Adams–Stokes attacks*. In acquired third-degree AV block, a permanent pacemaker is indicated.

Atrial Fibrillation

In atrial fibrillation, there are 350–600 atrial excitations per minute. Not every atrial excitation is transmitted to the ventricles, since the AV node functions as a frequency filter. The ventricular frequency depends on the number of conductions, where slow and rapid conductions are possible. Twenty percent of ventricular filling depends on proper atrial

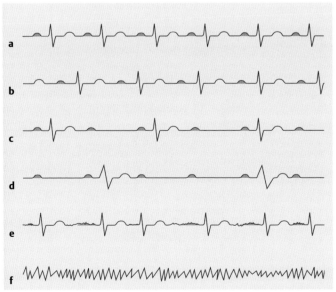

Fig. 6.25a–f ECG changes in cardiac arrhythmias. **a** Normal ECG. **b** First-degree AV block. **c** Second-degree AV block. **d** Third-degree AV block. **e** Atrial fibrillation. **f** Ventricular fibrillation.

contraction and 80% depends on the suction mechanism of the heart, so that atrial fibrillation normally has only slight effect on filling and ejection. However, where heart failure is present, atrial fibrillation can intensify the symptoms.

Where there is no organized atrial contraction, thrombi can form, particularly in the left atrium (Fig. 6.13), leading to thromboembolic complications such as stroke and acute occlusion of a limb artery (p. 126). For this reason, patients with persistent atrial fibrillation must be treated with anticoagulants.

Supraventricular Tachycardias

In certain anomalies of the excitation and conduction system, sudden onset of tachycardia can result. For instance, additional conduction pathways responsible for this permit circular excitation between atria and ventricles, so-called reentry tachycardias. Short-term treatment comprises vagal maneuvers, including carotid sinus massage and Valsalva maneuvers, and antiarrhythmic drug administration. If attacks of paroxysmal tachycardia are frequent and severe, long-term therapy is warranted by catheter ablation with a success rate of about 90% depending on the underlying arrhythmia.

Ventricular Tachycardias and Ventricular Fibrillation

Smooth transitions are possible between ventricular tachycardia (VT) with a frequency of over 100/min, ventricular flutter, and ventricular fibrillation. In ventricular fibrillation, the individual myocardial cells contract at an excitation frequency far above 300/min.

As a result of the chaos, no effective ventricular contraction is possible, so that ventricular fibrillation has the same effect, functionally, as cardiac arrest.

Usually it is patients with severe heart disease who suffer sudden cardiac death as a result of ventricular arrhythmias. A patient who can be successfully defibrillated and resuscitated receives an ICD as secondary prophylaxis.

Case Study: Ms. D.K., 69 years old, falls down during light housework and is not able to get up without help. She can no longer move her left arm and left leg. The ambulance immediately called by her husband brings the patient to the hospital.

As part of her history, she reports that she is taking medication for high blood pressure and occasional palpitations. Up to now, she has always been independent and active in her daily life.

Examination reveals left-sided hemiparesis and elevated blood pressure of 190/100 mmHg. Cerebral imaging shows embolic occlusion of the right median cerebral artery. The ECG shows previously undiagnosed atrial fibrillation as the cause of the event.

The clot is successfully dissolved by thrombolysis and the neurological symptoms are completely resolved. In the further course, long-term anticoagulation therapy with coumadin is prescribed to prevent further thromboembolism.

■ Cardiac-Circulatory Arrest

Causes

In more than 90% of cases, the causes are cardiac in nature.

Cardiac Causes

- In about 90%, ventricular fibrillation
- In about 10%, asystolic arrest, the actual cardiac arrest

Extracardiac Causes

- Shock of varying origins (p. 54)
- Respiratory causes such as aspiration and central respiratory disorders
- End stage of various diseases

Symptoms and Complications

Table 6.13 summarizes the signs of circulatory arrest.

Irreversible brain damage, even brain death, can set in within 3 minutes (p. 9)!

Resuscitation

The ABC rule for cardiopulmonary resuscitation that was valid until recent years has become the CAB rule. The first priority of the current recommendations (American Heart Association 2010), after cardiac arrest is confirmed, is immediate chest compressions without prior checking of pulse or respiration and defibrillation as early as possible by trained emergency personnel or by means of automated external defibrillation (AED), that is already available for first aid providers at some public places (**Fig. 6.26c**).

The rescue chain includes the following steps:
- Recognition of cardiac arrest and an immediate call to the emergency number 911
- Immediate commencement of resuscitation with emphasis on chest compressions with a frequency of at least 100 compressions/min (**Fig. 6.26a**)
- Compression and ventilation at a ratio of 30 : 2, independent of the number of helpers
- For mouth to nose, mouth to mouth or mask ventilation, hyperextend the head and pull the chin forward (**Fig. 6.26b**)
- Early defibrillation
- Extended resuscitation measures by trained personnel
- Interdisciplinary in-patient care

Table 6.13 Signs of cardio-circulatory arrest in the order of their appearance

Time	Symptoms
Immediately	Pulselessness
After 10–15 s	Unconsciousness
After 30–60 s	No breathing
After 2 min	Dilated, unreactive pupils (Also possible after medication)

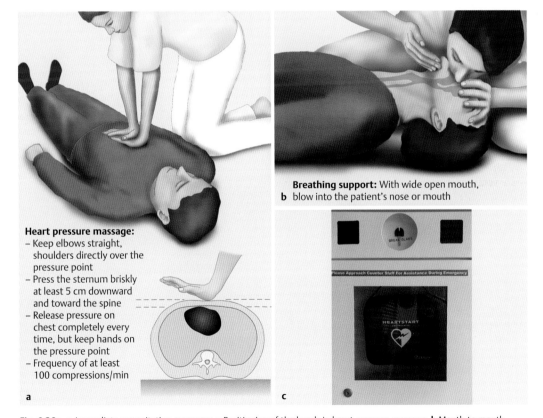

Breathing support: With wide open mouth, **b** blow into the patient's nose or mouth

Heart pressure massage:
- Keep elbows straight, shoulders directly over the pressure point
- Press the sternum briskly at least 5 cm downward and toward the spine
- Release pressure on chest completely every time, but keep hands on the pressure point
- Frequency of at least 100 compressions/min

a

c

Fig. 6.26a–c Immediate resuscitation measures. **a** Positioning of the hands in heart pressure massage. **b** Mouth-to-mouth breathing. **c** Automatic external defibrillator (AED) (© Cheng Poh Cheah, reprinted with kind permission).

> *Vigorous and expeditious chest compression CPR is the most important immediate measure that everyone should perform. If there is any doubt, lay persons may omit ventilation.*
> - *Basic measures, according to the CAB rule:*
>   - *Circulation, i.e., chest compressions*
>   - *Airway clearance*
>   - *Breathing support*
> - *Extended measures:*
>   - *Electrotherapy*
>   - *Medications, etc.*

Diseases of the Endocardium

■ Endocarditis

Inflammation of the endocardium and thus of the valves can have infectious and noninfectious causes, for example, autoimmune processes in rheumatic fever.

Rheumatic Fever

Rheumatic fever is a dangerous late complication after a streptococcal infection of the throat. It occurs when the antibodies formed attack not only the infectious agent but also the body's own structures.

> *Rheumatic fever occurs secondary to a streptococcal infection as a poststreptococcal disease.*

Whereas rheumatic fever has become rare in the West through the consistent use of antibiotics, in the developing world today it is still the chief cause of heart disease in juveniles.

Symptoms and Complications

About 1–3 weeks after a case of pharyngitis (sore throat), tonsillitis, or scarlet fever (p. 275), an abnormal immune reaction results in a secondary streptococcal disease affecting heart, joints, CNS, and skin. The symptoms include:
- General symptoms such as fever and joint pain
- Arthritis with variable involvement of the large joints
- Chorea minor with uncontrolled aggressive movements and disturbed speech
- Garland-shaped skin reddening in the area of the torso, which is called erythema marginatum or annulare
- Subcutaneous lumps

The threat of carditis determines the prognosis. It can involve all layers of the heart.
- In endocarditis, the heart valves are also affected. Inflammatory changes, especially in the aortic and mitral valves, can give rise to permanent valvular disease.
- Myocarditis favors cardiac arrhythmias and can lead to heart failure.
- Pericarditis can cause pericardial effusions and possible thoracic pain.

Diagnosis and Therapy

The diagnosis can be made on the basis of the clinical symptoms and knowledge of an earlier streptococcal infection, confirmed by laboratory values such as evidence of inflammatory parameters and streptococcus-specific antibodies.

Therapeutic measures during hospitalization include:
- Bed rest
- Antibiotic therapy with penicillin for a period of 10–14 days to combat remaining streptococci
- Anti-inflammatory therapy with ASA and, if necessary, glucocorticosteroids for severe cardiac involvement

Prognosis

The extent of cardiac involvement determines the prognosis; joint, CNS, and skin disorders are completely curable. About 50% of patients with rheumatic fever develop chronic rheumatic heart disease. Over the course of years, a valvular defect may arise, for example, mitral stenosis.

Prevention

Primary Prevention

For primary prevention of rheumatic fever, a detected streptococcal infection must be treated immediately and consistently with antibiotics, usually penicillin.

Secondary Prevention

The duration of secondary prevention with penicillin depends on the extent of cardiac involvement and lasts about 10 years beyond the acute disease phase. In chronic valvular disease, specific endocardial prophylaxis is required for diagnostic and surgical procedures, as presented in the context of infectious endocarditis.

Infective Endocarditis

Causes

If microorganisms, particularly bacteria and fungi, are spread by the blood circulation (bacteremia), they can colonize the previously damaged endocardium and cause an infective endocarditis. Frequent pathogens are:
- Streptococci (60%)
- Staphylococci (20%)
- Rarely, other bacteria or fungi

Patients at risk are:
- Patients with congenital heart disease
- Patients who have had rheumatic fever or previous endocarditis
- Patients with artificial heart valves

Symptoms and Complications

The following clinical signs can indicate infective endocarditis:
- Fever, shivers, and rigor
- General symptoms such as weakness, loss of appetite, weight loss, sweating, and joint pain
- Skin changes such as petechiae and lentil-sized painful reddish nodes, especially in fingers and toes

The most-feared complications are:
- Septic embolization that can lead to arterial occlusion and thus, for instance, to neurological deficits or embolic myocardial infarction
- Heart valve destruction and congestive heart failure

Diagnosis, Therapy, and Prognosis

Diagnostic indicators are:
- Heart murmurs
- Evidence of the characteristic lesion, the vegetation on the valve, which is a variably sized amorphous growth and can be precisely detected by transesophageal echocardiography
- Evidence of pathogens in blood cultures

Almost 30% of patients die despite intensive antibiotic therapy over a period of 4–6 weeks.

Prophylaxis of Endocarditis

> Because of the serious prognosis, all patients at risk receive a patient identification card that they must present at every visit to a physician. For diagnostic or therapeutic procedures that could lead to bacteremia, patients at risk must be protected with antibiotics. For instance, endocarditis prophylaxis can save a life in such simple dental procedures as calculus removal.

■ Valvular Heart Disease

Causes

Valvular heart disease can be congenital or acquired in the course of infective or noninfective endocarditis. Valvular defects can also be degenerative in origin.

Types

All heart valves can be subject to defect but as a rule it is the valves of the left heart, that is, the aortic and mitral valve, that are mainly involved. The defects are classified as valve stenosis and valve regurgitation.
- In *valvular stenosis* the valvular orifice is reduced and the valve opening is limited. The most frequent acquired valvular stenosis is aortic stenosis, which causes hypertrophy of the left ventricle and fluid congestion. In *advanced disease*, less blood is pumped into the systemic circulation.
- In *valvular regurgitation,* the valvular leaflets fail to close properly and a part of the blood volume is ejected backwards into the upstream section of the circulation. In mitral regurgitation, for instance, during systole, blood is regurgitated from the left ventricle back into the left atrium, which reacts by widening.

> Valve stenosis → Pressure stress → Hypertrophy
> Valve regurgitation → Volume stress → Dilatation

Symptoms and Complications

- Signs of impaired output, e.g., syncope with aortic stenosis
- Signs of heart failure
- Cardiac arrhythmias as a result of altered myocardial structure and its consequences, e.g., thromboembolism in atrial fibrillation (p. 107).

Diagnosis

Diagnostic indicators in addition to medical history are findings on auscultation and echocardiography:

- Murmurs heard on auscultation, arising when blood is forced through a valve that is too narrow or when blood regurgitates through a leaky valve
- Valvular disease and their hemodynamic effects imaged by echocardiography

Further diagnostic tools include:

- ECG to register cardiac arrhythmias and signs of hypertrophy
- Chest x-ray to detect any changes in heart silhouette and signs of congestion
- Heart catheterization studies to exclude CAD when valve surgery is planned and in case of inconclusive echocardiographic findings
- MRI to image complex heart and valve diseases

Therapy

In addition to conservative measures, therapy includes symptomatic measures such as:

- Therapy of heart failure
- Therapy of cardiac arrhythmias and their consequences
- Endocarditis prophylaxis

The indication for a surgical procedure must be evaluated and arrived at promptly in severe cases. The diseased valve is reconstructed or replaced with a prosthesis. The options are mechanical valves or bioprostheses (**Fig. 6.27a, b**).

- Bioprostheses (**Fig. 6.27a**) made from animal or human tissue rarely generate thrombi and anticoagulation is not necessary for long-term treatment. Unfortunately, their durability is lower compared to that of mechanical valve prostheses, so that bioprostheses are primarily used for older patients.
- Mechanical prostheses (**Fig. 6.27b**) have a longer durability than bioprostheses. However, since thrombi can form on the foreign surface, the patient must take oral anticoagulation for life. The clicking of the artificial valve can be heard with the unaided ear.

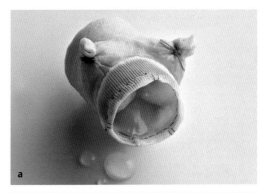

a

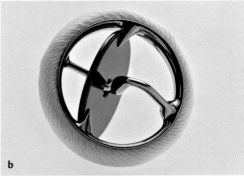

b

Fig. 6.27a, b Heart valves. **a** Biological heart valves from pigs. **b** Mechanical leaflet prosthesis (Medtronic). (Gerlach 2000.)

Case Study: A 78-year-old woman is admitted to the hospital after syncope with injuries (contusions of skull and ribs, hematomas). The patient cannot remember the event but she reports numerous episodes of vertigo. In general, she feels well, considering her age, and takes care of herself, but she has been avoiding physical exertion for years. She has no previous illnesses except gynecological diseases with surgery.

Physical examination shows a slender woman in good general condition, with a normal blood pressure at 110/80 mmHg. On auscultation there is a loud systolic murmur over the aortic valve region with transmission to both carotids. The second heart sound (closure of aortic valve) is no longer audible here.

In the ECG, indications of a left ventricular hypertrophy can be seen. Echocardiography reveals an aortic valve with severe calcification and a high degree of stenosis. Coronary angiography excludes significant coronary artery disease.

The patient is moved to the department of cardiac surgery where open heart surgery is performed and the diseased aortic valve is replaced by a biological valve prosthesis. The course was free of complications and the patient was discharged. She can now climb stairs again without difficulty. Oral anticoagulants are not required because the bioprosthesis entails no relevant thromboembolic risks.

Myocardial Diseases

Myocarditis

Definition and Causes

Myocarditis is an inflammatory disease of the heart, of infectious or noninfectious origin, which may involve the myocardium and the pericardium.

Fifty percent of all cases of myocarditis are caused by viruses such as Coxsackie, influenza and adenoviruses. It is assumed that at least 1% of all infections with cardiotropic viruses will lead to myocardial involvement. Streptococci and staphylococci can cause myocarditis and so can the pathogens of diphtheria and borreliosis. Fungal and protozoan infections are rare.

Noninfectious causes are:
- Illnesses of the rheumatic type, e.g., rheumatoid arthritis and collagenoses
- Irradiation of the mediastinum
- Certain medications
- Idiopathic origins

Symptoms

Manifestations of myocarditis range from an asymptomatic or mild course to a fatal outcome. The following symptoms are possible:
- Signs of heart failure
- Cardiac arrhythmias
- Signs of endo- or pericardial involvement, e.g., chest pain in pericarditis

Diagnosis

- ECG
- Rise in CK-MB, troponin, and inflammation markers
- Echocardiogram shows a decrease in contractility and possibly pericardial effusion
- Cardiac MRI provides imaging for inflammatory effects on myocardial areas
- Cardiac catheterization to exclude a coronary-ischemic cause and possibly take a ventricular biopsy sample

Therapy

If possible, causal treatment is implemented. Examples of this are antibiotic therapy in bacterial myocarditis and immunosuppressive therapy in autoimmune processes. In many cases, only symptomatic measures are available:
- Physical rest
- Treatment of complications, such as therapy for cardiac arrhythmias that may arise
- Application of a mechanical assist device to relieve stress on the heart in terminal heart failure
- HTX as a last resort

Physical rest is required for myocarditis!

Prognosis

In more than 80% of cases, patients with myocarditis recover fully. Sometimes harmless cardiac arrhythmias remain. Only a few patients present with a fulminant or progressive downhill course over a period of months to years leading to death or to dilated cardiomyopathy.

Cardiomyopathies

Classification

WHO Classification

All diseases of the heart muscle entailing cardiac functional disorders are classified as cardiomyopathies. According to the WHO classification, the cardiomyopathies are divided into five groups (**Fig. 6.28a–d**):
- Dilated cardiomyopathy (DCM, **Fig. 6.28**)
- Hypertrophic cardiomyopathies (HCM, **Fig. 6.28b, c**)
- Restrictive cardiomyopathies (RCM, **Fig 6.28d**)
- Arrhythmogenic right ventricular cardiomyopathy (ARVC)
- Unclassified cardiomyopathies

Primary and Specific Cardiomyopathies

Primary and secondary cardiomyopathies are distinguished on the basis of their etiologies. Primary cardiomyopathies are genetically determined or of unknown origin. If there is a prior cardiac or systemic disease, a secondary (specific) cardiomyopathy is present. Specific myocardial diseases imitate the classical cardiomyopathies morphologically, most often DCM, and can be caused, for example, by:
- Myocarditis
- Ischemia
- Valvular heart disease
- Arterial hypertension
- Alcohol and medications
- Neuromuscular diseases

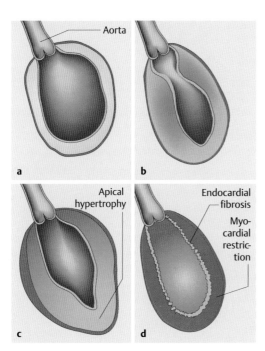

Fig. 6.28a–d Cardiomyopathies (CM). **a** Dilated cardiomyopathy (DCM). **b** Hypertrophic obstructive cardiomyopathy (HOCM). **c** Hypertrophic nonobstructive cardiomyopathy (HNCM). **d** Restrictive cardiomyopathy (RCM).

Dilated Cardiomyopathy

Consequences

The severely dilated heart is impaired chiefly in its systolic function. The patient shows symptoms of heart failure. Moreover, the dilatation promotes severe disturbances of cardiac rhythm, for example, ventricular fibrillation and the creation of thrombi, which can be the source of arterial and pulmonary emboli.

Diagnosis

Imaging procedures show the enlarged heart with its limited contractility. It may be that the diagnosis can be confirmed with a myocardial biopsy. Underlying diseases must be identified.

Therapy

In addition to treatment of the underlying diseases, the following symptomatic measures are necessary:
- Therapy for heart failure, HTX as a last resort (p. 97)
- Treatment of arrhythmias (p. 104)

- Oral anticoagulants (coumarins) for accompanying atrial fibrillation or very poor ventricular function, to avoid the formation of thrombi

Hypertrophic Cardiomyopathy

Further Classification and Consequences

Since the hypertrophied myocardium is less elastic, primarily the diastolic function is impaired. In some cases, the outflow of the left ventricle is narrowed so that a distinction is made between:
- Hypertrophic nonobstructive cardiomyopathy (HNCM, 75%)
- Hypertrophic obstructive cardiomyopathy (HOCM, 25%)

Frequently HCM will not be noticed. The most likely symptoms to occur are:
- Dyspnea
- Angina pectoris if the hypertrophied myocardium compromises the coronary arteries or if the perfusion of the severely thickened myocardium is insufficient
- Cardiac arrhythmias
- Vertigo and syncope

Diagnosis and Therapy

Diagnostic procedures and principles of therapy are comparable to those for DCM. The following considerations are particular to HOCM:
- Beta blockers are the therapy of choice.
- Substances that increase the contractile force are contraindicated.
- If necessary, an intervention must be applied to widen the outflow tract, e.g., by means of surgical myotomy or septum reduction by catheter-supported alcohol injection, for example, triggering a localized myocardial infarction in the area of the septum.

Restrictive Cardiomyopathy

Restrictive cardiomyopathy with fibrosis of the endocardium and myocardium is extremely rare in Western countries. The characteristic feature of the disease is abnormal diastolic function due to excessively rigid ventricular walls and impeded ventricular filling.

Pericarditis

Pericarditis is an inflammation of the pericardial layers. If the myocardium is also affected, the condition is called perimyocarditis.

Causes

- Microorganisms, especially viruses such as Coxsackie virus and adenoviruses
- Immunological processes, e.g., in rheumatic fever (p. 110) and postmyocardial infarction syndrome (Dressler syndrome)
- Invasive tumor growth, e.g., in breast and bronchial carcinoma or leukemia
- Surgery or trauma
- Accumulation of substances usually excreted in the urine, in case of renal failure
- Radiation therapy

Symptoms and Complications

The patient has sharp retrosternal pain that increases on lying down, during deep inspiration, and on coughing. If pericardial effusion develops, the pain decreases. Jugular venous distention indicates the following complications:

- Pericardial tamponade, which makes venous blood return to the heart impossible
- Constrictive pericarditis as a late complication, caused by a scarred and shrunken pericardium that primarily impedes ventricular filling and must often be eliminated by surgical intervention

Diagnosis

Diagnostic indicators are:

- Pericardial friction rub on auscultation that becomes softer or disappears in pericardial effusion
- Changes in the ECG
- Echocardiography to confirm the presence of effusion

Therapeutic Principles

- Therapy of underlying disease
- Physical rest
- Anti-inflammatory therapy with nonsteroidal antiphlogistics, glucocorticosteroids if necessary
- Therapeutic treatment of complications

Congenital Heart Disease in Adults

About 1% of all live-born children have a congenital malformation of the heart and circulation. Thanks to the treatment possibilities, especially cardiosurgical methods, over 80% of these now attain adulthood. Adult patients can then be found who are suffering from the consequences or complications of their congenital disease if these were not corrected, or only partially corrected, in childhood. Others can be completely asymptomatic if a timely complete correction was possible. Some congenital diseases are only diagnosed in adulthood if they have not previously caused any complaints.

Congenital heart diseases can arise as a result of endogenous or exogenous influences. Influences such as alcohol, medications, radiation, and certain infectious diseases such as rubella disrupt development of the embryonic heart. Chromosomal anomalies such as trisomy 21 or Turner syndrome are often accompanied by structural heart defects.

Table 6.14 and **Fig. 6.29a–f** show the classification of the most important congenital heart diseases into three groups.

Heart Diseases with Left-to-Right Shunt

In these malfromations blood flows through a short-circuit connection from the arterial to the venous system. Short-circuit connections can be localized at the atrium or the ventricle. In a persisting ductus arteriosus Botalli, blood from the aorta flows into the pulmonary artery. A left-to-right shunt leads to volume loading of the pulmonary circulation and the left heart. As the disease progresses, the right ventricle is subjected to pressure stress with right ventricular hypertrophy, right ventricular failure, and *pulmonary hypertension.*

In the *Eisenmenger syndrome,* the increased pressure in the pulmonary circulation or in the right heart exceeds the pressure in the left ventricle, thus leading to a shunt in both directions or to a shunt reversal. The resulting right-to-left shunt is accompanied by central cyanosis because some of the blood that has not been enriched with oxygen enters the systemic circulation. Surgical correction of a heart defect with left-to-right shunt should be carried out before pulmonary hypertension develops.

Table 6.14 Overview of the most important congenital heart diseases

Mechanism	Clinical picture	Frequency	Cyanosis	Life expectancy without correction (y)
Diseases with left-to-right shunt	Ventricular septal defect (VSD)	30%	Not primarily	20–40
	Atrial septal defect (ASD)	10%		40
	Patent ductus arteriosus Botalli	10%		30
Diseases without shunt	Pulmonary stenosis	7%	Not primarily	20–30
	Aortic stenosis	6%		20
	Coarctation of the aorta	7%		35
Diseases with right-to-left shunt	Fallot tetralogy	6%	Primarily	10
	Transposition of the great arteries	4%		<1

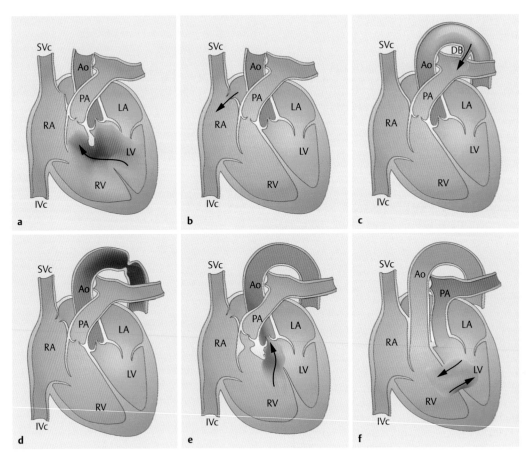

Fig. 6.29a–f Frequent congenital heart diseases. **a** Ventricular septal defect. **b** Atrial septal defect. **c** Persistent ductus arteriosus Botalli. **d** Coarctation of the aorta (aortic isthmus stenosis). **e** Fallot tetralogy. **f** Transposition of the great arteries. SVc: Superior vena cava; IVc: Inferior vena cava.

Heart Disease without Shunt

Malformations such as stenosis of the aorta or the aortic isthmus are accompanied by obstruction of the left ventricular outflow tract. The pulmonary stenosis leads to obstruction of the right ventricular outflow tract. Both left- and right-sided outflow tract obstruction leads to hypertrophy and later dilatation of the corresponding ventricle due to sustaining pressure stress. A late consequence is heart failure. Diagnosis and therapy of congenital valve stenosis is the same as for acquired valve stenosis (p. 111).

Aortic isthmus stenosis (coarctation of the aorta) is a localized narrowing of the descending aorta in the region of the origin of the left subclavian artery. There are two variants. In the form that is often only diagnosed in adult years, the narrowing is distal to the origin of the subclavian artery. The result is a blood pressure difference between the upper and the lower extremities. Hypertension in the upper half of the body can lead to headache, nose bleed, and pressure stress on the left ventricle resulting in the typical cardiac hypertension damage (p. 117). In contrast, the pressure in the lower half of the body is decreased and the femoral and foot pulses are severely weakened or lacking.

Heart Disease with Right-to-Left Shunt

In complex malformations with right-to-left shunts there is a short-circuit connection between the pulmonary and the systemic circulation. Only part of the blood low in oxygen flows through the pulmonary pathway; the other part is mixed directly with the oxygen-enriched blood of the body circulation. This leads to decreased oxygen saturation of the arterial blood and to central cyanosis ("blue babies"). Chronic oxygen deficiency is depicted by clubbing of the digits and toes, slow body development, attacks of hypoxemia, and syncope. Heart failure, thromboembolisms, and endocarditis are typical complications of these defects.

The most frequent malformation in this group is *Fallot tetralogy*, consisting of four main components:
- Pulmonary stenosis that restricts circulation in the lungs and determines the extent of the symptoms
- Ventricular septal defect
- An aorta "riding" over the ventricular septal defect so that left and right ventricles pump blood into the systemic circulation
- Right ventricular hypertrophy as a result of pulmonary stenosis

Corrective surgery should be performed as soon as possible to avoid symptoms and complications of chronic oxygen deficiency.

In *transposition of the large vessels*, pulmonary circulation is completely separated from the systemic circulation because the aorta arises from the right ventricle and the pulmonary trunk arises from the left ventricle. The newborn can live only if both circulations are connected by an additional septal defect or a patent ductus arteriosus. Surgical correction by switching the great arteries to the appropriate ventricles is performed in the first days of life.

Circulatory Diseases

■ Arterial Hypertension

Definition and Significance

According to the WHO, arterial hypertension exists when systolic values over 140 mmHg and diastolic values above 90 mmHg are measured repeatedly. The WHO definition and the classification of stages are given in **Table 6.15**.

About 20% of the population in Western industrialized countries have excessively high blood pressure and its frequency increases with the age of the population. Usually it is the result of too much food and not enough exercise and is part of the metabolic syndrome (prosperity syndrome, p. 222).

The importance of this disease is presented in the World Health Report 2002. As a result, every eighth death is related to arterial hypertension, which is thus the third most frequent cause of death worldwide.

Table 6.15 WHO Definition and stage classification of arterial hypertension

WHO Definition	Systolic blood pressure (mmHg)	Diastolic blood pressure (mmHg)
Optimal	<120	<80
Normal	<130	<85
High normal	130–139	85–89
Hypertension		
Stage I	140–159	90–99
Stage II	160–179	100–109
Stage III	>180	>110

Forms and Causes

In arterial hypertension, there is a distinction between essential or primary hypertension and secondary hypertension, in which the high blood pressure is the result of an underlying disease.

Essential or Primary Hypertension

In about 90% of patients, no disease underlying the high blood pressure can be determined. A multifactorial disease is assumed that is promoted by, among other things:
- Genetic disposition
- Lifestyle
- Constitution

Secondary Hypertension

In about 8% of patients, arterial hypertension is the result of kidney disease and in 1% it is caused by hormonal disorders or by vascular malformations such as coarctation of the aorta (**Fig. 6.29d**, p. 115).

Renal Hypertension

The pathophysiological background is the renin–angiotensin–aldosterone system (p. 85), which is normally activated by a drop in blood pressure but also in kidney disease.

Endocrine Hypertension

- Pheochromocytoma is a tumor, usually located in the adrenal cortex, that autonomously produces the stress hormones epinephrine and norepinephrine.
- In Cushing syndrome, arterial hypertension is caused by glucocorticosteroids (p. 239).
- In Conn syndrome, an excess of aldosterone is secreted, which raises the blood pressure by promoting sodium resorption and inhibiting diuresis (p. 239).

Symptoms

▌ *High blood pressure is unfortunately not painful.*

Patients with hypertension are often free of symptoms and their disease is not noticed until the symptoms of complications arise. However, the following signs should suggest arterial hypertension:
- Headaches that typically appear early in the morning at the back of the head
- Vertigo and ringing in the ears
- Nervousness
- Nosebleeds

Complications

In patients with high blood pressure, 50%–60% develop early arteriosclerosis with the corresponding secondary diseases (**Fig. 6.30**, p. 31). For this reason, arterial hypertension is considered a main vascular risk factor.

Cardiovascular complications, from which two-thirds of all hypertensive patients die, are frequent:
- Coronary artery disease (CAD, p. 98) as a cardiac manifestation of arteriosclerosis
- Left ventricular hypertrophy that is primarily elicited by chronic pressure stress
- Heart failure (p. 87)
- Abdominal aortic aneurysm and aortic dissection (p. 127)

Another possible complication is apoplexy. Strokes are fatal in 15% of patients and are caused by:
- Cerebral infarctions as a result of arteriosclerosis
- Massive hypertensive bleeding, which can occur during a high-pressure crisis

In addition, high blood pressure lasting for years causes chronic renal insufficiency (CRI). Thus 25% of patients requiring dialysis suffer from hypertensive nephropathy, which activates the RAAS and makes arterial hypertension chronic.

Values over 230/130 mmHg constitute a *hypertensive crisis*. The patient is under acute threat of:
- Cerebral hemorrhage
- Left ventricular failure
- Aortic dissection

Diagnosis

If repeated measurements of blood pressure and an ambulatory 24-hour blood pressure monitoring (p. 90) show that arterial hypertension is indeed present, the following questions must be answered by further diagnostic procedures:
- What are the underlying causes of the hypertension?
- Are there other vascular risk factors?
- Are complications already present such as target organ damage?

Therapy

Causal treatment is possible if underlying diseases that promote hypertension can be eliminated, for example, surgical removal of hormone-secreting tumors. However, usually only symptomatic treatment by basic therapy and medication remain as options.

Basic Therapy

Lifestyle modifications can effectively help in lowering blood pressure in all hypertensive patients and even regulate mild hypertension. In addition, lifestyle changes can have favorable impact on other vascular risk factors. The hypertensive patient is advised to:

- Normalize body weight
- Eat a balanced diet
- Limit use of coffee and alcohol
- Avoid smoking and passive smoking
- Restrict sodium intake
- Exercise regularly
- Learn and use relaxation techniques

Drug Therapy

Important antihypertensive drugs are:

- Diuretics
- Vasodilators such as ACE inhibitors or angiotensin-receptor blockers and calcium channel blockers
- Inhibitors of the adrenergic nervous system such as beta blockers

It is usually necessary to prescribe a combination of two or more of these in order to obtain normal pressure values.

Another important element in symptomatic therapy is treatment of the complications and of damaged target organs (**Fig. 6.30**), which will be described in the corresponding chapters.

■ Arterial Hypotension

When arterial hypotension is present, decreased blood pressure is measured. A systolic value of 100 mmHg is considered the lower normal limit. In contrast to arterial hypertension, hypotension does not lead to cardiovascular damage. Hypotension is only given disease status if it leads to complaints.

Forms and Causes

As in arterial hypertension, a distinction is made between essential or primary hypotension and symptomatic or secondary hypotension resulting from various underlying diseases or as a side-effect of medication. Possible causes for secondary hypotension are:

- Cardiovascular diseases, e.g., aortic stenosis, cardiac arrhythmias, pulmonary embolism, varicosis

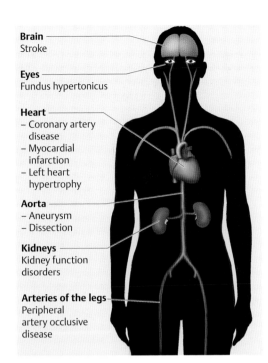

Brain
Stroke

Eyes
Fundus hypertonicus

Heart
– Coronary artery
  disease
– Myocardial
  infarction
– Left heart
  hypertrophy

Aorta
– Aneurysm
– Dissection

Kidneys
Kidney function
disorders

Arteries of the legs
Peripheral
artery occlusive
disease

Fig. 6.30 Complications and target organ damage in arterial hypertension.

- Hypovolemia, e.g., in case of bleeding, burns, diarrhea
- Endocrine disorders, e.g., hypothyroidism, Addison disease, hypophyseal insufficiency
- Neurogenic causes, e.g., diabetic neuropathy, alcoholic neuropathy, late-stage syphilis, Parkinson disease, cerebral infarctions
- Medications, e.g., antihypertensives, sympatholytics

Symptoms and Clinical Classification

The forms of hypotension can be clinically classified on the basis of their symptoms:

- Asymptomatic chronic hypotension
- Chronic hypotension with multiple symptoms
- Orthostatic dysregulation

Asymptomatic Chronic Hypotension

This form of hypotension is not considered a disease and does not require treatment. It is considered to be a normal, constitutionally determined variant of circulatory regulation and is often observed in trained endurance and high-performance athletes when the resting circulation is in a parasympathetic state.

Chronic Hypotension with Multiple Symptoms

In chronically or occasionally decreased blood pressure, various subjective complaints can arise that are due partly to insufficient circulation to the organs but also partly to unspecific disorders of general condition:

- Rapid tiring
- Lack of concentration
- Sleep disorders
- Irritability
- Vertigo
- Ringing in the ears, fluttering of the eyes
- Sensitivity to cold
- Lack of appetite, feeling of fullness
- Dyspnea, feeling of choking
- Painful "stitches" near the heart

It is often hard to differentiate these symptoms from psychovegetative disorders of general condition.

Orthostatic Dysregulation

In this form, changes in position, especially standing up or stooping, cause a decrease in venous blood return to the heart which results in a sudden drop in blood pressure. Corresponding symptoms are various, such as feelings of vertigo, empty feeling in the head, flickering eyes, insecurity in walking, collapse, and syncope.

Orthostatic hypotension is frequent in older people and patients with disorders of the autonomic nervous system, for example, in diabetic neuropathy and Parkinson disease.

Diagnosis and Therapy

A diagnosis is made when repeated blood pressure measurements show a decrease in blood pressure associated with subjective complaints. Orthostatic disorders are identified with the help of the Schellong test in which pulse and blood pressure are measured after the patient has been lying down for 10–15 minutes, 1 minute after standing up, and after 3, 7, and 10 minutes of standing freely.

The principal therapy for secondary hypotension is treatment of the underlying disease.

For symptomatic therapy, general measures are very important:

- Intake of fluids, increased intake of salt
- Training of circulation through exercise

- Massages, hydrotherapy such as Kneipp applications
- Standing up slowly after bed rest
- Use of compression stockings
- Crossing the legs while standing

For some patients with orthostatic dysregulation, additional vessel-toning medications may be indicated.

Functional Heart Disease

Functional heart disease represents a relatively frequent psychosomatic clinical picture chiefly found in people under 40 years of age. In about 15% of patients who consult a physician because they believe they have heart problems, no objective organic findings are observed. Other names for this disorder are cardiac neurosis, cardiophobia, and heart fear syndrome.

Symptoms

Patients are consumed with thoughts of suffering from heart disease. They maintain close contact with their physicians and complain of the following symptoms:

- Chest pain that is independent of stress and can radiate to the arms
- "Heart attacks" with tachycardia, fear, feelings of fainting, sweating, trembling
- Occasionally hyperventilation

Diagnosis and Therapy

The basic diagnostic program includes physical examination, ECG, stress ECG, chest radiography, laboratory screening including thyroid values, possibly echocardiography, and long-term ECG. After an organ illness has been excluded by means of these measures, the patient must be informed that the complaints are harmless. Possible treatment approaches are relaxation techniques and physical training as well as psychosomatic therapy, although it is effective in only about 50% of patients.

7 Vascular Medicine

Cardinal Symptoms in Vascular Medicine

Table 7.1 shows the principal cardinal symptoms in arterial and venous circulatory disorders.

Vascular Diagnosis

◼ Physical Examination

Inspection

Indications of arterial or venous circulatory disorders can already be found by inspection:

- Pale or livid skin color
- Reddish-brown hyper- or hypopigmentation (Stage II CVI; p. 129)
- Difference in circumference due to swelling or muscular atrophy
- Trophic disorders such as sparse or absent hair and pathological nail growth
- Necrosis or gangrene

Palpation

The following can be observed on palpation:

- Skin temperature, especially differences between sides
  - Cold extremities as a sign of an arterial circulatory disorder
  - Excess warmth as a possible indication of a venous circulation disorder or inflammation
- Pulses

Pulse Status

Figure 7.1a–c shows palpation techniques and the arterial pulses that can be felt. If more than 90% of an arterial lumen is occluded, no pulse can be palpated distal to the stenosis.

Auscultation

If more than 60% of an arterial lumen is obliterated, a vascular bruit is heard on auscultation.

Table 7.1 Important symptoms of disorders of arterial and venous circulation

Symptoms	Circulation disorder	
	Arterial	**Venous**
Pain	Improvement with lowering	Improvement with raising
Paleness (p. 43)	Yes	No
Cyanosis (p. 43)	No	Yes
Edema (p. 47)	No	Yes

◼ Imaging

Sonography

Vessels and morphological changes such as calcification, stenoses, thrombi, or aneurysms can be directly imaged by sonography.

- In Doppler sonography, the flow of blood is converted into an acoustic signal. It is used mainly to measure the speed of the blood flow, which allows the detection and evaluation of a vessel stenosis.
- The flow of blood can be visualized in color by means of color-coded sonography. This is now a standard element of vascular diagnosis because it is a noninvasive technique for visualizing stenoses and occlusions as well as reflux of blood in venous valve regurgitation.

Radiological Procedures

Vessels can also be imaged radiologically, by injection of a contrast agent.

- Phlebography for detection of venous circulatory disorders, especially thromboses
- Angiography, for detection of arterial circulatory disorders (**Fig. 7.2a, b**)
- Angio-CT and angio-MRI for tomographic views

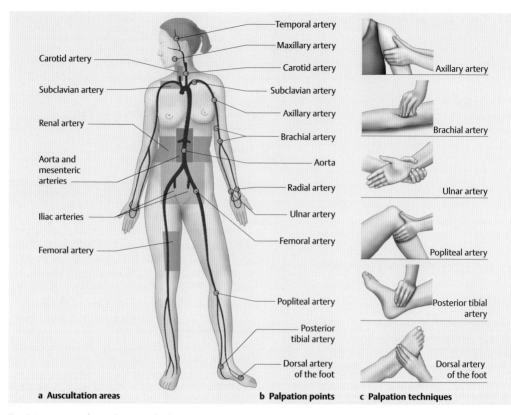

Carotid artery

Subclavian artery

Renal artery

Aorta and
mesenteric
arteries

Iliac arteries

Femoral artery

Temporal artery

Maxillary artery

Carotid artery

Subclavian artery

Axillary artery

Brachial artery

Aorta

Radial artery

Ulnar artery

Femoral artery

Axillary artery

Brachial artery

Ulnar artery

Popliteal artery

Posterior tibial
artery

Popliteal artery

Posterior
tibial artery

Dorsal artery
of the foot

Dorsal artery
of the foot

a Auscultation areas

b Palpation points

c Palpation techniques

Fig. 7.1a–c Areas of auscultation and palpation of the peripheral arterial pulses. **a** Auscultation areas. **b** Palpation points.
c Palpation techniques.

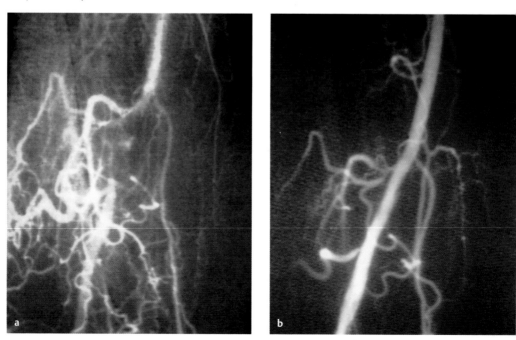

a

b

Fig. 7.2a, b Angiography in peripheral arterial disease (PAD). (Baenkler 1999.) **a** 2.5 cm-long obstruction of the femoral artery
with numerous collateral vessels. **b** Control angiography after successful percutaneous transluminal angioplasty.

Diseases of the Arteries

The following clinical pictures will be presented in this chapter:
• Peripheral arterial disease
• Acute occlusion of a limb artery
• Arterial disease of the cerebral arteries
  Aneurysms and aortic dissection

Peripheral Arterial Disease

Synonyms and Frequency

Synonymous terms for peripheral arterial disease (PAD) are:
• Peripheral artery occlusive disease (PAOD)
• Chronic occlusive disease of arteries in the extremities
• Intermittent claudication
• Smokers' legs

PAD can be found in about 11% of the male population; men are affected up to five times as frequently as women.

Causes

In 95% of cases, PAD is caused by arteriosclerosis, the pathological mechanism of which, including vascular risk factors, was discussed in detail in Chapter 31. Less frequent causes are inflammations and relapsing arterial embolisms.

Symptoms and Diagnosis

Walking-related pain is a cardinal symptom. For instance, the oxygen demand of the muscles can no longer be met during walking, resulting in ischemic pain distal to the stenosis, which causes the patient to stop. When the muscle is once more sufficiently perfused, the pain retreats and the patient can continue walking ("window shopper's phenomenon"). The degree of severity is defined by the distance the patient can walk. In advanced stages, the patient already experiences pain at rest, or the blood supply is so poor that the tissue dies.

Table 7.2 shows the clinical stages according to Fontaine–Ratschow, depending chiefly on the degree of stenosis, blood viscosity, and development of the collateral circulation. These are arterial vessels deriving from a main vessel and supplying the same perfusion region, which can adapt to the requirements if constantly demand is made on them, for instance in case of progressively narrowing or occlusion of the main artery.

Suspicion of PAD and its localization can already be entertained after a detailed medical history and physical examination (**Table 7.3**).

Table 7.2 Clinical stages according to Fontaine–Ratschow

Stage	Definition
I	Symptom free (75% of patients)
II	Intermittent claudication • IIa: Can walk over 200 m • IIb: Can walk less than 200 m
III	Pain at rest
IV	Necrosis, gangrene

Table 7.3 Classification by localization of one-stage diseases

Type (frequency)	Affected vessels	Absent pulses	Pain
Pelvic type (30%)	• Abdominal aorta • Iliac artery	From groin downward	• Hip • Thigh
Thigh type (50%)	• Femoral artery • Popliteal artery	From popliteal fossa downward	Calf
Peripheral type (20%)	• Posterior tibial artery • Anterior tibial artery • Peroneal artery • Dorsal artery of foot	Foot pulses	Sole of foot

Medical History
• History of pain
• Questions regarding vascular risk factors
• Questions regarding other cardiovascular diseases such as CAD

Physical Examination

The following changes may already be evident on inspection of the affected extremity:
• Skin pale or showing cyanotic mottling
• Sparse or absent hair
• Diminished nail growth
• Possible necrosis or gangrene (**Fig. 7.3**)
• Possible muscular atrophy

On palpation, the following can be found:
• Temperature differences: the affected side is colder.

- Pulse status: when more than 90% of the vessel lumen is occluded, no pulse can be detected distal to the stenosis (**Table 7.3**; **Fig. 7.1a–c**).

An arterial bruit can be heard on auscultation if more than 60% of the lumen is involved.

Functional Tests

The following studies are useful for diagnosis and observation of the progress of the disease, so that they can be used to document the outcome of treatment:

- Doppler pressure measurement

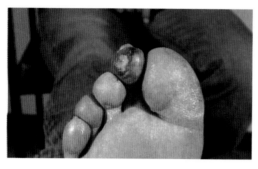

Fig. 7.3 PAD in stage IV: necrosis of second toe. (Baenkler 1999.)

- Measurement of distance walked
- Ratschow position test

In Doppler pressure measurement, the ankle brachial pressure index (ABI) is determined. The blood pressure at the ankle or the back of the foot (P_{ankle}) is measured with a specialized probe and compared with the pressure measured at the brachial artery (P_{ba}) Because of hydrostatic pressures, the healthy pressure at the ankle of a reclining patient is higher than the pressure in the arm ($P_{ankle} > P_{ba}$ = ABI ratio > 1). The values are interpreted as follows:

ABI ratio:	Interpretation
>1:	Normal value
<1:	Consistent with PAD
1–0.75:	PAD with compensation
0.75–0.5:	Moderate disease
<0.5:	Critical ischemia

Often, the physical therapist must determine the distance the patient can walk and conduct the Ratschow position test (**Fig. 7.4**).

In the position test, patients lift their legs vertically and move their feet until ischemic pain sets in. Then they sit and allow their legs to hang down while the examiner observes how long it takes for the skin to regain its color and the veins to fill.

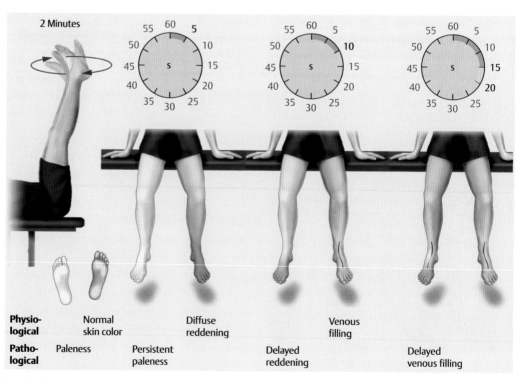

Physio-logical	Normal skin color		Diffuse reddening		Venous filling
Patho-logical	Paleness	Persistent paleness		Delayed reddening	Delayed venous filling

Fig. 7.4 Ratschow position test.

Normal values:
- Reddening (rubor) after 5–10 seconds
- Vein filling after 15–20 seconds.

Imaging

- Doppler and duplex sonography
- Angio-MRI
- Conventional angiography (**Fig. 7.2a, b**)

Therapy

> *An important component is causal treatment, i.e., vascular risk factors must be eliminated or minimized. This is achieved by lifestyle modifications and medical therapy.*

Symptomatic measures must be selected in accordance with the stage of the disease (**Table 7.4**):
- In stages I and II, formation of collateral vessels is promoted by walking exercise. Physical therapists instruct patients to walk 90% of the possible distance several times a day at determined intervals, i.e., to pause before ischemic pain sets in.
- In stages II–IV, the flow properties of the blood are improved by means of medication.

Table 7.4 Stage-dependent symptomatic therapy of PAD

Stage	I	II	III	IV
Walking	Yes	Yes	No	No
Medications	No	Yes	Yes	Yes
Revascularization	No	Partial	Yes	Yes

- In stages III and IV, sometimes in stage IIb, revascularization is indicated.

Revascularization

As in symptomatic CAD (p. 98), catheter-based interventions as well as surgical procedures are considered.

Catheterization is used for short stenoses: a balloon catheter introduced into the narrowed vessel is used to dilate the stenosis. Balloon dilatation is also known as *percutaneous transluminal angioplasty* (PTA). By simultaneous implantation of a support for the vessel, called a stent, the rate of restenosis can be reduced in certain vessel sections, for example, the iliac artery or the femoral artery (**Fig. 7.2b**).

Figure 7.5a–d shows the surgical options.
- Bypass surgery: extensive stenoses are bypassed with autologous veins.
- Grafts: depending on the size of the stenosed vessel, autologous veins such as the saphenous vein or plastic prostheses replace the narrowed section.
- Thromboendarterectomy (TEA): the internal wall of the vessel affected by arteriosclerosis is stripped.
- Amputation is a last resort.

> *Physical therapists must be aware of the following points in PAD patients:*
> - *Do not apply local heat or cold, since the affected vessels can react paradoxically.*
> - *Avoid pressure from position, clothing, etc.*
> - *Do not use compression stockings at Doppler pressure below 50 mmHg.*
> - *Keep the extremity low.*

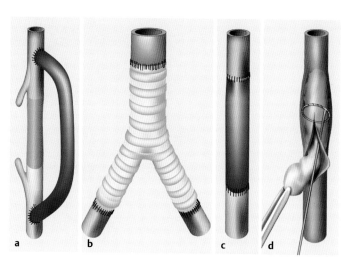

Fig. 7.5a–d Surgical procedure in PAD. **a** Bypass. **b** Implantation of a plastic prosthesis, here a Y-prosthesis. **c** Autovenous repair. **d** Thromboendarterectomy (TEA).

a b c d

■ Acute Occlusion of a Limb Artery

Acute occlusion of a peripheral artery is a life-threatening surgical emergency. In about 7% of patients, amputation of the affected limb becomes necessary and about 30% die in the acute phase.

Causes

In 30% of cases, acute occlusion is caused by an embolism. In 90%, the heart is the chief source of embolisms, for example, in atrial fibrillation (p. 107), endocarditis (p. 110), and aneurysms. Much less frequently, plaque material detaches from the walls of arteriosclerotic diseased vessels, most often the aorta.

In 40%, arterial thromboses develop in PAD, 20% of the occlusions affect operated arteries, for example bypasses. In rare cases, a trauma or external compression causes the occlusion.

> An acute occlusion of a limb artery is frequently a thrombotic complication of atrial fibrillation.

Symptoms and Complications

The symptoms can be summarized as "6 Ps."
- Pain: suddenly occurring, severe pain that improves when the limb is lowered
- Paleness: paleness distal to the occlusion
- Paresthesia: loss of sensation and false sensations that indicate nerve involvement
- Paralysis: paralysis of the affected extremity
- Pulselessness: absence of pulses distal to the arterial occlusion
- Prostration: shock (p. 54)

If the ischemia lasts longer than 6–12 hours, the muscles undergo deterioration or rhabdomyolysis. The disintegration products, together with shock, can cause acute renal failure (p. 209).

Diagnosis

The most important indications can be obtained from the medical history and the physical examination. In case of a doubtful pulse status, the diagnosis can be based on color and Doppler sonography. Angiography may occasionally be necessary.

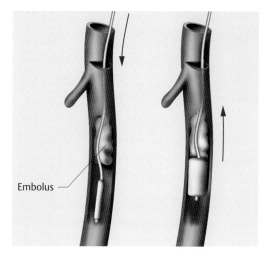

Embolus

Fig. 7.6 Removal of the embolus with a Fogarty catheter.

Therapy

Immediate measures:
- Keeping the extremity low
- Cotton bandage to protect against cooling
- Intravenous analgesics to prevent sympathetic vasoconstriction
- Intravenous heparin to prevent further thrombus formation
- Shock prophylaxis

> The following are strictly forbidden:
> - Propping up the extremity
> - Pressure
> - Local application of heat or cold

The patient must be immediately referred for vascular surgery, where the embolus is usually removed with a Fogarty balloon catheter (**Fig. 7.6**). For occlusions in the lower arm or lower leg, local lysis therapy is a possible alternative to embolectomy. To prevent another occlusion, the source of the embolism must be found and eliminated.

■ Arterial Disease of the Extracranial Cerebral Arteries

This disease affects the vessels between the aortic arch and the base of the skull (**Fig. 7.7**). It indicates the presence of systemic arteriosclerosis and can be simply detected by means of sonography. In patients with vascular risk factors, stenoses of the internal carotid artery are particularly frequent and can be the cause of a stroke.

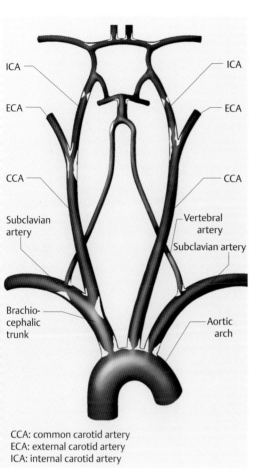

ICA

ICA

ECA

ECA

CCA

CCA

Subclavian
artery

Vertebral
artery

Subclavian artery

Brachio-
cephalic
trunk

Aortic
arch

CCA: common carotid artery
ECA: external carotid artery
ICA: internal carotid artery

Fig. 7.7 Most frequent sites of arteriosclerosis in extracranial cerebral arteries.

Therapy

Just as in treatment of CAD and PAD, causal treatment is the most important. That is, existing risk factors must be eliminated or minimized. Affected patients must also be screened for symptoms of coronary artery disease and peripheral vascular disease.

If neurological symptoms arise, the patient can profit from surgical carotid thromboendarterectomy (CTEA). In selected cases, catheterization with stent implantation can also be considered.

■ **Aneurysms**

Overview

Definition

An aneurysm is an abnormal local weakening and widening of the arterial wall.

Types

Figure 7.8a–c shows the three different types of aneurysm.
- *True aneurysm* (**Fig. 7.8a**). In a true aneurysm, the entire vessel wall is dilated. Eighty per cent of all aneurysms are true aneurysms that occur chiefly in the area of the abdominal aorta (p. 128) but can also form in the vessels supplying the brain.
- *Dissecting aneurysm* (**Fig. 7.8b**). If the intima is torn, there is bleeding into the vessel wall so that it is split longitudinally and a second, false vessel

Fig. 7.8a–c Types of aneurysm. **a** True aneurysm. **b** Dissecting aneurysm. **c** Spurious aneurysm.

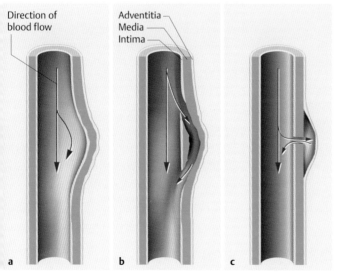

Direction of
blood flow

Adventitia
Media
Intima

a

b

c

lumen is formed in the media. The longitudinal split is called a dissection. Dissecting aneurysms, affecting the thoracic and abdominal aorta (see below) account for 15%–20% of aneurysms.

- *Spurious aneurysm* (**Fig. 7.8c**). A spurious aneurysm is a false aneurysm. Blood trickles into the surroundings through an injury to the vessel, for example a puncture produced during heart catheterization, and forms a hematoma enclosed by tissue.

Abdominal Aortic Aneurysm

About 1% of persons over 50 years of age suffer from an abdominal wall aneurysm that is a true aneurysm. This is almost always located below the branching of the renal arteries and in 30% of cases extends as far as the pelvic arteries.

Causes

An aneurysm of the abdominal aorta is caused by a vessel wall with arteriosclerotic alterations in combination with arterial hypertension.

Symptoms and Complications

At first, an aneurysm of the abdominal aorta remains unnoticed. When symptoms arise, they are signs of a threatening rupture:

- Abdominal or back pain
- Sensitivity to pressure
- Sensations of pulsation

Diagnosis and Therapy

Diagnosis is made on the basis of imaging:

- Sonography
- Angiography (**Fig. 7.9**)
- Tomographic procedures such as angio-CT and angio-MRI

The external diameter of the abdominal aorta is normally no more than 3.5 cm. Each symptomatic abdominal aortic aneurysm (AAA) must be treated. This can be done surgically or interventionally. In asymptomatic AAA, an external diameter of 6 cm or higher is an indication for surgery because from this size onward there is an abrupt increase in the risk of rupture. In the surgery, the abdominal aorta and both pelvic arteries are replaced, for example, by a Y-shaped prosthesis (**Fig. 7.5b**). Alternatively, a stent can be inserted. Both procedures have a surgical mortality of about 3%.

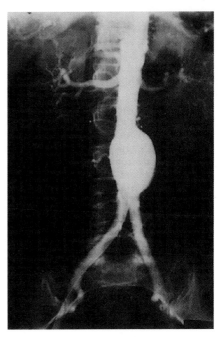

Fig. 7.9 Aneurysm of the abdominal aorta. Angiography shows the bulging of the aorta downstream of the branching of the renal arteries. (Greten 2005.)

Prevention

▮ *Systematic therapy of arterial hypertension.*

Aortic Dissection

In aortic dissection, the components of the aortic wall are separated longitudinally. This is a rare but life-threatening event. Without treatment, half of the patients die in the first 48 hours. Risk groups are:

- Patients with arterial hypertension in 80% of cases
- Patients with Marfan syndrome, an autosomal, dominantly inherited connective tissue disease

The Stanford classification recognizes two types, according to localization:

- Type A is the proximal type, affecting the aortic arch and the ascending aorta.
- Type B is the distal type, affecting the descending aorta.

Table 7.5 Complications of aortic dissection

Type	Complications
Type A (proximal type)	• Pericardial tamponade (p. 115). • Aortic valve regurgitation (p. 111) • Myocardial infarction due to compromise of the coronary arteries (p. 101) • Apoplexy due to obstruction of the cerebral vessels
Type B (distal type)	• Hematothorax (p. 166). • Bleeding into the mediastinum or abdomen • Renal insufficiency due to compromise of the renal arteries (p. 202) • Mesenteric infarction due to compromise of the vessels supplying the intestine

Symptoms and Complications

Devastating, retrosternal chest pain occurs in type A, while in type B the pain radiates in the back and abdomen. There are further complications in addition to rupture of the aorta, depending on the location of the dissection (**Table 7.5**).

Diagnosis

• Medical history and clinical data
• Visualization by imaging procedures such as transesophageal echocardiography and angio-CT or angio-MRI

Therapy and prognosis

• Lowering systolic blood pressure to values below 110 mmHg
• In proximal dissection, immediate surgery with implantation of a plastic prosthesis, possibly in combination with an artificial aortic valve
• In the distal type, stent implantation if necessary

Up to 30% of patients die in the hospital.

Diseases of the Veins

After discussing the anatomical and physiological basis, this chapter will present the following diseases:
• Varicose veins
• Thrombosis
  – Thrombophlebitis
  – Phlebothrombosis
• Chronic venous insufficiency (CVI)

■ Anatomical and Physiological Basis

Venous Systems

There are three venous systems in the leg (**Fig. 7.10a, b**):
• Superficial leg veins consisting of:
  – The great saphenous vein, which begins at the inner ankle and flows into the deep venous system below the groin
  – The small saphenous vein, which runs along the calf and, approximately at the level of the hollow of the knee, runs into the deep venous system
• Deep leg veins, which have venous valves and account for about 90% of the venous blood return
• Perforating veins that connect the superficial and the deep venous systems. The normal direction of flow from outside to inside is ensured by venous valves. The three important groups are:
  – The Dodd group on the inner side of the mid-thigh
  – The Boyd group at the inner side of the calf, directly under the knee
  – The Cockett group in the distal region of the inner lower leg

Venous Blood Return

The venous blood return has already been discussed on page 85.

■ Varicose Veins

Definition and Significance

• A varicose vein is a superficial vein that has become irreversibly expanded and torturous.
• Varicose veins affect about 20% of the population. This clinical picture must be taken seriously, since a varicosity can lead to thrombosis, chronic venous insufficiency, or leg ulcers.

Causes

In 95% of cases the varicose vein is primary or idiopathic and can be encouraged by the following factors:
• Genetic disposition
• Hormonal influence in women, since progesterone decreases the tonus of smooth muscles
• Standing or seated working conditions

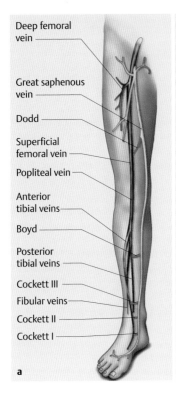

Deep femoral vein

Great saphenous vein

Dodd

Superficial femoral vein

Popliteal vein

Anterior tibial veins

Boyd

Posterior tibial veins

Cockett III

Fibular veins

Cockett II

Cockett I

a

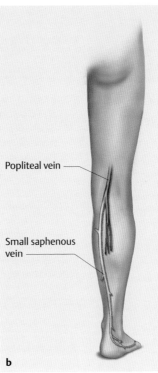

Popliteal vein

Small saphenous vein

b

Fig. 7.10a, b Venous system of the lower extremity. The superficial veins are white, the deep veins blue, and the perforating veins are denoted Dodd, Boyd, Cockett.

If return in the deep vein system is impeded, for example, after a thrombosis, venous blood return takes place via the superficial veins, resulting in a secondary varicosity.

Forms and Stages

A varicosity can affect both the large venous trunks and the small branches of the venous system (**Fig. 7.11a–c**). The most frequently occurring type is trunk varicosis, in which the bulging great saphenous vein along the inner side of the upper and lower leg and the distended small saphenous vein along the back of the lower leg become enlarged (**Fig. 7.11a**). The stages of trunk varicosis are shown in **Fig. 7.12**.

Other forms are:

- In reticular varicosis a network of distended veins with a diameter of 2–4 mm can be seen in the popliteal fossa as well as the outer side of the upper and lower leg (**Fig. 7.11b**).
- In starburst varices, the smallest veins under the skin are distended. Starbursts have a diameter of up to 1 mm and are localized chiefly on the dorsal thigh (**Fig. 7.11c**).

Symptoms

A varicosis can remain asymptomatic for a considerable time. Some patients complain of a feeling of heaviness or stretching in the legs as well as pain around the varices. The ankles can be swollen in the evening. These complaints are exacerbated by standing and by heat. They improve when patients move their legs or elevate them. The extent of the pain is not necessarily proportional to the actual status of the veins.

Complications

- Thrombophlebitis and phlebothrombosis (p. 131)
- Chronic venous insufficiency (p. 135)
- Leg ulcers

Diagnosis

- Patient history and physical examination
- Sonography

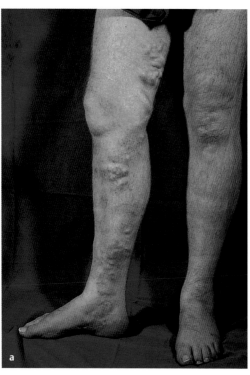

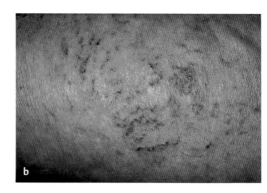

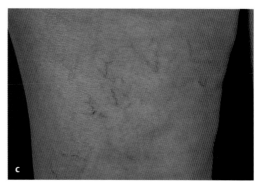

Fig. 7.11a–c Forms of varicoses. **a** Trunk varicosity of the great saphenous vein. **b** Reticular varices. **c** Starburst varices (Baenkler 1999).

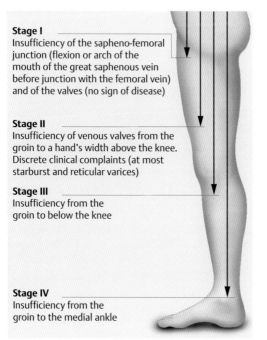

Stage I
Insufficiency of the sapheno-femoral junction (flexion or arch of the mouth of the great saphenous vein before junction with the femoral vein) and of the valves (no sign of disease)

Stage II
Insufficiency of venous valves from the groin to a hand's width above the knee. Discrete clinical complaints (at most starburst and reticular varices)

Stage III
Insufficiency from the groin to below the knee

Stage IV
Insufficiency from the groin to the medial ankle

Fig. 7.12 Stages of trunk varicosity of the great saphenous vein.

Therapy

Conservative Therapy

- Activation of the muscle pump
- Elevation of the legs
- Compression treatment with stockings of compression class II that exert a pressure of 30 mmHg
- Physical measures such as cold water treatments
- Sclerotherapy of starburst or reticular varices

Surgical Therapy

If the deep veins are patent, symptomatic varices can be removed surgically.

■ **Thrombosis**

In thrombosis, aggregates of platelets or clots form in the superficial or deep veins.
- *Thrombophlebitis* is an inflammation of a superficial vein in which the vein is blocked by a thrombus.
- *Phlebothrombosis* is thrombotic blockage of a deep vein, especially in the drainage area of the inferior vena cava.

Phlebothrombosis represents a great threat, since it carries with it the risk of pulmonary embolism (p. 163).

Thrombophlebitis

Definition and Causes

In thrombophlebitis, a superficial vein is inflamed and blocked by a thrombus. Thrombophlebitis at the legs usually arises from a previously existing varicosity and is triggered by additional immobilization or injuries. Inflammation of the superficial veins of the arms is usually iatrogenic, caused, for instance, by an indwelling venous catheter.

Symptoms and Complications

The affected vein is palpable as a coarse strand, painful on palpation (**Fig. 7.13**). In addition, there are local signs of inflammation. In contrast to deep venous thrombosis, the extremity is not swollen, since venous blood return is carried by the deep veins.

Possible complications:
- Spread of the process over the perforating veins to the deep veins, creating the risk of pulmonary embolism (p. 163)
- Infection

In rare cases, pulmonary embolism can result from thrombophlebitis.

Diagnosis

- Clinical
- Sonographic measures, especially to exclude phlebothrombosis

Therapy

- Mobilization to protect against deep vein thrombosis
- Compression
- Analgesic therapy with nonsteroidal antiphlogistics, cooling compresses, and salve bandages
- Treatment with anticoagulants in thrombophlebitis of the great saphenous vein or the small saphenous vein in the area of transition to the deep venous system

Patients with thrombophlebitis should walk a great deal.

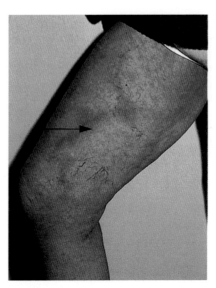

Fig. 7.13 Thrombophlebitis along the course of the proximal great saphenous vein. The reddened strand of vein is overly warm, roughly palpable, and painful to palpation. (Baenkler 1999.)

Phlebothrombosis

Since in phlebothrombosis a deep vein is completely or partially blocked, it is also known as a deep vein thrombosis (DVT). With an incidence of 160/100 000, DVT is a frequent illness. A serious complication is pulmonary embolism, responsible for approximately 15%–20% of hospital deaths.

Localization

More than 90% of DVTs are formed in vessels flowing into the inferior vena cava.
- Iliac vein: 10%
- Femoral vein: 50%
- Popliteal vein: 20%
- Veins of the lower leg: 20%

The left leg is affected in two-thirds of cases because the pelvic artery crosses and compresses the pelvic vein. The upper extremity is only rarely affected; a thrombosis in the subclavian vein or the axillary vein is called Paget–von Schroetter syndrome.

Causes: Virchow's Triad

As early as 1856, the pathologist Rudolf Virchow ascribed a thrombosis to retarded blood flow, changes in vessel walls, or changed composition of the blood.

Circulation

Factors that reduce the blood's flow rate can promote formation of a thrombus. The following are important causes:

- Immobility, e.g., caused by bed rest or a cast
- Distended vessels, e.g., varicose veins (p. 129)
- Previous thromboses leading to CVI (p. 135)
- Right heart failure (p. 87)
- Compression of vessels by long periods of sitting in a car or airplane or by a tumor

Vessel Walls

Surgery, trauma, and inflammation damage the vessel walls and in this way cause slowing and clotting of the blood.

> Without preventive measures, up to 60% of patients develop a deep vein thrombosis after hip replacement.

Blood

A change in the composition of the blood can also lead to a DVT. In addition to increased blood viscosity, for example, due to dehydration (exsiccosis) or increased platelet count (thrombocytosis), an increased clotting potential favors formation of a DVT. There is increased clotting potential as a result of:

- Congenital or acquired inhibitor deficiency (Protein S, Protein C or AT III deficiency; p. 242)
- APC resistance, in which activated Protein C (APC) cannot produce its effect
- Effect of sex hormones, e.g., when taking ovulation inhibitors ("the pill") or during pregnancy or shortly after giving birth

The importance of inhibitor deficiency and APC resistance is seen in **Table 7.6**. Decreased fibrinolysis, for example, because of plasminogen deficiency, is relatively rare (p. 242).

Other Risk Factors

Risk factors that cannot directly be classified with circulation, vessel wall, and blood factors are:

- Tumors (paraneoplasia, p. 33)
- Age > 65 years
- Smoking
- Severe infections and sepsis

Table 7.6 Importance of APC resistance or lack of inhibitors

Defect	Occurrence	Risk of thrombosis
APC resistance	30% of all DVT patients	Increased up to 200-fold
AT III deficiency	2% of all DVT patients	Increased up to 100-fold
Protein C deficiency	5% of all DVT patients	Increased up to 7-fold
Protein S deficiency	5% of all DVT patients	Increased up to 7-fold

> Smoking → Risk is 5 times greater.
> "The pill" → Risk is 3 times greater.
> Smoking and "the pill" → Risk is 15 times greater.

Symptoms

Venous congestion causes the following complaints distal to the thrombosis:

- Feelings of heaviness or stretching
- Dragging pains in the calves, popliteal fossa, or groin that improve when the affected leg is elevated
- Swelling and difference in circumference (**Fig. 7.14**)
- Cyanosis
- Excessive warmth

> - Only 10% of all patients exhibit all of these symptoms.
> - The absence of symptoms does not exclude the presence of thrombosis.

Complications

- Pulmonary embolism (p. 163)
- Postthrombotic syndrome with CVI (p. 135)
- Recurrence

Diagnosis

If there are indications in the medical history and clinical signs of a DVT, the diagnosis is confirmed with a physical examination, imaging, and laboratory tests.

Physical Examination

- Sensitivity to pressure along the course of deep veins
- Mayr sign: When the calf is compressed the patient complains of pain.

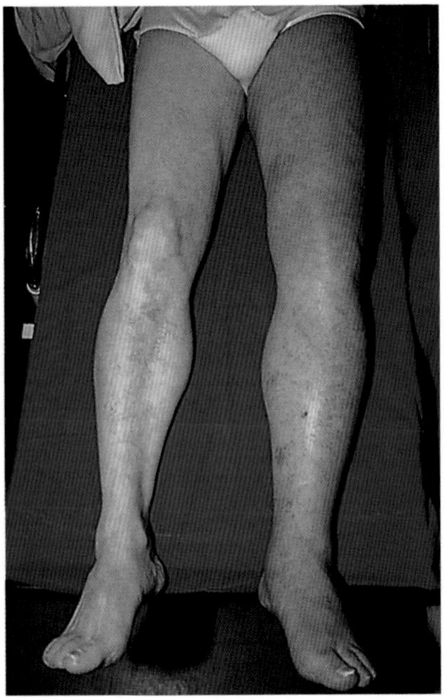

Fig. 7.14 Swelling and livid discoloration of the left leg with phlebothrombosis. (Kellnhauser 2004.)

- Homans sign: On dorsal extension of the foot, the patient complains of pain in the calf.
- Payr sign: The patient experiences pain on pressure to the sole of the foot.

> *Physical examination identifies only 50% of DVT cases.*

Imaging

- The diagnostic procedure of choice is compression sonography and, if necessary, color Doppler sonography.
- Phlebography, in which the veins are filled with a contrast agent and are visualized by radiography, is indicated only in doubtful cases.

Laboratory Measurements

Blood levels of D-dimers are determined. D-dimers are products of fibrin degradation that can be detected in the blood as a result of spontaneous fibrinolysis. They are elevated in cases of DVT and pulmonary embolism but also after surgery, in cases of inflammation, in the presence of tumors, and in pregnancy. Normal D-dimer values virtually exclude a DVT.

Therapy

The treatment is intended to prevent the expansion of the thrombus and the complication of pulmonary embolism. Moreover, the therapy aims at revascularizing the affected vessel.

General Measures

- Compression therapy is important, initially with elastic bandages and, after swelling has receded, with appropriate compression stockings.
- Immobilization with bed rest is required only in the rarest of cases, e.g., when the course is complicated, or in the early phase pulmonary embolism.

> *Usually patients with DVT are mobilized after introduction of anticoagulation and compression treatment.*

Drug Therapy

Mechanisms of action, side-effects, and contraindications of medications listed here are explained on p. 73.

- Administration of anticoagulants in therapeutic doses can decrease the risk of a pulmonary embolism by 60%.
- Lytic therapy is only rarely indicated, e.g., for complicated pelvic vein thromboses and fulminating pulmonary embolism.
- In order to prevent additional thromboses, oral anticoagulants, e.g., coumarin derivatives, are administered as secondary prophylaxis for at least 6 months.

Prophylaxis

Primary Prophylaxis

Nonpharmaceutical measures are necessary in addition to prophylactic subcutaneous injections of heparin or the application of other anticoagulants. These have the principal goal of minimizing risk factors and encouraging venous blood return (p. 85).

- Mobilization activates the muscle pump. **Table 7.7** shows how the flow rate is influenced by various measures. It is evident that standing without any other activity slows the blood flow.

> *Having a patient stand by their bed is not a useful measure for prevention of thrombosis.*

- Antithrombosis stockings compress the superficial veins. The blood reaches the deep veins via the perforating veins. Here the flow rate increases as a result of increased filling. The

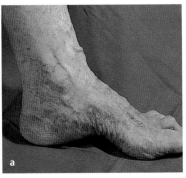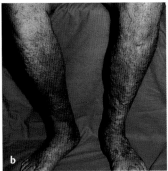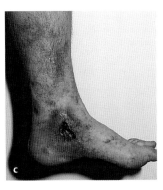

Fig. 7.15a–c Stages of chronic venous insufficiency (CVI). **a** *Corona phlebectatica*, edema, and cyanosis in stage I. **b** Additional reddish-brown hyperpigmentation and white atrophy in stage II. **c** Leg ulcer in stage III (Baenkler 1999).

Table 7.7 Effect of mobilization, elevation, and anti-thrombosis stockings on the flow rate in deep leg veins

Situation and measures	Rate of flow (%)
Reclining	100
Standing	60
Foot exercises	190
Recumbent bicycle	440
Foot end of bed raised 20°	250
Antithrombosis stockings	190

antithrombosis stockings can only achieve this effect when the patient is lying down. When the patient is standing, the pressure in the venous system increases as a result of gravity and the stockings can no longer overcome it.

▮ *Compression stockings are "bed stockings."*

Secondary Prophylaxis

If the patient already has a DVT, an additional thrombosis should be prevented by administration of oral anticoagulants. The secondary prophylaxis continues for 6 months if there are no risk factors. If risk factors such as AT III deficiency or APC resistance exist, coumarin derivatives are prescribed for an indefinite time.

▣ Chronic Venous Insufficiency

Chronic venous insufficiency (CVI) can cause ulceration of the lower leg via trophic disorders.

Pathological Mechanism

The chief cause is postthrombotic syndrome (p. 131). Moreover, varicosities (p. 129) and venous angiodysplasias, i.e., congenital defects of the venous valves, can lead to CVI. These factors cause the pressure in the venous system to rise. The small blood vessels become more permeable and blood components escape and deposit in the tissues. This results in edema, inflammatory reactions, and finally tissue loss.

Symptoms and Stages

The characteristic changes in veins and skin go through three stages (**Fig. 7.15a–c**).

Stage I

- Congestive edema is reversible.
- At the edge of the foot, dark blue skin veins called *corona phlebectatica* can be seen (**Fig. 7.15a**).

Stage II

- The edema is no longer reversible. Congestive eczema can result from the chronic edema.
- The lower leg exhibits reddish-brown hyperpigmentation.
- In addition there are areas of depigmented, atrophied skin, especially above the malleolae, known as white atrophy (**Fig. 7.15b**).

Stage III

- The third stage is marked by ulceration of the lower leg, often forming above the inner ankle, called venous leg ulcer or *ulcus cruris venosum* (**Fig. 7.15c**).

Diagnosis and Therapy

Diagnosis and therapy of stages I and II are the same as those for varicose veins (p. 129).

Principles of Treatment for Leg Ulcers

- First the ulcer must be cleaned—mechanically, enzymatically, or with special chemical agents.
- Once the ulcer is clean, the formation of granulation tissue (scar tissue) is encouraged, e.g., mechanically by debridement with a sterile scalpel.
- When the ulcer has filled in with granulation tissue, the formation of epithelial tissue is encouraged.

Lymphedema

Lymphedema is a pathological collection of lymph, mainly in the extremities. It is relatively rare, affects women much more frequently than men, and usually requires lifelong therapy by a physical therapist.

Pathological Mechanism

The tissues of the body are maintained by solutes and water that are forced out of the capillaries by hydrostatic pressure. Only 90% of the expressed fluid is reabsorbed directly into the bloodstream The remaining 10% returns to the venous system through the lymphatic circulation (p. 47). In disorders of lymph transport, this fluid remains and deposits in the tissue, causing a condition called lymphedema. A distinction is made between primary and secondary forms of this disorder.

Primary Lymphedema

Primary lymphedema is caused by malformations of the lymph vessels. This can be congenital or may appear in puberty.

Secondary Lymphedema

Secondary lymphedema develops out of underlying diseases and conditions such as:
- Infectious diseases such as erysipelas (p. 274)
- Tumor infiltration
- Postthrombotic syndrome
- Surgical removal of lymph nodes
- Radiation (p. 67)

Symptoms and Stages

Figure 7.16 shows a case of lymphedema. It is usually pale, painless, of normal temperature, and can affect fingers and toes as well. Lymphedema can present three stages:
- Stage I: Reversible edema
- Stage II: Irreversible edema
- Stage III: Lymphostatic elephantiasis

Therapy

Physical elimination of congestion by means of:
- Manual lymph drainage
- Intermittent compression treatment

After these measures, consistent compression therapy with bandages or stockings is mandatory.

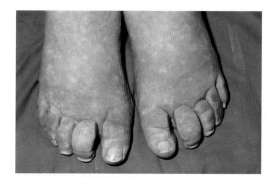

Fig. 7.16 Marked primary lymphedema with swelling of the anterior foot and toes (Greten 2005).

8 Pulmonology

Physiological Principles

■ Components of Pulmonary Function

The three components of pulmonary function are (**Fig. 8.1**):
• Ventilation
• Perfusion, i.e., blood flow
• Diffusion, i.e., gas exchange

Ventilation

Inspiration

Gases flow from regions of high pressure to regions of low pressure. Thus at inhalation, the intrapulmonary pressure must be lower than atmospheric pressure. The drop in pressure is produced by increasing the volume of the lungs. To do this, the diaphragm moves downward and the ribs are raised by contraction of the external intercostal muscles. During forced breathing, the auxiliary breathing muscles are also called into play.

Expiration

Unforced exhalation is a passive event. The diaphragm relaxes, the ribs return to their lower position, and the lungs follow their natural tendency to contract. As a result, the intrapulmonary volume falls and the intrapulmonary pressure rises under the influence of the ambient pressure. Air streams outward. In forced breathing, on the other hand, the expiratory breathing muscles are activated.

Pleura

The lung must be able to follow the breathing movements without being completely held fast to the diaphragm and the rib cage. This is enabled by the two pleural layers:
• The visceral pleura covers the lung.
• The parietal pleura lines the thorax.

Between the two pleural layers is a thin liquid film through which the lung adheres to the thorax and the diaphragm by surface tension. Except during

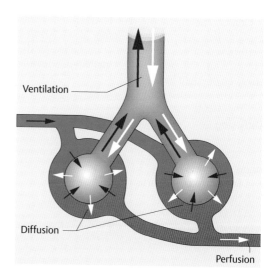

Fig. 8.1 Components of pulmonary function.

forced expiration, there is always negative pressure in the pleural cavity.

Clinical relevance: If, for example, air enters the pleural cavity as the result of a thoracic injury, the negative intrapleural pressure is eliminated and the lung collapses as a result of its elasticity. This condition is called pneumothorax (p. 166).

Perfusion

The lung is perfused by two vascular systems:
• The bronchial arteries, part of the systemic circulation, that supply oxygen-rich blood to the lungs
• The pulmonary arteries, part of the pulmonary circulation, that carry oxygen-poor blood from the right heart to the lungs, where it can be recharged with oxygen

Low-Pressure System

In connection with respiration, the pulmonary veins and arteries are of interest. They are part of the low-pressure system (p. 85) where pressures are only 5–20 mmHg. The myocardium of the right ventricle is correspondingly thin.

Ventilation–Perfusion Relationship

Physiologically, ventilated lung areas are well perfused. In order to maintain an effective ventilation–perfusion relationship, blood flow is reduced by vasoconstriction in lung parts with decreased ventilation.

Clinical relevance: The Euler–Liljestrand reflex explains how a ventilation disorder also leads to a perfusion disorder. Vasoconstriction increases the pressure in the pulmonary circulation, creating stress on the right heart.

Diffusion

The ideal conditions for diffusion through a membrane are:
- A large membrane surface
- A thin membrane
- A large concentration gradient
- A substance that "likes" to diffuse, i.e., that has a high diffusion coefficient

Alveoli and respiratory gases create favorable conditions for gas exchange in the lung.

Alveoli

- The lungs consist of about 300 million alveoli, i.e., small air sacks, each with a diameter of about 0.3 mm. This provides an exchange surface of 100 m^2 for diffusion.
- The alveolar membrane is only 1–2 μm thick and does not impede gas exchange.
- The alveoli are protected from collapsing by a very thin film of phospholipids, which is called *surfactant* and decreases the surface tension.

Respiratory Gases

Energy is generated in the tissues by oxidation of glucose. The resulting carbon dioxide is carried to the lungs by the blood and diffuses from the capillary to the alveolus in accordance with the concentration gradient. Oxygen diffuses in the other direction and is carried to the tissues in the bloodstream. The different partial pressures of O_2 and CO_2, which provide the driving force of diffusion, are shown in **Table 8.1**.

In spite of the small differences in concentration, enough CO_2 diffuses because CO_2 has a high diffusion coefficient. In fact, CO_2 diffuses 23 times as rapidly as O_2.

Clinical relevance: Deviations from normal values are classified as follows:

- **Hypoxemia:** *Decline in the partial pressure of O_2*
- **Hypercapnia:** *Increase in the partial pressure of CO_2*
- **Hypocapnia:** *Decline in the partial pressure of CO_2*

When gas exchange is impeded, CO_2 can still be exhaled fairly well at first because of its high diffusion coefficient; i.e., hypoxemia sets in first and hypercapnia only sets in later (respiratory insufficiency, p. 140).

Table 8.1 O_2 and CO_2 partial pressures (mmHg) in alveoli and blood

Partial pressure	O_2-poor blood	Alveoli	O_2-rich blood
pO_2	40	100	95
pCO_2	46	40	40

Blood pH

The pH value indicates the hydrogen ion (H⁺) concentration of a solution:

$$pH = -\log [H^+]$$

This definition makes it clear that:
- The pH value falls with rising H⁺ concentration. This leads to acidosis (**Fig. 8.2**).
- The pH value rises with decreasing H⁺ concentration. This leads to alkalosis.

The following chemical equation shows that the carbon dioxide generated in the tissue reacts with water to form carbonic acid. This is unstable and dissociates into bicarbonate and hydrogen ions:

$$CO_2 + H_2O \leftrightarrow H_2CO_3 \leftrightarrow HCO_3^- + H^+$$

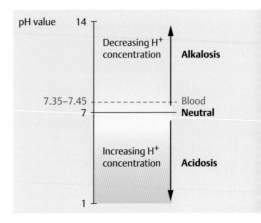

Fig. 8.2 pH value

CO_2 and H^+ ions are in equilibrium, so the pH value of the blood is dependent, among other things, on the CO_2 concentration:

$CO_2 \uparrow \rightarrow H^+ \uparrow \rightarrow pH \downarrow \rightarrow$ respiratory acidosis

$CO_2 \downarrow \rightarrow H^+ \downarrow \rightarrow pH \uparrow \rightarrow$ respiratory alkalosis

Regulation of Breathing

Breathing is controlled from the breathing center in the medulla oblongata. The breathing center reacts to numerous influences, especially to changes in the partial pressure of O_2 and CO_2 in the blood.

Chemical Breathing Stimulus

- Peripheral chemoreceptors in the aortic arch and the carotid artery measure the partial O_2 pressure in the blood and mediate the peripheral breathing stimulus. When the partial pressure of O_2 drops, a reflex stimulates breathing.
- Central chemical receptors in the medulla oblongata measure the partial pressure of CO_2 and the pH value of the spinal fluid, which are in equilibrium with the values in the blood. They mediate the central breathing impulse. When the partial pressure of CO_2 rises or the pH value falls, breathing becomes more rapid and deeper.

Figure 8.3a–c shows that rising partial pressure of CO_2 has the greatest influence on respiratory minute volume, so that CO_2 represents the strongest breathing stimulus. At the same time, it is clear that above a certain partial pressure of CO_2 the respiratory minute volume decreases, which is to say that CO_2 has a narcotic effect.

Clinical relevance: It is possible that patients with marked pulmonary diseases have a high partial pressure of CO_2 and have thus lost their central breathing stimulus (global respiratory insufficiency, p. 140).

Classification of Pulmonary Diseases

Pulmonary diseases can affect one or more of the functional components of the lung and thus lead to ventilation, perfusion, or diffusion disorders.

Ventilation Disorders

In a ventilation disorder, the lungs or individual areas of the lungs will be ventilated less efficiently. The differences between obstructive and restrictive ventilation disorders as well as their causes are presented in **Table 8.2**.

Perfusion Disorders

A direct effect on pulmonary circulation is exerted by:
- Disruption of arterial blood supply, especially in cases of pulmonary embolism (p. 163)
- Disruption of venous drainage, especially in left heart failure (p. 87)

A ventilation disorder can lead to a perfusion disorder via the Euler–Liljestrand reflex since in less well-ventilated sections of the lung the vessels are constricted in order to optimize the ventilation–perfusion relationship.

Perfusion disorders stress the right heart and can lead to a state of *cor pulmonale* (p. 142).

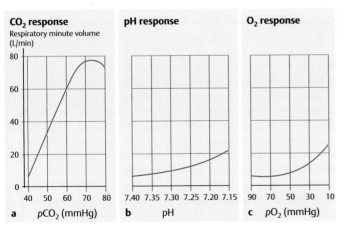

Fig. 8.3a–c Chemical respiratory stimuli: **a** CO_2 response; **b** pH response; **c** O_2 response.

CO_2 response
Respiratory minute volume (L/min)

pH response

O_2 response

a pCO_2 (mmHg)

b pH

c pO_2 (mmHg)

Table 8.2 Causes of ventilation disorders

Type of disorder	Definition	Localization of cause	Examples
Obstructive ventilation disorder	Airways are narrowed or obstructed	• Upper airways	• Malformations • Rhinitis (cold) • Foreign body aspiration • Epiglottitis • Sleep apnea syndrome (p. 165)
		• Lower airways	• Acute bronchitis (p. 148) • Chronic bronchitis (p. 148) • Pulmonary emphysema (p. 148) • Bronchial asthma (p. 153)
Restrictive ventilation disorder	Reduced elasticity of the lung–thorax–diaphragm system	• Pulmonary	• Status post partial resection of the lung • Pulmonary fibrosis (p. 160) • Pleural effusion (p. 167)
		• Extrapulmonary	• Deformities of the thorax, e.g., scoliosis, Bechterew disease • Neuromuscular diseases

Diffusion Disorders

Diffusion disorders disrupt gas exchange between alveoli and capillaries. Since CO_2 can diffuse significantly faster than O_2, the first effect is hypoxemia, a decrease in the partial pressure of O_2 in the blood, and then subsequently hypercapnia, an increase of the partial pressure of CO_2 in the blood. There are functional barriers between the alveoli and capillaries in:
• Pulmonary fibrosis (p. 160)
• Pulmonary emphysema (p. 148)
• Pneumonia (p. 155)
• Pulmonary edema (p. 87)

Cardinal Pulmonary Symptoms

Overview

Important cardinal pulmonary symptoms are:
• Dyspnea (p. 49)
• Cyanosis (p. 43)
• Chest pain (p. 50)
• Coughing and expectoration

Coughing and Expectoration

Coughing is a physiological protective mechanism to clear the airways, but it can also be a sign of pulmonary disease. Depending on duration, distinctions are made among:

• Acute cough lasting up to 3 weeks, e.g., in acute bronchitis, pneumonia, pulmonary embolism, and aspiration of a foreign body
• Spasmodic coughing as in bronchial asthma
• Chronic coughing lasting longer than 3 weeks, e.g., in chronic bronchitis, tumors, or bronchiectases.

In addition, a distinction is made between:
• Coughing without expectoration, also called dry or irritated cough
• Coughing with expectoration, also called productive cough.

Expectoration can involve bronchial secretions (sputum) or blood (**Table 8.3**).

> Chronic cough and bloody expectoration must be diagnostically clarified.

Complications of Pulmonary Diseases

In this section we will discuss complications that can occur in a number of pulmonary diseases:
• Respiratory insufficiency
• Pulmonary hypertension and cor pulmonale
• Atelectases
• Bronchiectases

Respiratory Insufficiency

Bronchopulmonary diseases can reduce respiratory efficiency to such an extent that there is a change

Table 8.3 Diagnostic indications provided by sputum quality

Sputum	Possible causes
Cough urge without expectoration	• Interstitial processes, e.g., in: – Interstitial pneumonia (p. 155) – Interstitial pulmonary disease and pulmonary fibrosis (p. 160) • Side-effects of medication, e.g. in ACE inhibitors
Thick, glassy secretion	Bronchial asthma (p. 153);
Serous secretion	Virus infection
Yellowish secretion	Bacterial superinfection
Hemoptysis	Sputum stained with a small amount of blood, e.g., in: • Bronchitis (p. 148) • Pneumonia (p. 155) • Bronchiectases (p. 143) • Bronchial carcinoma (p. 157) • Tuberculosis (p. 268)
Hemoptoe	Coughing up of large quantities of blood, e.g., in: • Bronchiectases (p. 143) • Tuberculosis (p. 268) • Central bronchial carcinoma (p. 157) • Trauma

in the blood gases. Blood gas analysis (BGA, p. 147) provides information as to whether there is a partial or a global respiratory insufficiency.
• Partial respiratory insufficiency:
  – Hypoxemia
  – The partial pressure of CO_2 is normal or diminished because of increased respiratory activity
• Global respiratory insufficiency:
  – Hypoxemia
  – Hypercapnia
  – Respiratory acidosis

> There is a difference between partial and global respiratory insufficiency.

In global respiratory insufficiency the central respiratory drive is absent (p. 139), whereas the peripheral respiratory drive is still activated by lack of oxygen. Uncontrolled administration of oxygen deprives the patient of the remaining respiratory drive and thus puts them in a life-threatening situation.

> In global respiratory insufficiency, oxygen is administered with BGA monitoring.

Symptoms

Partial Respiratory Insufficiency

• Dyspnea
• Tachycardia
• Possible central cyanosis (p. 43)
• Possible confusion and altered consciousness
• Possible clubbed digits resulting from chronic lack of oxygen (p. 49)

Global Respiratory Insufficiency

In addition to the symptoms of partial insufficiency there are headache, vertigo, and sweating as expression of hypercapnia. As the disorder progresses, CO_2 narcosis can develop (p. 139).

Therapy

Treatment of the underlying disease is a significant component of therapy. The goal of symptomatic therapy is to improve oxygenation and elimination of CO_2. In addition to physical therapy and respiratory therapy, treatment with oxygen and, if appropriate, the use of respiratory aids are options for symptomatic therapy.

Treatment with Oxygen

Patients with partial respiratory insufficiency can receive oxygen without danger, either through nasal prongs or via a face mask. Oxygen can also be administered at home over the long term.

In patients with global respiratory insufficiency, uncontrolled administration of oxygen is life-threatening because hypercapnia has already disabled the respiratory drive, so that now the drive is only activated by a lack of oxygen. If such patients receive uncontrolled oxygen, they are deprived of the remaining stimulus to breathing. In such cases, oxygen must be administered under meticulous BGA monitoring. If the pCO_2 continues to rise, respiratory support is required.

Use of Respiratory Support and Ventilation

Respiratory support is indicated when the patient can no longer exert the respiratory effort required for adequate gas exchange. Of the many procedures that support breathing, two important forms are described here:
• *Continuous positive airway pressure* (CPAP) using a CPAP mask can reduce the patient's respiratory effort and support spontaneous breathing. This procedure is indicated if the respiratory mus-

cles are exhausted and there is a threat of global respiratory insufficiency. The patient can use this noninvasive ventilatory procedure at home, for instance at night.

- If the patient no longer spontaneously breathes enough or if there is a gas exchange disorder that cannot be overcome in any other way, *controlled mechanical ventilation* in an intensive care unit is required. For this procedure, the patient is sedated and intubated with an endotracheal tube. The ventilation apparatus takes over the entire work of respiration.

Lung Transplantation

Lung transplantation (LTX) is the last resort for the most severe respiratory insufficiency resulting from a variety of irreversible diseases, for example, in advanced pulmonary fibrosis or mucoviscidosis.

■ Pulmonary Hypertension and Cor Pulmonale

Pathomechanism of Pulmonary Hypertension

The pulmonary circulation is part of the low-pressure system (p. 85). The myocardium of the right ventricle is of sufficient strength to overcome the low maximal pressure of 20 mmHg.

Any factor that reduces the overall vascular diameter of the pulmonary circulation raises the flow resistance of the pulmonary arteries and thus the pressure in the pulmonary circulation. This results in pulmonary hypertension, which places a stress on the right ventricle.

> *Total diameter ↓ → resistance to flow in the pulmonary arteries ↑ → pulmonary hypertension*

Cor Pulmonale

Enlargement of the right heart caused by stress resulting from a disorder in pulmonary function is called cor pulmonale. This can develop suddenly or over a long period. The clinical signs of right heart failure are given on page 87.

Acute Cor Pulmonale

When parts of the pulmonary arterial circulation are suddenly blocked by an embolus (p. 163), the pressure and thus the resistance to flow in the pulmonary circulation are abruptly increased. The right ventricle is not able to adapt to the new conditions rapidly enough and acute cor pulmonale results.

> *Pulmonary embolism → acute cor pulmonale*

Chronic Cor Pulmonale

Chronic cor pulmonale is often caused by ventilation disorders that lead to pulmonary vasoconstriction. The physiological background is the Euler–Liljestrand reflex (p. 137).

Through this mechanism, diseases like bronchial asthma, COPD, and pulmonary fibrosis develop a gradual increase of pressure in the pulmonary circulation, to which the right ventricle can adapt itself at first by hypertrophy. Chronic cor pulmonale can also develop in perfusion disorders such as relapsing small pulmonary embolisms.

> *Ventilation disorders → perfusion disorders → slow rise in pressure → chronic cor pulmonale*

■ Atelectasis

Definition and Causes

Atelectasis is defined as lung tissue empty of air but without inflammatory changes.

Primary atelectasis is present when sections of the lungs have never been ventilated. It can occur in newborn or premature infants if the lungs did not expand completely with the first breath, for example, when there is:

- Lack of surfactant (p. 137), especially in premature infants
- Aspiration of embryonic fluid
- Damage to the respiratory center

Secondary atelectasis is produced by the collapse of alveoli that have already been ventilated. Three different forms are distinguished (they are given in **Table 8.4** with examples):

- In *obstructive atelectasis*, also known as *resorption atalectasis*, the airways are blocked and the sections downstream of the obstruction can no longer be ventilated. The gas mixture that is still present is absorbed in time and the alveoli collapse.
- In *compression atelectasis*, pressure prevents adequate ventilation.
- *Relaxation atelectasis* results when the lung collapses as a result of pneumothorax (p. 166).

> *Postoperative pain therapy and physical therapy encourage diaphragmatic breathing and thus prevent formation of atelectasis.*

Complications

- Respiratory insufficiency
- Infections and abscesses

Diagnosis and Therapy

Chest radiography gives diagnostic information (**Fig. 8.4**). In addition to causal treatment such as removal of foreign bodies, the following symptomatic measures can be considered:

- Respiratory therapy
- Antibiotics for infections
- Segment or lobe resection in chronic atelectasis

Table 8.4 Types and causes of secondary atelectasis

Type	Causes
Obstruction atelectasis	• Bronchial carcinoma (p. 157) • Foreign bodies • Secretion
Compression atelectasis	• Reduced diaphragmatic breathing, e.g., postoperatively • Thoracic deformities, e.g., marked scoliosis • Pleural effusion (p. 167) • Pulmonary embolism resulting from reduction of surfactant (p. 163)
Relaxation atelectasis	• Pneumothorax (p. 166)

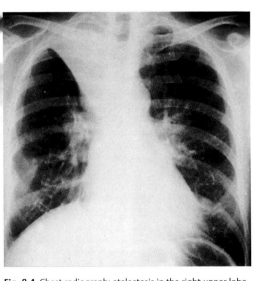

Fig. 8.4 Chest radiograph: atelectasis in the right upper lobe.

■ Bronchiectasis

Definition and Causes

Bronchiectases are irreversible pouch-shaped or cylindrical distensions of the bronchi, principally in consequence of an underlying pulmonary disease (**Fig. 8.5**). As a result of the chronic inflammation, the walls of the bronchi disintegrate and elastic fibers and smooth muscles are destroyed. Bronchial obstruction produces unphysiological pressures that distend the weakened airways.

Possible congenital causes are:
- Mucoviscidosis (p. 161)
- Immune deficiencies such as IgA deficiency
- Primary ciliary dyskinesia, an autosomal recessive disease in which the mobility of the cilia in the airways is reduced. The reduced mucociliary clearance favors bronchopulmonary infections.

Examples of acquired causes are:
- COPD (page 148)
- Bronchial stenosis caused by tumors and foreign bodies

Symptoms and Complications

The distended bronchi collect secretions that can be cleared by coughing after a change in position and

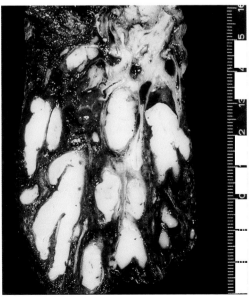

Fig. 8.5 Autopsy findings: extended bronchiectases filled with secretion. Healthy lung tissue is hardly recognizable. (Riede 2004.)

that present an ideal environment for microorganisms. Typical signs of disease are:
- A high volume of expectoration
- Three-layered, sweetish smelling sputum consisting of pus, slime, and foam

Some important complications are:
- Relapsing bronchopulmonary infections, lung abscesses, and fungal infestations
- Pulmonary bleeding
- Respiratory insufficiency

Diagnosis and Therapy

Bronchiectases can be visualized by imaging procedures, such as computed tomography, which has replaced bronchography. Therapy consists of both surgical and conservative measures:
- Segment or lobe resection in locally limited bronchiectases
- Mobilization of secretions
- Inoculations
- Where appropriate, bronchospasmolysis and specific antibiotic therapy

Pulmonological Diagnosis

■ Physical Examination

Inspection

Inspection reveals principally:
- The shape of the thorax, e.g., deformation of the thorax or barrel chest in hyperdistension
- The respiratory excursion, e.g., symmetry, thoracic or abdominal breathing
- Indications of dyspnea such as elevated respiratory rate, choosing a bodily position to facilitate breathing, and use of the auxiliary respiratory muscles
- Cyanosis, etc.

Percussion

Percussion of the thorax can determine the borders of the lungs in inspiration and expiration and thus the respiratory displacement. In a healthy person, this is 3–5 cm.

In addition, percussion yields a characteristic sound that is described as sonorous. Differences in sound on percussion reveal pathological deviations:

- A loud, deep sound on percussion is called hypersonorous and is the result of an elevated air content in the lungs, such as in pulmonary emphysema.
- A muted sound on percussion indicates infiltration, e.g., in pneumonia or pleural effusion.

Auscultation

Physiological Auscultation Findings

In a healthy person, auscultation with the stethoscope yields:
- A relatively loud, rough sound over the trachea and the large bronchi, caused by turbulent flow and called bronchial breathing
- On the periphery, a soft, low inspiratory sound caused by laminar flow, called vesicular breathing

Pathological Auscultation Findings

A weakened or absent breathing sound can occur, for example, in emphysema or pneumothorax. Stridor, wheezing, and crepitation are pathological breath sounds.
- Stridor is a whistling breath sound, occurring with constricted airways, that can be heard even without a stethoscope. If the upper respiratory airways are constricted by swelling, secretion, or foreign bodies, inspiratory stridor results, i.e., whistling on inhalation. Bronchial obstruction, on the other hand, leads to expiratory stridor.

> - *Inspiratory stridor in obstruction of the upper airways*
> - *Expiratory stridor in bronchial obstruction*

- Wheezing is a variable breath sound that can be heard as whistling, squeaking, or humming. It is caused by obstruction such as secretion and can sometimes be heard even without a stethoscope.
- Crackling is a background noise of breathing that can be heard with a stethoscope. It is caused by accumulated fluid, e.g., pulmonary edema or accumulation of secretions.

■ Pulmonary Function Test

The following procedures are used in a pulmonary function test:
- Spirometry
- Whole-body plethysmography
- Compliance measurement

Spirometry

Ventilation can be evaluated by means of spirometry. Both static values, as shown in **Fig. 8.6** and summarized in **Table 8.5**, and dynamic values can be determined with spirometry.

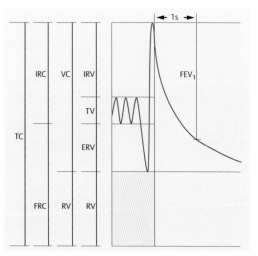

Fig 8.6 Lung volumes and capacities (TV = tidal volume; IRV = inspiratory reserve volume; ERV = expiratory reserve volume; RV = residual volume; VC = vital capacity; IRC = inspiratory reserve capacity; FRC = functional residual capacity; TC = total lung capacity; FEV$_1$ = forced expiratory volume in 1 second).

- The *one-second capacity* is determined with the *Tiffeneau test*. The patient inhales slowly and as deeply as possible and then exhales as rapidly as possible. The spirometer measures how much the patient exhales in the first second. In a person with healthy lungs, the forced expiratory volume in the first second (FEV$_1$) is equal to 80% of the vital capacity (VC). This value is lower in patients with obstructive ventilation disorders because of the constricted airways.

> One-second capacity or FEV$_1$ = 80% VC

- In the *bronchospasmolysis test*, the Tiffeneau test is repeated after inhalation of a bronchodilator. In this way it can be determined whether the previously demonstrated obstruction is reversible, e.g., in bronchial asthma (p. 153).
- The peak expiratory flow is measured with the *peak flow meter*. This is a simple device given to patients so that they can measure and monitor themselves. Normal values depend on sex, age, and height and are presented in **Fig. 8.7**.

Whole-Body Plethysmography

The whole-body plethysmograph is a closed chamber with a volume of about 1 m³ in which the patient is seated. In contrast to spirometry, the examination

Table 8.5 Lung volumes and capacities

Static size	Definition	Averages for men. Values in women are up to 20% lower
Tidal volume (TV)	Quantity of air that is inhaled and exhaled with each breath at rest	500 mL
Inspiratory reserve volume (IRV)	Additional amount of air that can be inhaled after unforced inspiration	~2500 mL
Expiratory reserve volume (ERV)	Additional amount of air that can be exhaled after unforced expiration	~1500 mL
Residual volume (RV)	• Amount of air remaining in the lungs after a maximal expiration • The RV cannot be measured spirometrically	• ~1500 mL • 20% TC
Vital capacity (VC)	• Maximal amount of air that can be exhaled after a maximal inspiration • TV + IRV + ERV	• ~4500 mL • 80% TC
Total capacity (TC)	• Amount of air in the lungs after a maximal inspiration • VC + RV • The TC cannot be measured spirometrically	~6000 mL
Functional residual capacity (FRC)	• Amount of air in the lungs after an unforced expiration • ERV + RV • The FRC cannot be measured spirometrically	~3000 mL
Inspiratory reserve capacity (IRC)	• Maximal amount of air that can be inhaled after unforced expiration • TV + IRV	~3000 mL

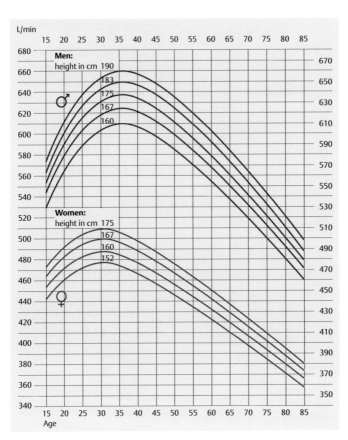

Fig. 8.7 Normal peak flow values.

does not depend on the patient's cooperation. In addition, values can be measured that cannot be recorded with spirometry:

- Residual volume, total capacity, and functional residual capacity
- Airway resistance, known simply as resistance

Lung Compliance

Compliance is a measure of the expansibility of the lung–thorax–diaphragm system. The quantity measured is the change in volume of the lung per unit of intrathoracic pressure difference. The patient must swallow a pressure probe that measures pressure in the esophagus at the beginning and end of inspiration. The difference corresponds to the intrathoracic pressure difference.

The normal value is 0.03–0.05 L/kPa. Lower values indicate decreased expansibility and thus a restrictive ventilation disorder. This examination is seldom used because it is unpleasant for the patient and equivalent information can be obtained by measuring the vital capacity.

Pulmonary Function in Ventilation Disorders

The different measurement results in obstructive and restrictive ventilation disorders are summarized in **Table 8.6**.

- The changed values in *obstructive ventilation disorders* can be ascribed to the fact that constricted airways interfere especially with exhalation, which is normally a passive process. Air remains in the alveoli, and this is called *air trapping* (**Fig. 8.8**). Thus an obstruction is expressed, in addition to increased resistance to flow, by decreased FEV$_1$ and increased residual volume.

Patients and physical therapists can determine the extent of the obstruction themselves, by measuring the expiratory peak flow with a peak flow meter.

- In *restrictive ventilation disorders*, the lung–thorax–diaphragm system is no longer as elastic as in a person with healthy lungs, so that the total capacity and all its constituent values decrease. Decreased compliance is also an expression of decreased expansibility.

Physical therapists can determine the extent of the restriction by measuring the vital capacity with a hand spirometer.

Table 8.6 Pulmonary function test in obstructive and restrictive ventilation disorders

	Obstruction	Restriction
Vital capacity	(↓)	↓
• FEV₁ • Peak-flow	↓	Normal
• TC • RV	↑	↓
Resistance	↑	Normal
Compliance	Normal	↓

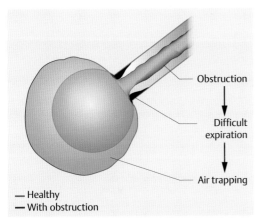

— Healthy
— With obstruction

Fig. 8.8 Air trapping. Since obstruction is chiefly an impediment to exhalation, air is trapped in the alveoli.

Blood Gas Analysis

Blood gas analysis (BGA) determines the partial pressures of the respiratory gases and the pH value of the arterial blood and the capillary blood. The measurement results provide an indication of the extent of respiratory insufficiency (**Table 8.7**).

Noninvasive Imaging

The following noninvasive imaging techniques are used in pulmonary diagnosis:
• Sonography to confirm pleural effusion and space-occupying lesions near the thoracic wall
• Conventional X-rays of the thorax, in order to:
 – Demonstrate infiltrates in pneumonia (p. 155)

Table 8.7 Blood gas analysis. Normal values and changes in respiratory insufficiency

Parameter	Normal value	Partial insufficiency	Global insufficiency
O₂ saturation	94%–98%	↓	↓
O₂ partial pressure	80–108 mmHg	↓	↓
CO₂ partial pressure	32–47 mmHg	Normal	↑
pH value	7.35–7.45	Normal	↓

 – Visualize space-occupying lesions, e.g., tumors (p. 157)
 – Recognize atelectases, i.e., nonventilated areas (**Fig. 8.4**)
 – Confirm the presence of pneumothorax (p. 166)
 – Diagnose a pleural effusion (p. 167)
 – Evaluate the position of the diaphragm, e.g., a lowered position in pulmonary emphysema (p. 148)
 – In cardiological diagnosis, recognize an altered heart contour or size, increased drawing of the pulmonary vessel, and pulmonary edema (p. 93)
• CT or MRI, principally to image the growth of space-occupying structures
• Angiography and perfusion and ventilation scintigraphy to demonstrate perfusion disorders, for example, in pulmonary embolism

Endoscopic and Bioptic Methods

Various endoscopic techniques are available to see directly into airways and pulmonary structures.
• The most important diagnostic procedure is bronchoscopy, with which it is possible to look into the large airways down to the segmental and subsegmental bronchi (**Fig. 8.9**). In addition, material for microbiological and fine-tissue studies can be obtained by means of:
 – Bronchoalveolar lavage (BAL), in which a physiological sodium chloride solution is infused into a lung segment and recovered after a few seconds
 – Forceps biopsy
• Thoracoscopy provides a view into the thoracic cavity.
• Mediastinoscopy provides a view into the anterior mediastinum.

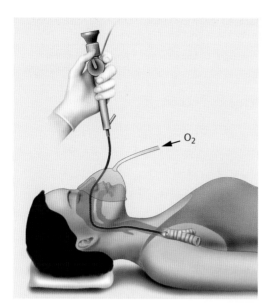

Fig. 8.9 Transnasal bronchoscopy with flexible broncho-
scope.

Thoracoscopy and mediastinoscopy are surgical-
endoscopic procedures performed under anesthesia
and permit removal of a specific tissue sample.

Acute Bronchitis

Definition and Causes

Acute bronchitis is an inflammatory disease of the
airways. It usually occurs as part of a cold, in association with rhinitis and inflammation of the sinuses
and larynx. Acute bronchitis is one of the most frequently occurring diseases, with peak seasons in
spring and fall. Among the causes are:
- Viruses in about 90% of cases
- More rarely, bacteria such as *Mycoplasma* and
  Chlamydia, with possible bacterial superinfec-
  tions
- Toxins such as gases, dusts, or radiation

Symptoms

The usual symptoms are the same as for colds, such
as fever, fatigue, headache, muscle and joint pain,
rhinitis, hoarseness, and coughing with retrosternal
pain. Usually the cough starts as a dry cough that
may later be associated with a whitish expectoration. Yellowish-green expectoration suggests a bacterial superinfection. In serious cases, the sputum

may contain a small amount of blood. Acute bronchitis may last from a few days up to weeks.

Diagnosis and Therapy

In uncomplicated viral bronchitis special diagnostic
procedures are usually not necessary. Diagnosis is
made on the basis of typical clinical symptoms.
  Treatment is symptomatic with:
- Physical rest
- Dilution of secretions by copious fluid intake and
  inhalation
- Antitussives, i.e., substances that inhibit coughing,
  such as codeine, to aid in sleeping
- Chest packs and sweat cures
- Antibiotics only for bacterial infection, or for
  patients with previous pulmonary disease or
  elderly or immunocompromised patients

Chronic Obstructive Pulmonary Diseases

The following synonyms for chronic obstructive pul-
monary disease are commonly encountered:
- Chronic obstructive pulmonary disease (COPD)
- Chronic obstructive lung disease (COLD)

The disease implies mainly two clinical pictures:
- Chronic obstructive bronchitis
- Obstructive pulmonary emphysema

Significance

One in six occupational disabilities are caused by
COPD. This is the most frequent cause of cor pulmonale and respiratory insufficiency. Thus COPD holds
fourth place in causes of death in the industrialized
world.

Chronic Bronchitis

WHO Definition and Frequency

According to WHO, a patient has chronic bronchitis if they have a productive cough, i.e., cough with
expectoration for at least 3 consecutive months a
year for 2 consecutive years.
  In the industrialized world, 10% of the population suffers from chronic bronchitis, making this
the most frequently occurring chronic lung disease.
Men are affected three times as often as women.

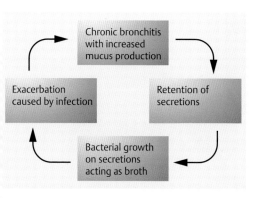

Fig. 8.10 Vicious spiral in chronic bronchitis.

Pathological Mechanism

Numerous exogenous and endogenous factors lead to mucociliary insufficiency in which the cilia of the airways are first paralyzed and then destroyed. Chronic bronchitis is usually caused by many years of cigarette smoking. Thus 90% of patients are smokers or ex-smokers and every second smoker over 40 years of age suffers from chronic bronchitis.

Additional exogenous factors are air pollution and relapsing infections that in the further course of the disease can lead to deterioration, i.e., an exacerbation of the disease (**Fig. 8.10**).

Endogenous factors include:
- Antibody deficiency syndrome such as congenital lack of IgA, in which the antibodies that occur naturally in the bronchial secretions are missing
- Primary ciliary dyskinesia, a congenital disease, in which the ciliated epithelium in the airways does not move
- Mucoviscidosis (p. 161)

The bronchial mucosa reacts to mucociliary insufficiency first by hypertrophy and increase in mucus production that blocks the airways and causes an *endotracheal obstruction*. Later the bronchial mucosa atrophies and with forced expiration the bronchi can collapse, a so-called *exobronchial obstruction*.

Symptoms and Complications

A persistent productive cough is a cardinal symptom. Later, complications define the clinical picture:
- Pneumonia and abscesses
- Bronchiectases
- Obstructive pulmonary emphysema
- Respiratory insufficiency
- Pulmonary hypertension and cor pulmonale

Pulmonary Emphysema

WHO Definition and Frequency

The WHO defines pulmonary emphysema as an irreversible distension of the air spaces distal to the terminal bronchioles as a result of destruction of their walls. Individual sections or an entire lung can be affected by the irreversible pouching of the alveoli. A distinction is made between localized emphysema and generalized emphysema.

In 10% of all autopsies, pulmonary emphysema is a significant cause of death.

Causes

Emphysema related to the physiological process of aging is called *primary atrophic emphysema*, whereas *secondary emphysema* develops out of a primary disease (**Table 8.8**).
- Obstructive ventilation disorders such as chronic bronchitis and bronchial asthma (p. 153) interfere primarily with expiration; air is held back distal to the obstruction of the passage. This air trapping distends the alveoli (**Fig. 8.8**).
- Due to scars arising postoperatively, after tuberculosis (p. 268) or in pulmonary fibrosis (p. 160), lung tissue shrinks and the adjacent areas are overdistended.
- Overdistension of lung tissue can also be the direct consequence of partial resection of the lung or thoracic deformities, e.g., massive scoliosis or kyphosis.
- Even in a healthy lung, neutrophilic granulocytes release proteases. These can attack lung tissue and must therefore be neutralized by protease inhibitors such as alpha$_1$-antitrypsin (AAT). Pulmonary emphysema develops when proteases are present in excess. Bronchopulmonary infections and cigarette smoking lead to an imbalance through which the protease inhibitors are inactivated. A congenital AAT insufficiency is the cause of the disease in 2% of cases.

Symptoms and Complications

The *pink puffer* (**Fig. 8.11**) and the *blue bloater* (**Fig. 8.12**) are two clinical pictures between which there is a smooth transition. They serve to describe the spectrum of symptoms.

Table 8.8 Causes of secondary pulmonary emphysema

Cause	Examples
Obstruction	• Chronic bronchitis • Bronchial asthma (p. 153) • Mucoviscidosis (p. 161)
Scars	• Pulmonary fibrosis (p. 160) • Status post tuberculosis (p. 268) • Status post partial lung resection
Overdistension	• Thoracic deformities, e.g., scoliosis • Status post partial lung resection
Disequilibrium between proteases and inhibitors	• Infections → proteases ↑ • Smoking → protease inhibitors ↓ • Alpha$_1$-antitrypsin deficiency

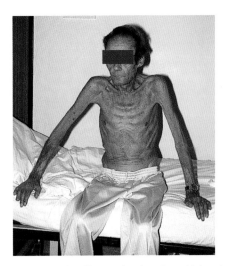

Fig. 8.11 Pink puffer: a cachectic patient with barrel chest who uses auxiliary breathing muscles in resting dyspnea. (Baenkler 1999.)

Pink Puffer

In the pink puffer, the emphysema is dominant and this patient is also called the emphysema type. The pink puffer is a rather gaunt type in whom a barrel chest points to excessive distension:
- The ribs are horizontal in the inhalation position, and so there is less difference between the circumference of the thorax in inspiration and the circumference in expiration.
- The diaphragm is also in inspiration position. It is flattened by the overdistended lungs and when it contracts, paradoxically, the lower edge of the ribs contracts—so-called thoracic wall–diaphragm antagonism.

Additional symptoms are:
- Marked dyspnea but hardly any cyanosis
- Possibly a dry cough
- Partial respiratory insufficiency that can also become global insufficiency

Blue Bloater

The bronchitis component is dominant in the blue bloater; this patient is also called the bronchitis type. The blue bloater tends to be obese and exhibits:
- Marked cyanosis with polyglobulia (p. 43), but hardly any dyspnea
- Productive cough as part of the chronic bronchitis
- Global respiratory insufficiency
- Early cor pulmonale

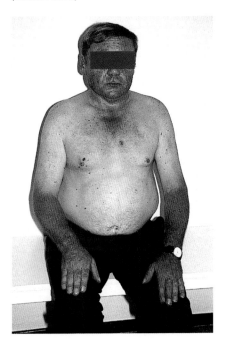

Fig. 8.12 Blue bloater: an obese patient with cyanosis and suggestion of clubbed digits but without resting dyspnea. (Baenkler 1999.)

> *Important complications of both COPD pictures are:*
> - *Respiratory failure*
> - *Acute exacerbations*
> - *Extrapulmonary symptoms such as weight loss, muscular atrophy, and osteoporosis*

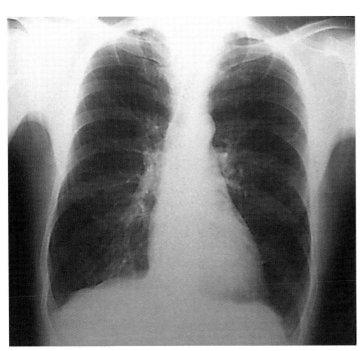

Fig. 8.13 Chest radiograph of a COPD patient with marked pulmonary emphysema: the transparency of the lung to X-rays is increased, the ribs are in horizontal position, and the diaphragm is flattened. (Baenkler 1999.)

COPD

Diagnostic and therapeutic principles of chronic bronchitis and pulmonary emphysema are discussed together below.

Diagnosis

Indicative symptoms in the medical history:
- Productive cough
- Dyspnea
- History of cigarette smoking

> Chronic bronchitis is an exclusion diagnosis. The same symptoms can be caused particularly by bronchial carcinoma, which must be excluded by further diagnostic steps.

The physical examination shows:
- Crackling sounds and wheezing with predominant bronchitic components
- Barrel chest, weakened breath sounds and hypersonorous sounds on percussion in pulmonary emphysema
- Possible signs of right heart failure such as jugular vein engorgement and peripheral edema with decompensated cor pulmonale (p. 87)

Imaging procedures such as chest radiography (**Fig. 8.13**) or CT yield, among other things, indications of overdistension:
- Lung increasingly transparent to radiation
- Barrel chest
- Diaphragm in low position
- Possible infiltrates with exacerbated infection
- Possible large emphysema bubbles
- Possible signs of right heart stress
- Exclusion of pulmonary foci, e.g. bronchial carcinoma

The pulmonary function test provides information about the extent of the obstruction and overdistension (p. 144).

Important laboratory tests are:
- BGA
- Determination of alpha$_1$-antitrypsin
- Evidence of microorganisms in the sputum

COPD stages

See **Table 8.9**.

Therapy

Treatment of COPD has the following objectives:
- Reducing symptoms

Table 8.9 Degree of severity of COPD according to GINA (Global Initiative for Asthma 2006)

Degree of severity		FEV$_1$ (% nominal)	Symptoms
0	Risk group	Normal	Coughing and expectoration
I	Slight	>80	
II	Moderate	50–80	Additional dyspnea
III	Severe	30–50	
IV	Very serious	<50	Additional complications: • Respiratory insufficiency • Cor pulmonale
		<30	Very serious even with no complications

Table 8.10 Therapy of stable COPD according to GINA (Global Initiative for Asthma 2006)

Grade	Therapy recommendation
0	Eliminate exogenous triggers
I	• Eliminate exogenous triggers • Inhalable bronchodilators as needed
II	• Eliminate exogenous triggers • Inhalable bronchodilators as needed • Long term: – Long-acting bronchodilators – Physical therapy
III	Try inhalable glucocorticosteroids
IV	In addition: • If needed, long-term O$_2$ therapy • If needed, noninvasive ventilation • If needed, surgical measures

- Increasing capacity
- Improving quality of life
- Minimizing exacerbations
- Preventing complications
- Retarding progression
- Reducing mortality

Table 8.10 summarizes the stage-dependent therapy for stable COPD.

Conservative Therapy

General Measures
Exogenous causes such as smoking and occupational toxins must be eliminated.

Medication
- Inhaled beta$_2$-sympathomimetics and anticholinergics are the most important bronchodilators. Short-acting preparations are used for immediate therapy; long-acting substances are used for long-term therapy.
- Inhaled glucocorticosteroids have an anti-inflammatory action and increase the sensitivity of the beta$_2$-receptors in the airways. Not all patients respond to this.
- Antibiotics are administered for exacerbated infections.

Long-Term O$_2$ Therapy
Long-term O$_2$ therapy over a period of 16–18 hours a day is used at partial oxygen pressures below 55 mmHg. At present, it is the only available therapy proven to extend the life expectancy of affected patients.

Assistive Breathing Devices
Where there is a tendency to global insufficiency, noninvasive CPAP mask ventilation can be helpful (p. 140).

Rehabilitation
Rehabilitation programs for COPD patients are useful from stage II onward and include:
- Physical therapy
- Dietary counseling
- Psychological counseling
- Social medical care

Options for treatment by physical therapy include:
- Relaxation techniques
- Respiratory therapy, especially for improvement of ventilation and mobilization of secretions
- Physical training to improve capacity. The effect is more sustainable the longer the training is pursued.

Surgical Therapy

- If large emphysema bubbles are compressing healthy lung tissue, the surgical removal of these bubbles may be a useful treatment. The procedure is called *bullectomy*.
- Lung transplantation is the last resort in young patients.

Bronchial Asthma

Definition and Frequency of Occurrence

Bronchial asthma is an inflammatory disease of the airways in which the bronchial system is sensitive to numerous stimuli, leading to attacks of airway obstruction.

Bronchial asthma is the most frequent chronic disease in children. Half of affected patients become asymptomatic after puberty. The prevalence in children is about 10% and in adults about 5%.

Frequency and Pathogenesis

Local inflammatory mechanisms that can be triggered by allergic or nonallergic stimuli cause bronchial obstruction by:

- Bronchospasm
- Mucosal edema
- Secretion of dense mucus

Allergic Asthma

Allergic sensitization can often be seen especially in children. A characteristic finding in allergic asthma, also called *extrinsic asthma*, is a connection in the patient's history between allergen exposure and symptoms. Often there are additional signs of allergy of the atopic type (p. 27). The most frequent triggers of allergic asthma are:

- Pollen
- Household dust mites
- Animal hair
- Mold

Contact with allergens causes a type I allergic reaction (p. 27). Under the action of IgE antibodies, mediators such as histamine are released from the mast cells, leading to bronchospasm within a few minutes and after a few hours to an inflammatory reaction with edema of the bronchial mucosa, with formation of mucus.

Nonallergic Asthma

Nonallergic or *intrinsic asthma* usually appears between the 40th and 50th years of life with an airway infection. In all affected individuals, the bronchial mucosa is hyperreactive. An asthma attack can be triggered by the following nonspecific stimuli:

- Infections
- Environmental pollutants
- Climatic conditions such as cold or ozone
- Medications
- Physical stress
- Psychological stress

Mixed Forms

Most patients suffer from a mixed form of extrinsic and intrinsic asthma:

- *10% are purely allergic, extrinsic asthma*
- *10% are purely nonallergic, intrinsic asthma*
- *80% are mixed forms*

Symptoms and Complications

Attacks of dyspnea and fear of suffocation are the cardinal symptoms.

- Difficult and prolonged exhalation is accompanied by an expiratory breath sound of whistling, wheezing, or buzzing.
- In order to use the breathing muscles better, patients sit upright and brace their arms.
- Often there is a racking urge to cough, sometimes with dense, glassy expectoration.
- In a severe asthma attack, there is restlessness, tachypnea, tachycardia, and respiratory insufficiency with possible cyanosis.
- Since expiration is particularly impeded by the obstruction, the lungs become hyperdistended (air trapping) with a depressed diaphragm and horizontal position of the ribs. The hyperdistension can persist for days after the attack, especially in young, slim asthma patients.
- An asthma attack lasting for hours and days is called *status asthmaticus*. This condition cannot be dispelled by beta-sympathomimetics. This is a life-threatening emergency requiring intensive care.
- Rare complications are pneumothorax and secretory atelectases.

Degree of Severity

Bronchial asthma is divided into four degrees of severity, depending on frequency of attacks, and these stages determine the therapy (**Table 8.11**).

Diagnosis

- Patient history and physical examination
- Pulmonary function test to confirm bronchial obstruction (FEV_1 ↓, peak flow ↓, airway resistance ↑, p. 144); the bronchospasmolysis test shows that these changes are reversible.

Table 8.11 Degrees of severity of bronchial asthma according to GINA (Global Initiative for Asthma 2006)

Grade	Frequency	Daytime symptoms
1. Intermittent		<1 time/week
	75%	
2. Persistent, slight		<1 time/day
3. Persistent, moderate	20%	Daily
4. Persistent, severe	5%	Constant

Table 8.12 Classification of peak flow measurements according to the traffic-light scale

Color	Peak-flow value (% of personal best value)	Severity
Green	80–100	Free of symptoms
Yellow	60–80	Increasing symptoms and thus need for expanded therapy appropriate to scale
Red	<60	• Life-threatening • Emergency medications • Contact physician

- Allergen test where there is suspicion of allergic genesis; provocation inhalation test with the suspected allergen; prick test or intracutaneous test; RAST test to prove specific IgE antibodies (p. 27).
- Laboratory tests may indicate the cause, e.g., leukocytosis, elevated CRP in infection, elevated IgE in allergic asthma; blood gas analysis.
- Chest radiography with indications of hyperdistension, right heart stress, and possible complications such as pneumothorax
- ECG shows tachycardia and possible right heart stress.

All tests can give normal results in symptom-free intervals.

Self-Monitoring

A condition of optimal treatment is patient education in which patients learn to record and evaluate the extent of the obstruction by means of peak flow measurement. Patients measure the highest peak flow value in a symptom-free interval, corresponding to their personal best value. All subsequent measurements are then compared with this target value according to the traffic light scheme (**Table 8.12**).

Therapy

Long-Term Therapy

Causal treatment is possible only to a limited extent. The most important measure for the hyperreactive bronchial system is protection from irritants, and for allergic asthma it is elimination of allergens. In nonallergic asthma, the only causal treatment option is to avoid respiratory infections or to treat them effectively.

The objective of symptomatic therapy is to make it possible for patients to continue a normal life with their disease. General therapeutic measures include respiratory therapy, in which the patient learns, for example, to breathe through pursed lips in order to avoid bronchial collapse by creating upstream respiratory resistance. Psychosomatic therapy and climate management, with vacations in irritant-free regions such as the mountains, can be helpful.

Drug treatment is determined according to the degree of severity of the disease.

- *Anti-inflammatory medications:* Glucocorticosteroids (p. 77) administered by topical inhalation are the principal pillar of asthma therapy, since they have the strongest inhibitory effect on inflammation and potentiate the sensitivity of beta receptors. Long-term treatment with topic glucocorticosteroids reduces symptoms and diminishes the frequency of exacerbations and the hyperreactivity of the bronchial system. It decreases the loss of pulmonary function. In an acute asthma attack the drug must be administered systemically.
- *Bronchodilators:*
  - Beta$_2$-sympathomimetics cause bronchodilation by stimulating beta receptors of the bronchial muscles. They are administered by inhalation in the form of short-acting preparations for immediate therapy and in the form of long-acting substances as long-term therapy in fixed combination with an inhalable glucocorticosteroid.
  - Theophylline is used when treatment with beta stimulators is not sufficient. It produces bronchospasmolysis, stabilization of mast cells, central respiratory stimulation, and stimulation of the breathing muscles. An overdose can be reached quickly, with adverse side-effects such as tachycardia, sleeplessness, restlessness, nausea, vomiting, and diarrhea.
  - Leukotriene receptor antagonists such as montelukast block inflammation mediators and can be given prophylactically in reasonable cases from stage 2 onward. However, only about 50% of patients benefit.
- Antibiotics are indicated for infectious asthma.

Therapy of Severe Asthma Attacks and Status Asthmaticus

- *Inform the emergency physician who accompanies the patient to an intensive care unit.*
- *Exert a calming influence.*
- *Put the patient into a seated position that eases breathing.*
- *Encourage breathing through pursed lips.*
- *Administer oxygen and, if appropriate, introduce breathing aids or controlled ventilation.*
- *Medication:*
  - *Short-acting beta$_2$-sympathomimetics by inhalation, three puffs every 30 minutes.*
  - *Intravenous glucocorticosteroids are indispensable.*

Prognosis

Over 50% of children experience spontaneous improvement and healing of allergic asthma after puberty. In adults, cure is less frequent. Good patient education and consistent drug therapy can make a decisive improvement in quality of life and prognosis and can minimize complications. According to the Centers for Disease Control and Prevention, there were 1.1 deaths/100 000 due to asthma in 2007.

Pneumonia

Definition and Significance

Worldwide, pneumonia is in third place in the statistics for cause of death. In the industrialized world, it is the most frequently occurring infectious disease leading to death.

Pneumonia is an acute or chronic inflammation of the lung tissue that can affect the alveolar space and the interstitium. Depending on the pattern of effects, a distinction is made between:

- *Lobar pneumonia* in which an entire lobe of the lung is affected (**Fig. 8.14**)
- *Bronchial pneumonia*, also called focal pneumonia, which affects the small bronchi and the surrounding alveoli
- *Interstitial pneumonia*, in which the principal tissue inflamed is the connective tissue surrounding the alveoli

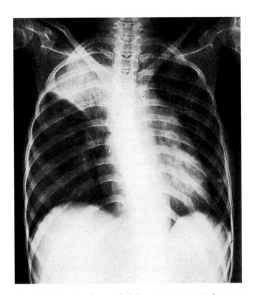

Fig. 8.14 Chest radiograph: lobar pneumonia in the upper right lobe. (Gerlach 2000.)

Table 8.13 Infectious causes of pneumonia

Pathogen	Species
Bacteria	• Pneumococci • Staphylococci, also MRSA (p. 273) • *Haemophilus influenzae* • Mycoplasms • Chlamydiae • *Legionella pneumophila* (p. 270);
Viruses	• RS (respiratory syncytial) viruses • Paramyxoviruses (p. 268) • Picornaviruses • Cytomegaloviruses (p. 278)
Fungi	• *Candida* species • *Aspergillus* species
Protozoa	• *Pneumocystis jiroveci*

Causes

- In this section, emphasis is on infectious causes. The most important pathogens are summarized in **Table 8.13**.
- Noninfectious agents such as allergic, chemical, and physical irritants as well as circulatory disorders usually cause interstitial pulmonary disease and may lead to pulmonary fibrosis (p. 160).

Symptoms

The characteristic signs of disease are different for typical and atypical pneumonia (**Table 8.14**).

Table 8.14 Important differences between typical and atypical pneumonias

	Typical pneumonia	*Atypical pneumonia*
Important pathogens	Pneumococci	• Chlamydiae • Mycoplasms • Legionellae • Viruses • *Pneumocystis jiroveci*
Localization	Lobes of the lung	Interstitium
Onset	Sudden	Insidious
Cardinal symptom	• High fever • Coughing and expectoration	Dyspnea
Auscultation	Crackling sounds	No secondary sounds

Typical Pneumonia

Typical pneumonia is a lobar pneumonia, usually caused by pneumococci. It begins violently with:
• High fever and rigor
• Productive cough and red-brown sputum from the second day
• Dyspnea
• Chest pain with accompanying pleuritis (p. 167) that can radiate into the upper abdomen

Atypical Pneumonia

Chlamydia, *Mycoplasma*, *Legionella*, and viruses cause interstitial pneumonia that begins slowly. *Pneumocystis jiroveci* causes opportunistic atypical pneumonia in immunocompromised patients (AIDS, p. 283). The symptoms are:
• Moderate fever
• Dry cough
• Dyspnea as a cardinal symptom

Complications

• Concomitant pleuritis with pleural effusion (p. 167); possible pleural empyema, i.e., accumulation of pus in the pleural cavity
• Lung abscesses
• Sepsis
• Respiratory insufficiency that may require intensive care and ventilation
• Consequences of immobility, e.g., thrombosis (p. 131)
• Exacerbation of previously existing heart failure (p. 87)

Diagnosis

The chief objective of diagnostic measures is to detect pulmonary infiltration and identify the pathogen.
• On physical examination, crackling sounds on inspiration and bronchial breathing are observed. In interstitial pneumonia the findings on auscultation are usually unremarkable.
• The chest radiograph shows different characteristic shadows in lobar pneumonia, bronchial pneumonia, and interstitial pneumonia.
• The pathogen can be identified in the sputum, in secretion obtained by bronchoscopy, and possibly in the blood. However, negative findings on examination do not exclude pneumonia since direct detection of the pathogen is successful in at most two-thirds of cases.

Therapy

Hospitalization is required in older patients (>65 years), concomitant diseases, complications, and inadequate provision for home care. Otherwise outpatient treatment is possible.

General Measures

• Physical rest
• Thrombosis prophylaxis (p. 131)
• Mobilization of secretions by respiratory therapy, inhalation, adequate liquid intake, and mucolytics, whose effectiveness is controversial
• Antipyretic measures such as cold leg compresses or administration of acetaminophen or similar drugs
• If necessary, administration of oxygen

Antibiotic Therapy

The antibiotic is selected according to the expected bacterial spectrum. Thus community-acquired pneumonia is caused by different pathogens than hospital-acquired, nosocomial pneumonia. Moreover, there are typical pneumonia pathogens for each age group and each immune status. If the patient still has a fever after a few days, a different antibiotic must be prescribed. In uncomplicated cases, the antibiotic therapy lasts for about 2 weeks.

> **Case Study:** Mr. M.L., 55 years old, comes to the hospital with a high fever, resting dyspnea, and productive cough. He has a history of marked cigarette smoking (40 cigarettes a day for more than 30 years) and chronic productive cough. At present, the sputum is yellowish. His physical capacity has already been reduced for some time, but the previous night he experienced resting dyspnea for the first time. Clinically, the patient presents in visibly reduced general condition with resting dyspnea, tachypnea, prolonged expiration and cyanotic lips. His body temperature is 39.5 °C. On auscultation, dry crackling sounds are heard over all sections of the lungs. BGA shows global respiratory insufficiency. Inflammatory parameters are elevated. On the chest radiograph there are signs of pulmonary emphysema and the beginnings of infiltration in the right middle lobe.
> Mr. M.L. is diagnosed with COPD exacerbated by infection with pneumonia of the right middle lobe. Treatment is with antibiotics and measures to reduce obstruction. The respiratory situation requires initial noninvasive mask ventilation. With concomitant physical therapy the symptoms improve and the patient can be transferred to a normal ward. After a total of 10 days, he is discharged with stage-appropriate COPD therapy.

Bronchial Carcinoma

Definition and Significance

Bronchial carcinomas are malignant tumors originating in the bronchial epithelium. The high incidence of 53/100 000 US inhabitants per year makes lung cancer, at 25%, the most frequent form of all carcinomas. In men, who are affected three times as often as women, it is the most frequent cause of cancer death. The disease usually manifests itself between the ages of 55 and 60, but 5% of patients are younger than 40 years.

Risk Factors

Eighty-five percent of bronchial carcinomas are the result of smoking. Passive smoking increases the risk by a factor of 1.3–2. Other carcinogens are asbestos, radon, arsenic, and chromate compounds.

A positive family history and scarring in the lungs after surgery or after tuberculosis also increase the disease risk.

Classification

The following forms are distinguished on the basis of location and extent:
- Central bronchial carcinoma close to the hilum (70%)
- Peripheral bronchial carcinoma
- Diffuse bronchial carcinoma

The histological findings determine the therapy plan and prognosis. Fifteen percent of all patients have small-cell lung cancer (SCLC), the tumor with the worst prognosis. In non–small-cell lung cancer (NSCLC), a distinction is made among:
- Squamous cell carcinoma, the most frequent form at 40%
- Adenocarcinomas, occurring in 35% of patients and the most frequently occurring forms in non-smokers and women
- Large-cell carcinoma, affecting only 10% of patients

Symptoms and Complications

There is no typical early symptom, so that in many patients the disease is diagnosed too late. Typical signs of disease are:
- Cough
- Dyspnea
- Thoracic pain
- Weight loss
- Decrease in physical capacity

Hemoptysis—bloody expectoration—is often a late symptom.

> Any cough lasting longer than 4 weeks despite treatment must be questioned.
> Chronic bronchitis is a diagnosis by exclusion.

Poststenotic pneumonia can develop, expressed chiefly by coughing and fever.

Signs of Infiltration

- Paresis of the recurrent laryngeal nerve: Vocal cord paralysis leads to hoarseness.
- Paresis of the phrenic nerve: The phrenic nerve innervates the diaphragm and the consequence of phrenic nerve paresis is a diaphragm fixed in the raised position.
- Pleural effusion
- Upper venous congestion: A tumor that compresses the superior vena cava impedes venous blood return. The patient has engorged jugular veins.
- Pancoast syndrome: A carcinoma of the tip of the lung can grow into the first rib, the first thoracic vertebra, the brachial plexus, and the subclavian vein. If the cervical sympathetic trunk is disturbed, a Horner syndrome develops with contracted pupils (miosis), drooping upper lid (ptosis), and apparently depressed eyeball (enophthalmus).

If the tumor infiltrates neighboring structures, it is usually already inoperable.

Paraneoplastic Syndrome

Paraneoplastic syndromes (p. 34) occur especially in small-cell lung cancer.
- Some tumors can produce hormones, usually adrenocorticotropic hormone (ACTH), which stimulates cortisone production by the adrenal glands, leading to Cushing syndrome (p. 239).
- Paraneoplastic neuropathy and myopathy cause neurological symptoms such as paralysis.
- One third of all patients have too many platelets (thrombocytosis) with the associated risk of thrombosis.

Metastasis

Lymphogenic metastasis occurs early in bronchial carcinoma. In patients with small-cell lung cancer, metastases are frequently already present when the diagnosis is first made. The chief locations for metastases are:
- Liver
- Brain
- Adrenal glands
- Skeleton, especially the spinal column

Diagnosis and Staging

- Chest radiography (**Fig. 8.15**), CT
- Bronchoscopy with cytology and biopsy (**Fig. 8.16a–c**)
- Possibly diagnostic mediastinoscopy or thoracoscopy to obtain tumor tissue
- Staging
- Preoperative pulmonary function tests

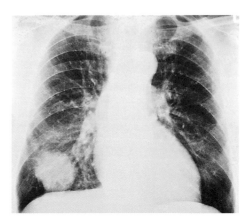

Fig. 8.15 Chest radiograph: round focus in the right lower lobe that proved on biopsy to be bronchial carcinoma. (Gerlach 2000.)

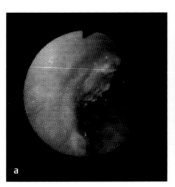 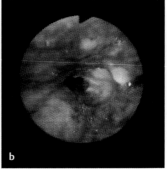 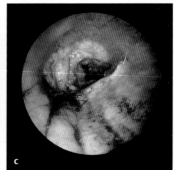

Fig. 8.16a–c Bronchoscopic findings in bronchial carcinoma. (Baenkler 1999.)

Staging of the bronchial carcinoma is presented in **Table 8.15**.

Table 8.15 Brief classification of bronchial carcinoma stages

Stage	Definition
T1	• Tumor diameter <3 cm • No infiltration of pleura and main bronchus
T2	• Tumor diameter >3 cm
T3	• Tumor of any size with infiltration of chest wall, diaphragm, pericardium, or mediastinal pleura • Atelectasis
T4	• Tumor of any size with infiltration of mediastinum, heart, trachea, esophagus, and large vessels or metastases in the affected lung • Pleural or pericardial effusion

Therapy

The type of treatment depends on histological findings and tumor stage. Non–small-cell T1 and T2 tumors can be surgically removed with curative intent. **Figure 8.17a–f** shows the usual approaches and resection procedures.

T3 and T4 tumors are treated palliatively, like small-cell bronchial carcinomas that have already disseminated (developed metastases) at the time of diagnosis. The following measures are available:
• Tumor resection with palliative intent
• Radiation therapy
• Chemotherapy
• Bronchoscopic measures such as laser therapy or implantation of a stent to keep the airways open
• Puncture of a pleural effusion
• In relapsing pleural effusions, possibly pleurodesis, in which substances are introduced into the pleural cavity that provoke a massive inflammation and are intended to make the pleural sheets adhere
• Pain therapy

Prognosis

In spite of the best clinical care, half of all patients die within a year after diagnosis. The 5-year survival rate of all patients is only 15%.

Prophylaxis

Cessation of smoking and avoidance of passive smoke as well as safety and health provisions for workers inevitably exposed to carcinogens, decreases the

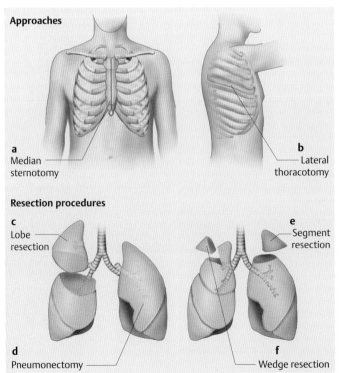

Fig. 8.17a–f Thoracic surgery: usual approaches and resection procedures. **a** Median sternotomy. **b** Lateral thoracotomy. **c** Lobe resection. **d** Pneumonectomy. **e** Segment resection (segmentectomy). **f** Wedge resection.

Approaches

a
Median sternotomy

b
Lateral thoracotomy

Resection procedures

c
Lobe resection

e
Segment resection

d
Pneumonectomy

f
Wedge resection

incidence of lung cancer. Ten years after cessation of smoking, the risk of lung cancer is decreased by half.

Case Study: Mr. M.K., a 52-year-old construction worker, has been experiencing increasing shortness of breath for the last 2 months. He has been smoking about 40 cigarettes a day for the past 30 years.

The clinical examination of heart and lungs on admission yields no pathological findings. Chest radiography shows a shadow with unclear borders in the area of the right hilum and in the right upper lobe of the lung. Bronchoscopy shows that the bronchus of the upper lobe is obstructed by foreign tissue. Histological examination of the tissue sample results in a diagnosis of small-cell lung cancer. Examinations for staging do not yet show metastasis.

The patient receives several cycles of combined chemotherapy as well as prophylactic skull irradiation and finally irradiation of the tumor. In the clinical course, the tumor is no longer visible on radiography, CT, or bronchoscopy. Mr. M.K. has a good quality of life over the next 12 months before dying of extensive tumor generalization.

Interstitial Pulmonary Diseases and Pulmonary Fibrosis

Definition and Frequency of Occurrence

Interstitial pulmonary disease has an underlying origin of chronic inflammation of the pulmonary interstitium that also affects the alveolar and capillary membranes. The inflammatory process causes an increase of connective tissue, from which pulmonary fibrosis develops. The final state is a functionless honeycomb lung with restrictive ventilation disorder and diffusion disorder.

Causes

In 50% of cases, the pulmonary fibrosis is idiopathic. In the remaining patients, the cause is one of the following:
- Chronic infection, e.g., *Pneumocystis jiroveci* pneumonia and viral infections
- Inhaled agents listed, together with the resulting diseases, in **Table 8.16**
- Noninhaled agents, especially medications and radiation used in oncological therapy
- Circulation-induced lung damage in chronically congested lung as a result of left heart failure and shock lung

- Systemic diseases such as:
  - Sarcoidosis (p. 162)
  - Rheumatic arthritis (p. 256)
  - Scleroderma (p. 262)

Table 8.16 Inhalable triggers and resulting clinical pictures

Inhaled trigger	Clinical picture
Inorganic dusts	Pneumoconiosis
• Quartz	Silicosis
• Asbestos	Asbestosis
Organic dusts	
• Fungal spores in hay	Farmer's lung
• Bird guano	Bird fancier's lung

Symptoms and Complications

Typical signs of disease are:
- Increasing dyspnea and tachypnea
- Shallow breathing
- Dry cough

With time, the following develop:
- Increasing respiratory insufficiency
- Cor pulmonale

Diagnosis

- Patient history, e.g., possible indications of causes
- Physical examination, e.g., the typical auscultation finding that is called "Velcro crackle"
- Chest radiography shows, among other things, denser lung tissue (**Fig. 8.18**).
- Pulmonary function test indicates a restrictive ventilation disorder (p. 142).
- Lung biopsy to confirm the diagnosis
- Search for causes

Therapy

- If the cause is known, causal treatment is instituted if possible.
- Idiopathic pulmonary fibrosis is treated with glucocorticosteroids and possibly immunosuppressants.
- Lung transplantation is a last resort.

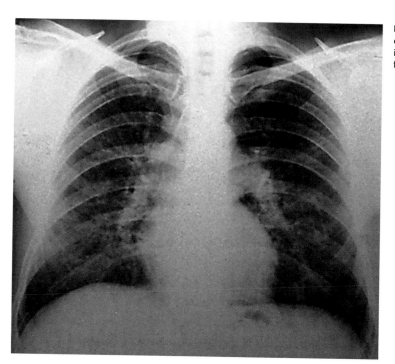

Fig. 8.18 Chest radiograph: distinct infiltrations of both lungs in a 44-year-old farmer with farmer's lung. (Baenkler 1999.)

Systemic Diseases with Principal Manifestations in the Lungs

■ Mucoviscidosis

The disease also known as cystic fibrosis (CF) is the most frequent hereditary metabolic disease in the white population. In the United States and in Central Europe, there is one case per 2500 births each year.

Cause

The cause is an autosomal recessive gene defect on chromosome 7 (p. 13). The consequence is disturbed chloride ion transport at the cell membranes of all exocrine glands with production of an unphysiologically thick secretion.

Tracheal and bronchial mucosa, pancreas, bile ducts, and intestinal mucosa are affected, as well as salivary glands, sweat glands, and gonads. Clinically, the principal manifestations of the disease are in the respiratory and gastrointestinal tracts.

Consequences

Pulmonary Manifestations

The thick mucus blocks the airways and leads to obstruction. In addition, this secretion forms a good breeding ground for harmful bacteria such as staphylococci and pseudomonads. This results in relapsing bronchitis and pneumonia. Chronic inflammatory irritation can cause bronchiectases; the constant obstruction of the airways encourages atelectasis or obstructive pulmonary emphysema (p. 148). When emphysema bubbles next to the pleural cavity burst, a spontaneous pneumothorax results (p. 166). In the long term, the changes in the lungs lead to increasing respiratory insufficiency and cor pulmonale.

Intestinal Manifestation

In newborns, a meconium ileus can be the first sign of illness. An intestinal obstruction can also develop as a result of the pathologically thick intestinal secretions.

Maldigestion is characteristic of all affected patients (p. 173). The thick mucus coats the glandular ducts of the liver and pancreas so that the digestive enzymes can no longer reach the small intestine. Nutritional elements, especially lipids, are not sufficiently broken down into their absorbable components and thus cannot be taken up by the intestinal mucosa. The result is voluminous, malodorous diarrhea, so-called lipid stools. Distended abdomen, malnutrition, and weight loss are the consequences.

In 10%–20% of affected individuals, in addition to the exocrine insufficiency there is also endocrine pancreatic insufficiency, i.e., the chronically inflamed pancreatic tissue ceases production of hormones. The result is insulin-dependent diabetes mellitus. In rare cases, the backup of secretions in the bile ducts can cause liver cirrhosis.

Diagnosis

- Evidence of increased trypsinogen, i.e., precursors of a pancreatic enzyme in the serum
- Sweat test for evidence of altered electrolyte composition
- Genetic analysis, which can also be carried out prenatally

Therapy

At present, genetic therapy is still being tested, so that only symptomatic treatment is available. The objective of the therapy is to improve the prognosis.

Therapy of the Pulmonary Manifestations

- Mobilization of secretions by respiratory therapy, inhalation, adequate liquid intake, and mucolytics, whose effectiveness is controversial
- Inoculations in compliance with the US Centers for Disease Control and Prevention (CDC)
- Treatment of complications, e.g., antibiotics for infections, long-term oxygen therapy for respiratory insufficiency
- Lung transplantation as a last resort

Therapy of the Intestinal Manifestations

- Substitution of pancreatic enzymes in the diet
- High-energy diet rich in lipids
- Supplementation of fat-soluble vitamins A, D, E, and K
- Treatment of complications, e.g., insulin for diabetes mellitus, surgery for intestinal obstruction

Prognosis

The prognosis has improved thanks to improved symptomatic treatment options. The average life expectancy is 32 years. The principal cause of death is unmanageable respiratory infections. The 5-year survival rate after bilateral lung transplantation is about 60%.

■ Sarcoidosis

Sarcoidosis (Besnier–Boeck disease) is a systemic disease in which, for unexplained reasons, the T-lymphocyte function is impaired. First T cells and monocytes infiltrate the tissues. Inflammatory nodes, called granulomas, and scars leading to irreversible organ defects are formed. This process can occur in all organs, but in 90% of cases it manifests in the lungs. Prevalence rates for sarcoidosis can only be estimated because it can easily escape diagnosis. Prevalence rates in the US range from less than 1 to 40 cases per 100 000 population. The predominant age of appearance is the third and fourth decades of life.

Courses and Prognosis

Acute Sarcoidosis

Up to 10% of cases are the acute form, also known as *Löfgren syndrome.* Young women in particular develop the typical triad:
- Arthritis, chiefly affecting the ankles
- Erythema nodosum, i.e., nodular, painful skin changes, especially in the lower leg
- Swelling of the lymph nodes in the mediastinum

Acute sarcoidosis heals spontaneously within a few weeks to months.

Chronic Sarcoidosis

Of greatest importance are the pulmonary manifestations, which can range from isolated asymptomatic hilar lymph node enlargement to pulmonary fibrosis (p. 160). Involvement of the following organs is less frequent:
- Skin (20%)
- Eyes (25%)
- Nervous system (5%), e.g., facial paralysis and meningitis
- Heart (5%), e.g., cardiac arrhythmias

Frequently the radiological finding is made by chance, when there are no complaints. Twenty percent of patients exhibit permanently decreased pulmonary function and 5% of patients die as a result of chronic sarcoidosis.

Diagnosis

- *Imaging:* typical findings appear on chest radiography and CT.
- *Laboratory:* the serum level of angiotensin-converting enzyme (ACE) is often elevated.
- The diagnosis should be confirmed histologically.

Therapy

If necessary, acute sarcoidosis is treated with nonsteroidal antiphlogistics. Glucocorticosteroids are seldom necessary in the acute form, but in chronic sarcoidosis they are the treatment of choice. Immune suppressants may also be necessary.

Acute Pulmonary Failure

Acute pulmonary failure (ARDS, acute respiratory distress syndrome) occurs in patients who have previously had healthy lungs if certain damaging factors cause a severe inflammatory reaction in the lungs.

Triggers and Course of the Disease

The most frequent triggers are:
- Pneumonia
- Sepsis
- Aspiration of gastric contents or water
- Inhalation of toxic gases
- Shock
- Polytrauma

Characteristically there is first an escape of fluids from the pulmonary capillaries into the interstitium and the alveolar space. An interstitial and then alveolar, noncardiogenic pulmonary edema develops. In the course of the disease, proliferative processes are initiated that lead to generalized irreversible pulmonary fibrosis in the late stage.

Symptoms and Diagnosis

- An early symptom is an increase in respiratory rate with dyspnea increasing within hours.
- Initially, blood gas analysis shows hypoxemia; later, in addition, hypercapnia, i.e., global respiratory insufficiency.
- Within 12–24 hours, radiography shows widespread spotty shadows in both lungs.
- Additional important diagnostic criteria are the presence of a trigger and the acute onset.

Therapy and Prognosis

The decisive therapeutic measure is to gain control over the underlying triggering disease or at least to prevent its progress. Symptomatic measures serve to win time for causal treatment. Since hypoxemia typically cannot be satisfactorily corrected by oxygen inhalation, mechanical ventilation is required.

Among a large number of intensive care measures, positional therapy is very important. Since gravity draws the edematous fluid into the lower parts of the lungs and the affected areas are no longer ventilated and perfused, the already critical oxygenation is additionally aggravated (atelectasis, p. 142). Turning the patient to another position, especially from supine to prone, temporarily counteracts this mechanism.

If these measures are not sufficient to sustain gas exchange and there is a danger of life-threatening hypoxemia, extracorporeal gas exchange procedures must be considered, which are performed by specialized hospitals only.

Depending on the underlying disease, ARDS mortality ranges from 30% to over 60%.

Pulmonary Embolism

Pulmonary embolism is a life-threatening disease that arises from the obstruction of a pulmonary artery. Up to 2% of all hospitalized patients develop a pulmonary embolism, and this accounts for 15%–20% of all hospital deaths.

Causes

The principal source of embolism is deep vein thrombosis (DVT, page 131). Especially in sudden physical exertion such as getting up in the morning and exercising or pressing, for example, during defecation, fragments of the thrombus can work loose and move via the inferior vena cava and the right heart into the arterial pulmonary circulation where they are trapped in the narrower vessels.
- Most cases (95%) are due to thromboembolism.
- Rarer causes include air embolism, fat embolism in fractures, inflow of amniotic fluid, septic material, or tumor fragments.

Only 25% of all patients with DVT exhibit symptoms before they throw an embolus. Failure to confirm the presence of a DVT does not argue against a pulmonary embolism.

Symptoms

There are no typical disease symptoms. The symptoms listed can be ordered by their frequency of occurrence:

- Sudden onset of dyspnea, tachypnea, and tachycardia (90% of patients)
- Chest pain (70%)
- Anxiety, sense of oppression (60%)
- Cough (50%), possibly bloody sputum (10%)
- Sweating (30%)
- Loss of consciousness (15%)
- Shock (15%)

Complications

Acute Cor Pulmonale

Obstruction of parts of the pulmonary arterial circulation decreases the overall cross-section of the vessels and increases the resistance. The result is pulmonary hypertension, which places stress on the right ventricle with resulting cor pulmonale.

Pulmonary Infarction

Since lung tissue is supplied by both the pulmonary and bronchial arteries, pulmonary infarctions occur in only 10% of cases. They are accompanied by bloody sputum.

Further Complications

- Infarct pneumonia
- Pleuritis with pain on breathing and pleural effusion
- Atelectases, since the production of surfactant is limited
- Relapses of embolism in about 30% of cases if there is no anticoagulation

Diagnosis

The following indicators will help to establish the diagnosis:

- Patient history with risk factors for DVT
- Clinical signs
- Evidence of dysfunction of the right ventricle through echocardiography; characteristic ECG changes only in 25%
- Compression sonography of the legs may identify deep vein thrombosis
- Evidence of decreased perfusion through angio-CT or ventilation–perfusion scintigraphy
- Evidence of biomarkers such as D-dimers or troponin

D-dimers are fibrin degradation products that can be detected in the blood as a result of spontaneous fibrinolysis. They are elevated in cases of DVT and pulmonary embolism but also after surgery, in cases of inflammation, in the presence of tumors, and in pregnancy. Normal D-dimer values virtually exclude a DVT. In case of acute right heart dysfunction, cardiac troponin is released from damaged heart muscles. An increased troponin serves as a marker for an impaired prognosis.

Degree of Severity

Unfortunately, there is no uniform classification. **Table 8.17** shows the classification according to Goldhaber as slight, moderate, and massive embolisms in relation to symptoms, perfusion defects, and hemodynamic importance.

> *A small embolism can be a harbinger of a large, lethal embolisms; 70% of lethal pulmonary embolisms progress in bursts.*

Therapy

Emergency Therapy

- Absolute bed rest, upright position
- Sedation and pain relief
- Oxygen via mask; intubation and ventilation for massive pulmonary embolism
- Administration of a heparin bolus of 10 000 IV
- Treatment for shock, if appropriate
- Resuscitation, if appropriate (p. 108)

Specific Therapy

Anticoagulation with drugs such as heparins is always the therapy of choice. Depending on the degree of severity, systemic thrombolysis may be indicated (**Table 8.17**). If this treatment cannot stabilize the patient hemodynamically, mechanical fragmentation of the embolus or surgical removal—embolectomy—must be considered as the last resort.

Prophylaxis

- DVT prophylaxis as primary prophylaxis
- Secondary prophylaxis: After pulmonary embolism, anticoagulants, for example, coumarin derivatives, are administered orally for at least 6 months in order to prevent relapse.

Table 8.17 Degrees of severity of pulmonary embolisms (modified according to Goldhaber; RV = right ventricular)

Degree of severity	Symptoms	Perfusion defect	RV dysfunction	Therapy	Lethality
Slight embolism	80% asymptomatic	<30%	None	Anticoagulants	Usually not lethal
Moderate embolism	• Dyspnea • Pain	30%–50%	Present	Anticoagulants, possibly thrombolysis	3%–15%
Massive embolism	• Dyspnea • Pain • Symptoms of shock	>50%	Present	Heparin and (!) thrombolysis	>15%

Case Study: The 42-year old Mr. L. comes in with a fever of 38.4 °C, breathing-related right chest pain, and dyspnea on exertion and coughing attacks. One week ago he noticed a pulling pain in his right calf that improved spontaneously. Before this, he had been on a study trip to Italy during which he spent 10 consecutive hours on a plane. There are no known previous illnesses. He has been smoking 20 cigarettes a day for 15 years.

Physical examination shows a respiratory rate of 24/min, normal blood pressure, tachycardia, and discrete increase in circumference of the right leg with painful pressure on the sole and the back of the calf. Increased breath sounds are noted with slight secondary sounds at the base of the right lung. Blood gas analysis shows slight hypoxemia and signs of hyperventilation. There are distinctly elevated signs of inflammation and D-dimers in the serum.

Compression sonography indicates an ascending leg vein thrombosis with a long thrombus in the right femoral vein. The chest radiograph shows a triangular infiltrate in the right lower field.

Angio-CT shows thrombotic filling defects in the region of the right lower lobe artery.

The ECG shows sinus tachycardia, the echocardiogram shows no important signs of right heart dysfunction.

A diagnosis of subacute pulmonary embolism of the right lower lobe artery with complicating infarction pneumonia is made. The cause is a right-sided deep vein thrombosis resulting from immobilization on a long journey. In addition, there is a new diagnosis of APC resistance (p. 129).

Mr. L. is given anticoagulation treatment; both legs are wrapped in elastic bandages. The pneumonia is treated with antibiotics.

He is discharged 1 week after admission with an oral anticoagulant and a fitted compression stocking.

Sleep Related Respiratory Disorders

Definition and Significance

The most frequently occurring sleep-related breathing disorder is *obstructive sleep apnea syndrome* (OSAS), in which the upper respiratory airways in the nasopharyngeal space collapse during sleep, causing repeated pauses of breathing. Patients are characterized by irregular snoring and breathing gaps during the night and marked tiredness during the day. About 2% of women and 4% of men between 30 and 60 years of age are affected by clinically significant OSAS. Eighty percent of sleep apnea patients are obese. There is a close correlation with diseases of the cardiac circulatory system.

Central breathing disorders, caused by absent or reduced respiratory drive without obstruction of the airways, are less frequent. They occur primarily in patients with heart failure.

Pathophysiology and Consequences

During sleep, the tonus of the pharynx decreases, which causes varying degrees of constriction of the upper respiratory airways, up to complete obstruction with apnea. Ear, nose, and throat disease such as polyps, enlargement of palatal tonsils, and deviation of the nasal septum favor the development of sleep apnea.

The apnea produces life-threatening hypoxemia, which elicits a waking reaction through activation of the sympathetic system and more intense respiration. The upper respiratory airways open with a loud snoring sound, causing the patient to hyperventilate and develop tachycardia. The sequence of breathing disruption and consequent waking is repeated through the night; the patient suffers a sleep deficit and is tired during the day, has a lower physical capacity, and becomes liable to accidents. In the long term, the increased sympathetic activity produces arterial hypertension and coronary artery disease. Through a number of different effects, heart failure develops or becomes worse.

Diagnosis

Sleep-related respiratory disorders can be detected through the patient's history and outpatient-based screening or monitoring systems that register the nocturnal oxygen saturation profile and the frequency of apneic phases. A more comprehensive examination, *polysomnography,* can be carried out in the sleep laboratory.

Therapy

The basic therapy for OSAS includes:
- Sleep hygiene, i.e., maintaining regular sleep times, avoidance of tranquilizers and sleeping medicines, performing relaxing evening activities, abstinence from alcohol
- Normalization of weight
- Elimination of possible impediments to breathing by an ENT physician
- Nocturnal CPAP ventilation, in which the respiratory passages are kept open by means of constant positive airway pressure

Diseases of the Pleura

◼ Pneumothorax

Definition and Types

An accumulation of air in the pleural space is called pneumothorax. The opening up of the pleural space counteracts the physiologically low pressure and the affected lung collapses under the tension of its tissue elasticity.
- *Open pneumothorax:* The pleural space is connected to the outside air through an opening in the thoracic wall.
- *Closed pneumothorax:* Inhaled air enters the pleural space through a defect on the respiratory tract such as a burst emphysema bubble.

On the basis of their etiology, a distinction is made between:
- Spontaneous pneumothorax:
  - Most frequently idiopathic in young, slim men, e.g., through bursting of an alveolus near the pleura
  - Secondarily to previous pulmonary disease

- Traumatic pneumothorax, e.g., through puncture wounds, rib fractures
- Iatrogenic pneumothorax, e.g., after pleural puncture, subclavian catheter, positive pressure ventilation, or thoracic surgery

Symptoms

Typical symptoms are stabbing pain on the affected side of the chest together with dyspnea and sometimes tachypnea and an urge to cough. Asymmetrical movement of the thorax with slow following of the affected side is characteristic. However, a pneumothorax can also be asymptomatic.

Complications

A dangerous complication is *tension pneumothorax,* which develops in about 3% of cases, especially in traumatic forms (**Fig. 8.19a, b**). This arises when the injured site forms a valve mechanism that lets air in but not out. This increasingly pushes the mediastinum toward the healthy side, impeding respiration accordingly. In addition, with increasing intrathoracic pressure, the venous blood return to the heart is impaired and this decreases the cardiac output. Tension pneumothorax thus rapidly leads to shock and a life-threatening emergency.

◼ *Tension pneumothorax is a life-threatening complication.*

Other important complications are:
- Infections
- Bleeding into the pleural cavity, called hemothorax
- Relapsing pneumothorax, which arises in up to 30% of cases of spontaneous pneumothorax

Diagnosis

In addition to the patient's history with indications of early spontaneous pneumothorax, previous chest trauma, or medical intervention, the following examinations provide indicative information:
- Percussion yields a hypersonorous pounding sound; on auscultation the respiratory sounds on the affected side are weak or absent.
- An X-ray of the thorax shows the accumulation of air in the pleural cavity, e.g., in the case of a small pneumothorax, a border of air around the lung, in an extensive pneumothorax, the collapse of the affected lung (**Fig. 8.20**). In tension pneumothorax, the mediastinum and the heart are displaced toward the healthy side as the diseased half of the thorax is hyperdistended.

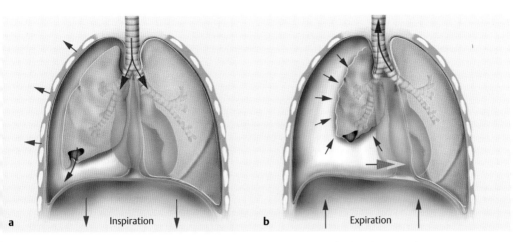

a   Inspiration   b   Expiration

Fig. 8.19a, b Development of tension pneumothorax. Upon inspiration, air enters the pleural cavity and cannot exit on expiration. Pressure rises on the affected side and the mediastinum is displaced toward the healthy side. **a** Inspiration. **b** Expiration.

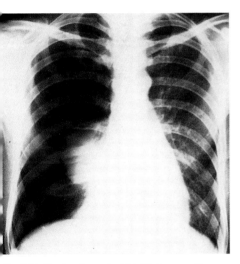

Fig. 8.20 Chest radiograph: right-sided pneumothorax; the lung has collapsed into a densely shadowed structure near the hilum. (Gerlach 2000.)

Therapy

- An uncomplicated, i.e., asymptomatic pneumothorax can first be simply observed. Small accumulations of air in the pleural space are spontaneously reabsorbed.
- In large or symptomatic pneumothorax, the air is removed by suction and negative pressure is restored. This is usually done using a drainage catheter that is introduced through the second or third intercostal space into the medioclavicular line and, through slight negative pressure or suction, gives the collapsed lung the opportunity to

recover by slow expansion. This usually requires 3–5 days.
- Direct treatment of the pleural defect with medicated patching, called *pleurodesis*, or surgical therapy is possible with the use of video-assisted thoracoscopy. This permits reduction of the relapse rate for spontaneous pneumothorax.
- Tension pneumothorax is an emergency. The pressure in the pleural cavity must be immediately relieved by puncture.

Pleuritis and Pleural Effusion

Definition and Types

Pleuritis is an inflammation of the pleural membranes, called *pleuritis sicca* when there is no effusion and *pleuritis exudativa* when effusion is present. Pleuritis sicca usually precedes pleuritis exudativa.

An accumulation of fluid in the pleural cavity is called a pleural effusion. Depending on the composition of the effusion, a distinction is made between transudate and exudate.

Transudates contain little protein and few cells. They are formed when the equilibrium between filtration and reabsorption in the pleural cavity is disrupted. This is the case when:
- Hydrostatic pressure is elevated, e.g., in left heart failure.
- Oncotic pressure is decreased through lack of proteins, e.g., in renal diseases or liver cirrhosis.

Exudates contain large amounts of protein and many cells. They occur as a result of altered pleural permeability, for example, in:
- Infections, e.g.: pneumonia and tuberculosis
- Inflammations of noninfectious origin, e.g., due to radiation
- Toxic damage
- Tumors

Symptoms

In pleuritis sicca there is breathing-related chest pain, and with larger effusions there is dyspnea. Sometimes symptoms of an underlying disease are present, for example, pneumonia or heart failure.

Complications

Parapneumonic or traumatic pleural effusion, for example, after diagnostic procedures and surgery, trauma, or esophageal perforation, can progress to *pleural empyema* as a result of infection. The lethality of this infected, purulent effusion is significant. Figures range between 1% and 20%. Chronic pleuritis can lead to *pleural scar tissue.*

Diagnosis

- In pleuritis sicca, clinical findings include pleural rub that can be heard with the stethoscope. The sound on percussion over a pleural effusion is damped and there are no breath sounds.
- Sonography is the most sensitive method for detecting an effusion.
- Chest radiography shows a homogeneous shadow running laterally and upward (**Fig. 8.21**).
- Puncture of the effusion permits diagnostic work-up of the material obtained for biochemical, cytological, and microbiological composition.
- With thoracoscopy and endoscopic guidance biopsies from altered areas of the pleura or lungs can be obtained.

Therapy and Prognosis

Treatment of the underlying disease is important. For the rest, the therapy is similar to therapy of pneumothorax: Symptomatic effusions are punctured and, in relapses, removed by thoracic drainage. Pleurodesis is helpful in relapsing malignant effusions. The prognosis depends on the underlying disease.

■ Pleural Tumors

Pleural mesotheliomas are *primary tumors* of the pleura, usually caused by asbestos. It has been estimated that incidence may have peaked at 15 per 1 000 000 in the United States in 2004, but since the tumors appear 15–50 years after exposure to asbestos, an increasing frequency of occurrence may be expected.

Secondary tumors are metastatic colonizations in the pleura originating in carcinomas of the lung, esophagus, breast, stomach, and thyroid gland. This is the so-called *pleural carcinosis.* In *lymphangiosis carcinomatosa* of the pleura, the tumor colonization takes place in the lymphatic vessels of the pleura, for example, in bronchial carcinoma.

There is no cure; therapy is palliative with puncture for relief drainage of effusions, pain therapy, and administration of oxygen.

Other Pulmonary Diseases

- Influenza (p. 268)
- Tuberculosis (page 268)
- Legionellosis (p. 270)
- Diphtheria (p. 270)

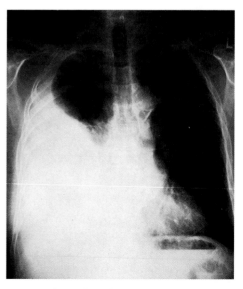

Fig. 8.21 Chest radiograph: right-sided pleural effusion. (Gerlach 2000.)

9   Gastroenterology

Anatomical and Physiological Principles

The following structures will be introduced:
- The digestive tract that extends from the esophagus to the rectum (**Fig. 9.1**)
- Digestive glands that excrete their secretions into the duodenum though the papilla of Vater (**Fig. 9.2**):
  - Liver
  - Pancreas

■ Digestive Tract

The mechanical and enzymatic breakdown of food begins in the mouth and continues in the stomach and duodenum. The smallest components of food can be absorbed in the jejunum and ileum. The processes that take place in the gastrointestinal tract are summarized in **Table 9.1**. **Figure 9.3** shows the basic structure of the wall of the digestive canal; these vary according to the function of the individual sections.

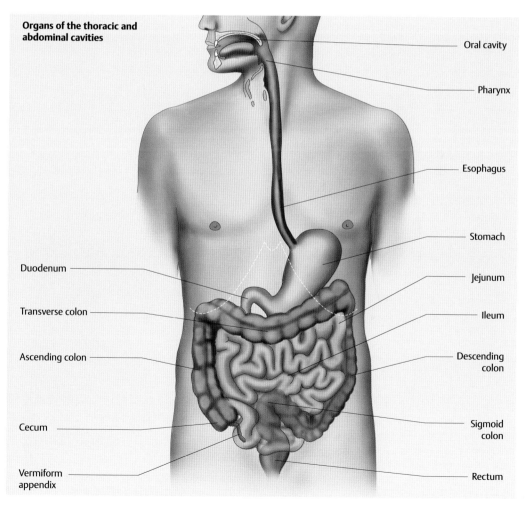

Organs of the thoracic and abdominal cavities

Oral cavity

Pharynx

Esophagus

Stomach

Duodenum

Jejunum

Transverse colon

Ileum

Ascending colon

Descending colon

Cecum

Sigmoid colon

Vermiform appendix

Rectum

Fig. 9.1 Overview of the position of the individual organs of the digestive tract.

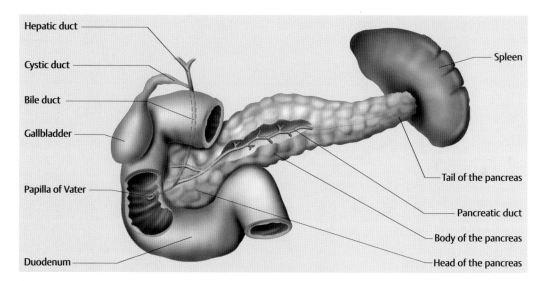

Fig. 9.2 The head of the pancreas is embedded in the duodenum. The bile duct (ductus choledochus) and the pancreatic duct (ductus pancreaticus) run into the duodenum together via the papilla of Vater.

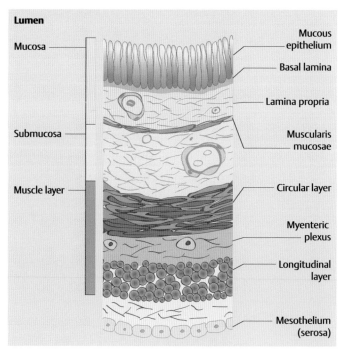

Fig 9.3 Basic structure of the wall of the digestive tract.

Liver

An overview of liver function shows that liver cells are the most versatile cells in the body.

• *Carbohydrate and lipid metabolism:* Under the control of hormones coming from the pancreas, the liver maintains a constant blood sugar level by producing and storing glycogen when there is an excess of glucose in the blood. This stored glycogen can be mobilized again when there is a need for it. When the liver cells are saturated with glycogen, carbohydrates are transformed to triglycerides and stored in the form of body fat. Stored lipids and amino acids, in turn, can be transformed into glucose. Moreover, the liver produces cholesterol, which plays an important role in the

Table 9.1 Sections of the digestive tract

Section (length)	Function
Mouth	• Mechanical breakdown of food • Amylase → breakdown of carbohydrates
Esophagus (25 cm)	• Transport of chyme
Stomach (25–30 cm)	• Storage • Mechanical breakdown of food • Pepsin, hydrochloric acid → Breakdown of proteins

Duodenum (25–30 cm)	• The bile duct and the pancreatic duct enter in the area of the papilla of Vater (**Fig. 9.2**)
	• Bile acid → breakdown of fats
	• Pancreatic enzymes:
	  – Amylase → breakdown of carbohydrates
	  – Lipase → Breakdown of fats
	  – Trypsin → Breakdown of proteins

Jejunum (about 2 m) and Ileum (about 3 m)	Increase in surface area through folds and villi to 100 m² for absorption of: • Breakdown products and other components of food • Fluid
Colon (about 1.5 m)	• Absorption of fluid

structure of cell membranes and the synthesis of hormones.
- *Protein metabolism:* The liver is the principal location for formation of amino acids and proteins, e.g., albumin, clotting factors, and enzymes. It also breaks down amino acids and proteins. The ammonia that results from this process is transformed into urea, which is excreted in the urine.
- *Inactivation and detoxification:* Steroid hormones such as estrogen and cortisone are inactivated by the liver. In addition, the liver deactivates substances foreign to the body, especially alcohol and pharmaceuticals.
- *Production of bile:* Liver cells produce bile, a substance consisting largely of water, bile acids, bilirubin, and cholesterol. Bile acid is necessary for the digestion of fat.

Gallbladder and Bile Ducts

Figure 9.2 shows the extrahepatic bile ducts through which the bile flows to the gallbladder and into the duodenum. The gallbladder serves to store the bile.

Hepatic Circulation

Blood is brought to the liver through two vessels:
- The *hepatic artery* supplies the liver with 500 mL/min of oxygen-rich blood.
- The *portal vein* brings 1000 mL/min of nutrient-rich blood from the intestine to the liver.

■ Pancreas

The pancreas lies retroperitoneally at the level of the first two lumbar vertebrae and is composed of three parts:
- The head of the pancreas, embedded in the duodenal C loop and lying very close to the bile ducts (**Fig. 9.2**)
- The body of the pancreas
- The pancreatic tail

On microscopic examination, a difference can be seen between exocrine and endocrine portions of this gland.

Exocrine Function

The exocrine pancreas consists of glands that daily produce about 2 liters of pancreatic secretions containing digestive enzymes. These secretions are carried via the pancreatic duct and released into the duodenum through the papilla of Vater.
The digestive enzymes are:
- Amylase to break down carbohydrates
- Lipase to break down fats
- Trypsin to break down proteins. The pancreas produces the precursor, trypsinogen, which is only activated when it reaches the duodenum, in order to prevent the organ from digesting itself.

Endocrine Function

Distributed throughout the organ are small hormone-producing groups of cells, the islets of Langerhans, that secrete their product directly into the blood:

- A cells produce glucagon.
- B cells produce insulin (for effect, see p. 214).
- Somatostatin, gastrin, and various polypeptides are also produced.

Cardinal Gastroenterological Symptoms

Important cardinal gastroenterological symptoms are:

- Abdominal pain (p. 50)
- Nausea and vomiting (p. 50)
- Dysphagia (difficulty swallowing)
- Bleeding
- Malassimilation syndrome
- Changed stool habits
- Icterus (p. 44)

■ Dysphagia

In swallowing disorders, there is a feeling of having to overcome an obstacle to swallowing. Sometimes the patient also reports a feeling of retrosternal pressure or pain.

Causes

The chief causes of dysphagia are summarized in **Table 9.2**. In *achalasia*, the motility of the esophagus is disrupted such that the muscle at the entrance to the stomach is unable to relax, with the result that food cannot enter the stomach. The esophagus is distended above the obstacle.

> Any swallowing disorder must be diagnostically clarified since, after 40 years of age, esophageal cancer is the most frequent cause.

Complications

In addition to the complications of the underlying disease, there is a danger of aspiration and aspiration pneumonia (p. 155).

Table 9.2 Differential diagnosis of dysphagia

Localization	Important examples	Page
Pharynx	• Inflammation	
	• Tumors	
Esophagus	• Foreign bodies	
	• Esophagitis	177
	• Tumors, suspicion of esophageal cancer	178
	• Diverticula	189
	• Hiatal hernias	190
	• Achalasia	
	• Spasms	
	• Scleroderma	262
CNS	Disorders of the swallowing reflex, e.g., in:	
	• Apoplexy	
	• Trauma	p. 54, 55
	• Loss of consciousness	
	• Sedation and anesthesia	
Other	• Neuromuscular diseases	
	• Tumors that compress the esophagus externally	
	• Psychogenic causes	

■ Gastrointestinal Bleeding

Depending on the source of the bleeding, the patient is examined for upper and lower gastrointestinal bleeding (GI bleeding).

- Upper GI bleeding: The source of the bleeding is the esophagus, stomach or duodenum.
- Lower GI bleeding: The source of the bleeding is the jejunum, ileum or colon.

Distended blood vessels (varices), ulcers, and tumors can always lead to gastrointestinal bleeding. Important examples are summarized in **Table 9.3**.

Symptoms

- *Hematemesis:* Vomiting blood, usually in upper GI bleeding.
- *Coffee grounds emesis:* A special form of hematemesis in which the blood is denatured by contact with stomach acid.
- *Tarry stools (melena):* During the long passage through the gastrointestinal tract, the blood is denatured, which results in tarry stools. Tarry stools occur in GI bleeding from the upper GI tract and upper regions of the lower GI tract.
- *Hematochezia:* Passage of bright red blood from the anus, often in or with stool. This occurs in lower or massive upper GI bleeding.

Table 9.3 Differentiation between upper and lower GI bleeding

GI bleeding	Frequency (%)	Localization and important examples	Page	Symptoms
Upper	90	• Esophagus		• Hematemesis (vomiting blood)
		– Bleeding from esophageal varices	195	• Melena (tarry stools)
		– Esophagitis	175	
		– Esophageal cancer	178	
		• Stomach		
		– Erosive gastritis	179	
		– Gastric ulcer	180	
		– Stomach cancer	181	
		• Duodenum: Duodenal ulcer	180	
Lower	10	• Jejunum and Ileum		• Hematochezia (bloody stools)
		– Enteritis	183	• Sometimes melena (tarry
		– Crohn Disease		stools)
		– Mesenteric infarction		
		• Colon		
		– Crohn Disease	185	
		– Ulcerative colitis	185	
		– Colon polyps	189	
		– Colorectal cancer	185	
		– Hemorrhoids		

• *Occult bleeding:* Chronic, unnoticed loss of blood that is often caused by tumors.

■ Malassimilation Syndrome

Definition and Causes

Malassimilation syndrome is present when the breakdown or absorption of nutrient components is impeded. The differences between *maldigestion*, in which the components of nutrients are insufficiently broken down, and *malabsorption*, in which the breakdown products cannot be taken up because of a small-intestine disorder, are presented in **Table 9.4**. In malassimilation, one nutrient component selectively or all the components can be affected.

Consequences

Malassimilation syndrome is characterized by:
• Chronic diarrhea, possibly voluminous shiny, gray, fatty stools (steatorrhea)
• Swollen abdomen, because nutrient components ferment in the intestine
• Loss of weight and failure to thrive in children
• Deficiency states such as:
  – Anemia and its consequences, e.g., paleness and fatigue (p. 246)
  – Hypoglycemia
  – Protein deficiency edema (p. 47)

– Vitamin deficiencies caused by insufficient absorption of fat-soluble vitamins, especially visual disturbances due to vitamin A deficiency, osteomalacia due to vitamin D deficiency (p. 228), and a tendency to hemorrhage due to vitamin K deficiency (p. 242)

■ Changed Stool Habits

Normal stool frequency ranges from three bowel movements a week to three bowel movements per day. Constipation and diarrhea are pathological deviations. Their differential diagnoses and consequences will be discussed in this chapter.

Constipation

Constipation is defined as fewer than three bowel movements per week, usually associated with hard stools.

More than 10% of the population in industrialized countries suffer from *chronic-habitual constipation* that can be ascribed to fiber-poor food, insufficient fluid intake, lack of exercise, and suppression of the urge to defecate. Many affected individuals attempt to relieve the constipation with laxatives. However, when these are taken regularly, the resulting electrolyte imbalance itself promotes constipation. Additional causes are summarized in **Table 9.5**.

Table 9.4 Definition and causes of maldigestion and malabsorption

Disorder	Definition	Causes	Page
Maldigestion	Components of food are not (sufficiently) broken down	• Decreased pancreatic enzyme activity, e.g., in:	
		– Chronic pancreatitis	198
		– Pancreatic cancer	200
		– Mucoviscidosis	161
		• Reduced concentration of bile acid, e.g.:	
		– Cholestasis, i.e., bile congestion	
		– Loss of bile acid if it cannot be resorbed in the terminal ileus	197
		• Decreased enzymatic activity in the mucosa of the small intestine, e.g., in lactase deficiency	183
		• Status post stomach resection	
Malabsorption	Breakdown products are not (sufficiently) absorbed	• Decreased surface area for absorption, e.g., in:	
		– Severe Crohn disease	183
		– Status post resection of small intestine	
		• Damage of the surface area for absorption, e.g., in:	271
		– Infectious diseases	182
		– Gluten sensitive enteropathy	250
		– Infiltration, e.g., lymphoma	
		• Disorders of the intestinal circulation, e.g., in:	87
		– Intestinal angina	
		– Right heart failure	

Table 9.5 Differential diagnosis of constipation

Causes and important examples	Page
Chronic habitual constipation	
Irritable bowel syndrome	188
Situational constipation, e.g.: • Fever • Confinement to bed • Change of diet	
Medications, e.g.: • Opiates • Laxatives	
Electrolyte imbalance, e.g.: • Hypokalemia • Hypercalcemia	
Organic intestinal diseases, e.g.: • Colon polyps • Colorectal cancer • Diverticulitis • Hernia • Painful hemorrhoids	189 185 190 190
Hormonal changes, such as: • Hypothyroidosis • Pregnancy	236
Neurogenic disorders, e.g.: • Autonomic diabetic neuropathy • Parkinson disease • Multiple sclerosis	215

Consequences

• Since a high pressure must be developed during a bowel movement, patients with constipation tend to suffer from evaginations of the intestinal wall (diverticuli, p. 190) and distended anal veins (hemorrhoids).
• There is some question whether prolonged passage time of stool promotes development of colorectal cancer (p. 185).

Diarrhea

A patient with diarrhea has more than three bowel movements a day. The stool is soft to liquid and the amount exceeds 250 g. Diarrhea results when:
• Osmotically active substances remain in the intestinal lumen and bind fluids, e.g., in malassimilation syndrome
• Damaged intestinal mucosa give off increased amounts of fluid into the lumen, e.g., in infectious diseases
• Peristalsis is increased, e.g., in hyperthyroidosis or irritable bowel syndrome

A distinction is made between acute and chronic diarrhea, the latter of which lasts for longer than 3 weeks (**Table 9.6**).

Table 9.6 Differential diagnosis of diarrhea

Course	Causes	Page
Acute	• Infectious diseases	271
	• Food poisoning by bacterial toxins	
	• Medications, e.g., laxatives, cyto-statics, and antibiotics	
Chronic	• Malassimilation syndrome	173
	• Chronic inflammatory intestinal diseases	183
	• Food allergies	
	• Colon polyps	189
	• Colorectal cancer	185
	• Autonomic diabetic neuropathy	215
	• Hormonal disorders, e.g.:	
	– Hyperthyroidism	235
	– Gastrinoma	200
	– Vipoma	200
	• Chronic intestinal infections, e.g., with amebas	
	• Irritable bowel syndrome	188

Paradoxical Diarrhea

When the last section of the large intestine is obstructed, for example, by colon polyps or colorectal cancer, intestinal bacteria liquefy the stool and there is alternation between constipation and diarrhea.

Complications

In severe diarrhea there is a risk of the consequences of water and electrolyte loss in elderly and children, for example:
• Circulatory failure leading to volume deficiency shock (p. 54)
• Cardiac arrhythmias (p. 104)
• Acute kidney failure (p. 209)
• Thrombosis (p. 131)

| Great loss of water and electrolytes can result in life-threatening complications.

Gastroenterological Diagnosis

■ Imaging

Important imaging techniques for elucidation of diseases of the digestive tract are:
• Sonography
• Radiological procedures, including computed tomography (CT)

Abdominal Sonography

• External evaluation of the liver, gallbladder, pancreas, spleen, kidneys, and abdominal aorta is possible by means of *abdominal sonography.* In addition, fluid accumulation in the abdominal cavity, such as ascites, blood, and pus, can be visualized.
• Imaging of the blood vessels is possible with *Doppler* or *duplex sonography* (p. 121).
• In certain conditions, the ultrasonic probe can be introduced into the esophagus, stomach, duodenum, or colon. *Endosonography* can be used to determine how deep a tumor extends.

Radiological Procedures

• An *x-ray image of the abdomen* is indicated where there is suspicion of gastrointestinal perforation or of ileus (intestinal occlusion). In perforation, accumulation of air under the diaphragm can be seen (**Fig. 9.4**). Typical for the ileus is the existence of gas–fluid levels in the intestinal loops (**Fig. 9.5**).
• Barium swallowing and barium enema are used for *contrast imaging* of the digestive tract. This procedure is used to visualize tumors, ulcers, fistulas, and diverticula (evagination of the walls) (**Fig. 9.6**, **Fig. 9.7**).
• *Angiography* is used to evaluate the blood supply of the digestive organs.
• The primary use of *CT* is the search for tumors and metastases.

■ Endoscopic Procedures

The upper digestive tract and the large intestine can be directly observed with inserted endoscopes:
• *Esophagoscopy* for examination of the esophagus
• *Gastroscopy* for examination of the stomach
• *Duodenoscopy* for examination of the duodenum
• *Colonoscopy* for examination of the large intestine
• *Sigmoidoscopy* for examination of the sigmoid colon
• *Rectoscopy* for examination of the rectum
• *Proctoscopy* for examination of the section of the intestine close to the rectum

If there is a significant finding, biopsy material is removed with forceps for histological work-up.

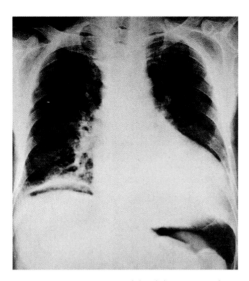

Fig. 9.4 Noncontrast image of the abdomen. In perforation of the stomach, a sickle-shaped air layer is seen under the diaphragm. (Gerlach 2000.)

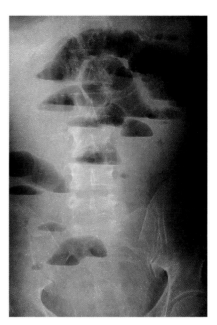

Fig. 9.5 Ileus. The standing noncontrast image of the abdomen shows typical horizontal air–fluid levels and air-filled intestinal loops. (Kellnhauser 2004.)

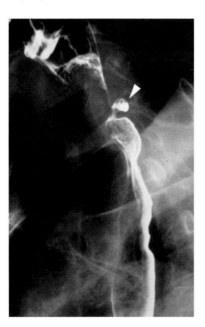

Fig. 9.6 Radiograph with contrast agent. With a barium swallow, a Zenker diverticulum can be demonstrated (p. 190). (Gerlach 2000.)

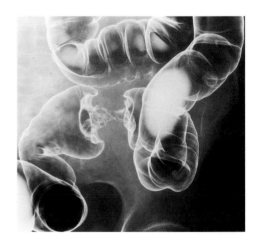

Fig. 9.7 Radiograph with contrast agent. With a barium enema, a contrast agent gap can be seen that is caused by a colorectal cancer. (Gerlach 2000.).

Endoscopic Retrograde Cholangiopancreatography

The bile duct and pancreatic ducts can be visualized by a combination of endoscopy and contrast radiography. In *endoscopic retrograde cholangiopancreatography* (ERCP), the papilla of Vater is found by duodenoscopy and a contrast agent is injected into the duct system in a direction counter to the flow (**Fig. 9.8**). **Figure 9.9** shows the radiograph that was subsequently made.

Stones and tumors are diagnosed with ERCP. In addition, small therapeutic procedures can be undertaken, such as:

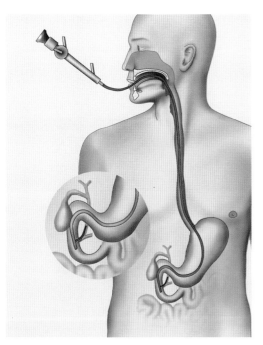

Fig. 9.8 Endoscopic retrograde cholangiopancreatography (ERCP), in which contrast agent is injected into bile and pancreatic ducts.

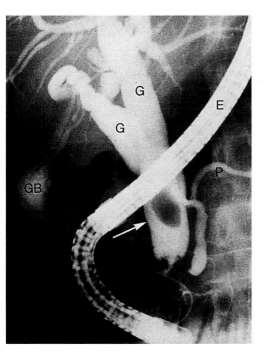

Fig. 9.9 In ERCP, congested, widened bile ducts (G) can be seen with a bile duct stone (arrow). E = endoscope, P = pancreatic duct, GB = gallbladder. (Gerlach 2000.)

- Papillotomy, in which the papilla of Vater is widened to extract an incarcerated gallstone
- Implantation of a stent in a bile duct to keep it open in the presence of a bile duct tumor.

Diseases of the Esophagus

■ Esophagitis

Inflammation of the esophageal mucosa can be caused by:
- Chemical noxae such as reflux of gastric juice (reflux esophagitis, see below), alcohol, and medications
- Physical noxae such as mechanical irritation caused by gastric probes and radiation
- Infection with yeasts or herpes virus, usually occurring only in immunosuppressed patients

Reflux Disease and Reflux Esophagitis

Frequency and Causes

In about 20% of the population, acid stomach contents flow back into the esophagus. This irritates the mucosa to such an extent that up to 50% of patients suffering from reflux develop reflux esophagitis. The background of this is insufficiency of the lower esophageal sphincter due to unclear causes. There is secondary increased reflux in:
- Hiatus hernia (p. 190)
- Scleroderma (p. 262)
- Status post surgical procedures
- Pregnancy

Symptoms and Complications

Cardinal symptoms are burning retrosternal pain occurring principally at meals and when the patient is lying down, called *heartburn.*
Additional typical signs of disease are:
- Burping, possibly with a salty aftertaste
- Difficulty in swallowing
- Regurgitation, i.e., bringing up of chyme (food which has been acted upon by gastric juices but has not yet been passed on into the intestines)

Over the course of years and decades, the following complications can arise:
- Scar tissue stenoses
- Ulcers
- Tissue changes known as Barrett syndrome

- Esophageal cancer arising from the tissue changes, in about 1% of patients with esophagitis (p. 178)

Diagnosis

- Patient history and clinical picture
- Esophagoscopy in which biopsy material is collected
- Monitoring in Barrett syndrome in intervals of three to four years.

Therapy

Low-grade complaints can be improved by means of the following general measures:
- Avoiding lavish meals
- Avoiding acid food, fatty food, alcohol, coffee, chocolate, onions, garlic, and peppermint
- Avoiding medications that decrease the tonus of the lower esophageal sphincter, e.g., nitrates
- Avoiding a horizontal position up to 4 hours after eating and sleeping with the upper body elevated by 10–20 cm
- Avoiding tight clothing
- Weight reduction

If these measures are not sufficient, medication is instituted to reduce or inhibit the acid production of the stomach, for example, proton pump inhibitors.

In advanced esophagitis or in case of insufficient compliance, anti-reflux surgery may be indicated. Fundoplication according to Nissen has proved successful. In this process, a cuff of the gastric fundus is wrapped around the distal esophagus in order to increase pressure on the sphincter of the lower esophagus. This procedure can be carried out laparoscopically and produces satisfactory results in 80% of cases.

■ **Esophageal Cancer**

In contrast to the situation in Asia and Africa, esophageal cancer is relatively rare in the industrialized world, with an incidence of 7/100 000. Men are affected in significantly higher numbers, with the main age of onset at 55 years. The prognosis is bad; the average life expectancy is 8 months after appearance of the first symptoms.

Causes

Important carcinogens are concentrated alcohol, hot drinks, smoking, nitrosamines, and aflatoxins, which are the toxins in some species of mold. The

principal esophageal diseases with an increased risk of cancer are:
- Reflux esophagitis that has led to permanent cell changes (Barrett syndrome, p. 177)
- Scars resulting from alkali burn
- Achalasia (p. 172)

Irradiation of the mediastinum, for example, in patients with breast cancer, can also promote esophageal cancer.

Clinical Picture

Signs of the disease are uncharacteristic and occur relatively late:
- Difficulty in swallowing, if more than two-thirds of the lumen is blocked
- Weight loss
- Retrosternal pain or back pain
- Hiccups in infiltration of the vagus nerve
- Hoarseness in infiltration of the recurrent nerve
- Consequences of aspiration when airway fistulas have developed
- Signs of metastases in lung, liver, and bones. These arise relatively late.

Esophageal cancer is the most frequent cause of swallowing difficulties after the 40th year of life.

Diagnosis and Therapy

- Patient history and clinical picture
- Esophagoscopy with biopsy
- Staging, to determine the extent of the tumor, e.g., endosonography, CT, and bronchoscopy

After the diagnosis has been histologically confirmed and the extent of the illness is known, therapy can be planned.

Curative Therapy

Only patients in whom the tumor has not yet attacked structures outside the esophagus can be operated on. They are only 30% of those affected. In the surgical procedure, the esophagus is almost completely removed (subtotal esophagectomy); it is usually replaced by pulling the stomach upward. More than 5% of patients die during surgery; more than 70% die in the next 5 years.

Palliative Therapy

The most important objective is to facilitate normal eating for as long as possible:

- Argon beam laser therapy, to eliminate stenoses
- Plastic tube or metal stent, implanted endoscopically
- Nutrition via PEG tube (percutaneous endoscopic gastrostomy, **Fig. 9.10a–d**) when food will no longer pass the tumor on swallowing.

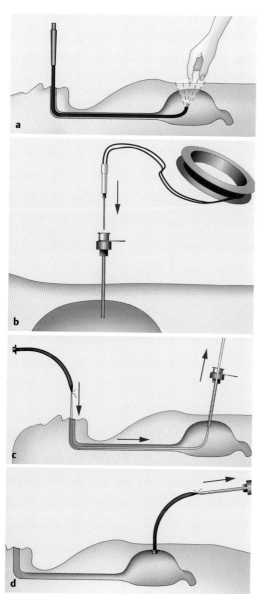

Fig. 9.10a–d Percutaneous endoscopic gastrostomy: PEG application. **a** The endoscopically introduced light source shows the position of the stomach on the outside. **b** The pull string is introduced into the stomach through the abdominal wall. **c** The probe is attached to the string and pulled into the stomach. **d** The probe is pulled out through the abdominal wall and anchored.

Diseases of the Stomach and Duodenum

■ Gastritis

Classification and Causes

The large number of possible classifications demonstrate that inflammation of the gastric mucosa is difficult to classify.

A distinction is made between acute and chronic gastritis on the basis of the time course. But since the disease can progress asymptomatically, it is often impossible to determine the time of onset. Moreover, the clinical relevance is doubtful, since it is impossible to draw conclusions about the extent of the tissue damage from the time course of the disease.

The *histological findings* show whether the gastritis is erosive or nonerosive:

- In erosive gastritis, tissue damage can already be seen endoscopically but it is limited to the surface layer of the gastric mucosa, the *lamina propria*. Since the damage to the mucosa can lead to hemorrhage, this form is also known as hemorrhagic gastritis.
- In nonerosive gastritis, the endoscopic view of the mucosa often looks normal. Inflammatory infiltrates are only noticed upon histological examination.

The *ABC classification* gives an overview of the etiology (causes of the disease):

- 5% of patients have type-A gastritis, caused by autoimmune processes. Autoantibodies attack the parietal cells of the gastric corpus, which, in addition to hydrochloric acid, produce *intrinsic factor*. If this substance is missing, vitamin B_{12} cannot be absorbed by the small intestine. As a consequence of vitamin B_{12} deficiency, formation of blood is limited and the result is pernicious anemia (p. 246).
- About 85% of patients have bacterially caused antrum gastritis. This type B gastritis is caused by *Helicobacter pylori* (HP), a pathogen that occurs more frequently with advancing age. Thus, there is evidence of HP in 50% of gastritis patients over the age of 50.
- About 10% have type C gastritis, caused by chemical agents such as refluxing bile and nonsteroidal antirheumatics (NSARs).

ABC classification:
- *A: Autoimmune processes*
- *B: Bacteria*
- *C: Chemicals*

Unfortunately, the ABC classification does not account for the following causes of gastritis:
- Stress, e.g., from treatment in intensive care
- Insufficient circulation caused by venous congestion, e.g., in right heart failure (p. 87).

Symptoms and Complications

Uncomplicated gastritis is often unsymptomatic, but possible signs are loss of appetite, nausea, vomiting, upper abdominal pain, feeling of fullness, and distension. The following complications can occur:
- Hemorrhage in erosive gastritis
- Development of gastric ulcers (*ulcus ventriculi*, p. 180)
- Stomach cancer with HP and autoimmune gastritis (p. 181)
- Pernicious anemia with autoimmune gastritis

Diagnosis

The diagnosis is confirmed endoscopically and histologically. HP can also be detected in the biopsy material obtained by gastroscopy.

The confirmation of HP is also possible by means of the noninvasive [^{13}C]urea breath test. This test makes use of the fact that HP produces an enzyme that breaks down urea. The patient is given a test meal with ^{13}C-labeled urea, which is broken down in the stomach if HP is present. The breakdown products first go to the blood and are then exhaled. If an increased amount of ^{13}C compared with the baseline is measured in the exhaled air, colonization with HP is indicated. The breath test is particularly suited for therapy monitoring if a repetition of the gastroscopy is not indicated.

Therapeutic Principles

- Noxae that can attack the gastric mucosa, such as coffee, alcohol, and certain medications, must be avoided. Food restriction is advisable in acute forms.
- The underlying disease must be treated, causes must be eliminated. For instance, where there is HP infection, antibiotics are initiated to eliminate the organism. At the same time, medications known as proton pump inhibitors are adminis-

tered. These raise the pH of the stomach, thus creating unfavorable conditions for HP.
- Therapy for complications, such as endoscopic hemostasis

■ Gastroduodenal Ulcer Disease

Definition and Frequency of Occurrence

An ulcer is a defect in the mucosa that reaches down at least as far as the muscularis mucosae. Surface defects are called erosions.

The morbidity is declining. At present, about 0.8% of the population in industrialized nations suffers from gastroduodenal ulcer disease. A distinction is made between gastric ulcer and duodenal ulcer, which with an incidence of 150/100 000 individuals is three times as frequent as gastric ulcer.

Causes

An ulcer can develop when there is an imbalance between factors that protect the mucosa and factors that attack it. Colonization by *Helicobacter pylori* is aggressive against the mucosa. Thus in HP gastritis (p. 179), the risk of ulcers rises by a factor of 4. In 75% of all patients with gastric ulcer and 99% of all patients with duodenal ulcer, the test for HP is positive. Thus an ulcer can be considered a complication of HP gastritis; genetic predisposition and exogenous factors play a role.
- Production of gastric acid is increased under physical and psychological stress, for instance when the patient is undergoing intensive care. This gastric acid is aggressive against the mucosa.
- Nonsteroidal antirheumatics (NSARs) and glucocorticosteroids have the adverse side-effect of reducing production of protective mucus.
- Patients with blood group O as well as patients with gastrinoma (p. 200) or hyperparathyroidism (p. 228) are more frequently affected.
- Cigarette smoking promotes the development of ulcers.

Symptoms and Complications

Eighty percent of patients complain of symptoms such as loss of appetite, nausea, a feeling of fullness, and epigastric pain. In the case of gastric ulcer these symptoms occur after meals, whereas in duodenal ulcer there is pain on an empty stomach. Especially ulcers caused by NSARs can be asymptomatic

and only noticed as a result of acute complications (**Fig. 9.11a–d**). Possible acute complications are:
- Bleeding ulcer
- Perforated ulcer, i.e., perforation with acute abdomen (p. 50)
- Penetrating ulcer, i.e., penetration into other organs, e.g., pancreas

In addition the following late complications can result:
- Stomach cancer (p. 181)
- On rare occasions, stenosis of the pyloric orifice

Diagnosis

The diagnosis is confirmed by endoscopic histology. In biopsy material, the presence of HP colonization can be detected.

Therapy

Gastroduodenal ulcer disease is treated conservatively. HP eradication therapy, that is, combined antibiotics and proton pump inhibitors are important in this process. This therapy can promote healing of the ulcer. In the case of ulcers without the presence of HP, other causes, as listed above, must be found and treated appropriately .

Thanks to advances in pharmacology, surgical treatment of ulcers is a thing of the past.

■ Stomach Cancer

Stomach cancer is the fourth most common cancer worldwide. Roughly 2% (25 500 cases) of all new cancer cases in the United States are stomach cancer, but it is more common in other countries, e.g., in Japan and China. It is the leading cancer type in Korea, with 20.8% of malignant neoplasms. Men are affected twice as often as women and onset is usually after the age of 50 years.

Causes

It is believed that at least 50% of all stomach cancers are caused by *Helicobacter pylori* infection, which increases the risk of cancer by a factor of 5. In addition, genetic factors and the following elements of lifestyle and eating habits are considered to be at fault:
- Very salty, smoked, or pickled food, as it contains large amounts of nitrate, which is transformed into the carcinogen nitrosamine
- Foods low in vitamins
- High alcohol consumption
- Cigarette smoking

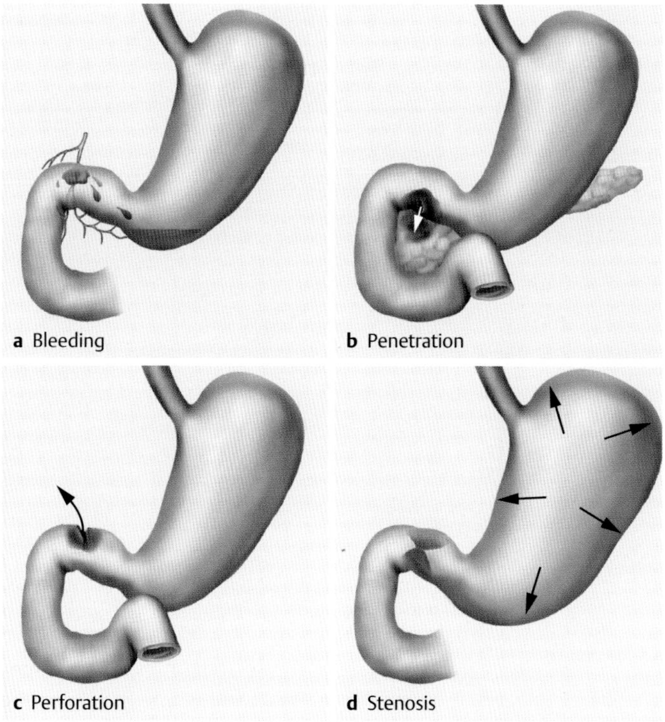

Fig. 9.11a–d Complications of ulcers.
a Bleeding. **b** Penetration. **c** Perforation.
d Stenosis.

a Bleeding

b Penetration

c Perforation

d Stenosis

Diseases with an increased risk of cancer are primarily:
- Type A and type B gastritis (p. 179)
- Stomach polyps
- Status post partial stomach resection

Symptoms and Metastasis

The disease often progresses as far as the late stage without symptoms. Loss of appetite, weight loss, decreased physical capacity, diffuse upper abdominal pain, and urge to vomit can be signs. An advanced tumor may bleed, obstruct the entrance or exit of the stomach, or be noticed as the result of metastases.
- When the diagnosis is made, about 70% of patients already have lymph node metastases. The Virchow lymph node, which can be palpated on the left side above the clavicle, is typical.
- Distant metastases usually colonize the liver, lungs, bones, and brain.
- Progressing metastasis can attack neighboring organs—esophagus, duodenum, colon, pancreas, and peritoneum.
- A Krukenberg tumor is formed by drop metastases to the ovaries.

Diagnosis and Therapy

The tumor is confirmed by gastroscopy and biopsy. Imaging procedures such as endosonography and CT show the extent to which the tumor has already spread. After the staging examinations, the therapy can be planned.

Thirty percent of patients can be surgically treated with curative intent. Current procedures are subtotal or total gastrectomy. **Figure 9.12a, b** shows examples of how a substitute stomach can be constructed after gastrectomy.

Diseases of the Small and Large Intestines

■ Gluten-Sensitive Enteropathy

Gluten-sensitive enteropathy is a malabsorption disease caused by gluten, or rather by the gluten component gliadin. In genetically predisposed persons, gluten in wheat, barley, oats, and rye elicits an abnormal immune response directed against the mucosal villi of the small intestine. This causes a reversible disappearance of the villi and the absorptive surface of the small intestine is significantly decreased. Depending on the patient's age at onset, a distinction is made between:
- *Celiac disease*, which can be recognized as early as the first or second year of life when the child starts eating cereals
- *Domestic (nontropical) sprue* with onset in the third or fourth decade of life

New diagnostic methods have shown that gluten-sensitive enteropathy occurs more frequently than previously thought. The average worldwide prevalence is about 1/270.

Consequences

In the classical course of the disease, patients show symptoms of malabsorption, particularly:
- Chronic diarrhea
- Deficiency syndromes, especially weight loss (**Fig. 9.13**), iron deficiency anemia, and osteomalacia (p. 228)
- Abdomen distended by the fermentation products of the unabsorbed intestinal contents

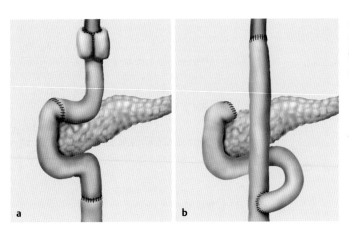

Fig. 9.12a, b Formation of a substitute stomach after gastrectomy. **a** Section of jejunum. **b** Elevation of jejunum (Roux-en-Y): digestive juices enter the jejunum via the blind end of the duodenum.

a   b

Up to 10% of patients develop malignant tumors after long-lasting course of disease, especially lymphomas and colon cancer.

Diagnosis and Therapy

The first diagnostic signs appear in the patient history and the physical examination. The diagnosis is confirmed by:

- Biopsy of the small intestine, in which the villous atrophy becomes visible
- Identification of transglutaminase antibodies in the serum

With a strictly gluten-free diet, the villi of the small intestine regenerate and patients become free of symptoms. However, they must consistently avoid all cereal products for the rest of their lives.

▪ Lactose Intolerance

Approximately 1 in 9 people in the United States (30 million people) are milk sugar intolerant as a result of congenital or acquired lack of lactase. They are lacking the mucosal enzyme of the small intestine that splits the disaccharide lactose into glucose and galactose. Lactose itself cannot be absorbed. It moves to the large intestine and is broken down into CO_2, H_2, and lactic acid. Lactose intolerance should not be confused with the rarer condition of allergy to milk, which is directed against the proteins lactalbumin and casein.

Symptoms

Signs of maldigestion appear after the patient has consumed milk products, especially bloating, cramping abdominal pain, and diarrhea.

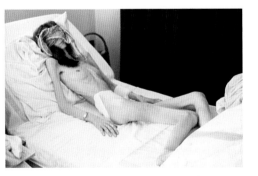

Fig. 9.13 Cachectic patient with gluten-sensitive enteropathy. (Greten 2005.)

Diagnosis and Therapy

Tests that are carried out when the patient's history raises suspicion:

- Lactose intolerance test in which, after ingestion of a test portion of lactose there is no rise in blood glucose
- H_2 breath test, which measures the increased H_2 concentration produced by the activity of intestinal bacteria

Proof of low lactase activity by means of a small-intestine biopsy is often no longer necessary.

Consequences for therapy:

- Avoid milk and milk products.
- Try lactose-poor and lactose-free milk.
- Try enzyme substitution.

▪ Chronic Inflammatory Intestinal Diseases

The chronic inflammatory intestinal diseases (CIDs) include *Crohn disease* and *ulcerative colitis*, which are distinguished from each other largely by localization, symptoms, and potential complications (**Fig. 9.14a,b**). It is estimated that as many as one million Americans suffer from inflammatory intestinal diseases.

Crohn Disease

Up to 150/100000 individuals suffer from Crohn disease, which manifests chiefly between the 20th and 40th years of life. The following factors promote its onset:

- Genetic disposition
- Barrier defects in the mucosa
- Overshoot in the inflammatory reaction to intestinal bacteria

Crohn disease can progressively affect the entire digestive tract. It is particularly frequent in the region of the last loop of the small intestine and is therefore also known as terminal ileitis. The inflammatory process affects all layers of the wall.

| *In Crohn disease there is a discontinuous involvement of the entire digestive tract and all layers of the walls.*

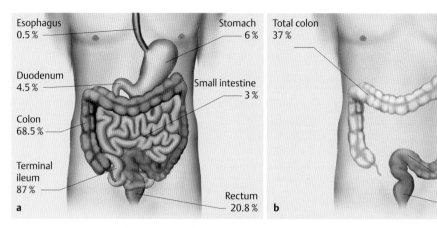

Fig. 9.14a, b Pattern of involvement in chronic inflammatory intestinal diseases. **a** Crohn disease that can affect the entire digestive tract in patches. **b** Ulcerative colitis that begins in the rectum and spreads continuously over the whole large intestine.

Symptoms

The disease progresses by discontinuous attacks. Significant symptoms are:
- Weight loss
- Abdominal pain
- Fever
- Diarrhea, with up to six bowel movements per day being common
- Signs of malabsorption if the small intestine is affected

Complications

Since all layers of the wall are affected, fistulas can form. Fistulas are connections between different sections of the intestine, between the intestine and other hollow organs, or between the intestine and the skin. Intestinal stenoses and abscesses are also possible. The risk of colorectal cancer is increased after several years of ongoing disease.

Extra-intestinal complications are:
- Joint involvement such as arthritis or spondylarthropathy (p. 259)
- Eye involvement
- Skin involvement
- Liver involvement

Malabsorption, fistulas, stenoses, and systemic complications are possible in Crohn disease.

Ulcerative Colitis

With a prevalence of 200/100 000 individuals, ulcerative colitis is somewhat more common than Crohn disease. Its genesis is not clear.

The inflammatory process, limited to the surface mucosa, rises continuously from the rectum and in more than 30% of patients involves the entire colon. Other sections of the gastrointestinal tract are not affected.

Continuous inflammation of the mucosa starts at the rectum and can affect the entire large intestine.

Symptoms

Ulcerative colitis is associated with spasmodically occurring abdominal pain, fever, and loss of weight. In contrast to the course of Crohn disease, the following occur:
- Bloody diarrhea
- Up to 30 bowel movements per day

Extra-intestinal symptoms such as joint, skin or eye involvement are less frequent than in Crohn disease.

Local Complications

- Massive bleeding
- Toxic megacolon with danger of perforation
- Colorectal cancer in 15% of patients after about 20 years of illness (p. 185)

Bleeding, megacolon and malignant degeneration are possible in ulcerative colitis.

Diagnosis and Principles of Therapy in CID

The diagnosis is confirmed by endoscopic histology. Conservative therapeutic measures are:
- Diet in an acute attack
- Anti-inflammatory medications
- Immunosuppressants
- Substitutes for some foods
- Psychosomatic therapy

In the case of local complications such as stenoses, fistulas, and abscesses, surgical interventions are indicated.

Colitis patients have a high risk of cancer, for which reason, after more than 8 years of illness, regular colonoscopies with biopsies are performed. In early degeneration or where the disease cannot be controlled conservatively, the large intestine is removed (colectomy). Whereas ulcerative colitis can be cured with a colectomy, Crohn disease is not at present curable.

■ Appendicitis

More than 5% of the population will undergo surgery in their lifetime because of acute inflammation of the vermiform appendix. This makes appendicitis one of the most frequent indications for abdominal surgery.

Appendicitis is thought to occur when the appendix is occluded by the intestinal contents, so that intestinal bacteria find an ideal breeding ground where they can promote an inflammation.

Symptoms and Complications

Abdominal pain, usually diffuse at onset, is a cardinal symptom. Often pain in the upper abdomen or in the region of the navel is reported, moving to the right lower abdomen in a few hours. Possible additional symptoms are:
- General feeling of unwellness
- Loss of appetite
- Nausea and vomiting
- Fever higher than 38.5 °C, often with a rectal–axillary temperature difference of more than 0.8 °C

In severe cases, perforation (penetration) can lead to peritonitis and the patient exhibits the picture of an acute abdomen (p. 183).

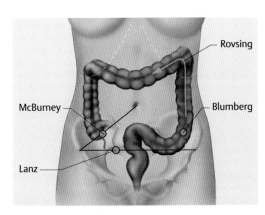

Fig. 9.15 Location of pain in appendicitis.

Diagnosis

- Patient history and clinical picture
- Palpation of the abdomen (**Fig. 9.15**):
  - Muscular defense
  - Pain on pressure to the McBurney point and the Lanz point
  - Pain in the right lower abdomen after sudden release of pressure on the abdomen on the left side (Blumberg sign, rebound tenderness)
  - Pain on retrograde pressure along the colon (Rovsing sign)
- Laboratory values that indicate inflammation, such as increased ESR (erythrocyte sedimentation rate) and leukocytosis
- Sonography showing thickened appendix wall

Therapy and Prognosis

Surgical removal of the vermiform appendix is called appendectomy; it can be open or performed laparoscopically. If the indication for surgery is established promptly, lethality is less than 0.2%.

■ Colorectal Cancer

Frequency

Colorectal cancer (CRC) is the second most frequently occurring malignant tumor in the Western industrialized world, after bronchial cancer. The incidence is more than 40/100 000 inhabitants per year, and the trend is rising. Currently, there are approximately 140 000 new cases of colorectal cancer per year in the United States, about 51 000 persons die from this disease.

Causes

In 75% of patients, living habits in particular are held responsible for the disease:

- Diet rich in fat and meat but poor in fiber
- Overweight
- Smoking and drinking alcohol

The risk of cancer increases with age. In individuals older than 40 years, the incidence doubles every 10 years and amounts to an average of 6%. Members of the following risk groups fall ill at a rate above the average:

- Patients with colorectal adenomas, so-called polyps (risk of disease 1%–50%, depending on the type and size of the adenoma; p. 189)
- First-degree relatives of CRC patients (risk of disease 10%–30%)
- Patients with ulcerative colitis (risk of disease 15%; p. 183)
- Patients with familial adenomatous polyposis (FAP; p. 189), in whom the large intestine is covered with polyps. FAP is inherited by autosomal dominant transmission and is an obligate precancerosis, i.e., affected individuals will definitely develop cancer. For this reason, after the age of 12 years they must have regular colonoscopies and after puberty they must undergo colectomy.
- Patients with hereditary nonpolyposis colon cancer syndrome (HNPCC), which is also inherited by autosomal dominant transmission and carries a 75% risk of CRC. These patients often develop other malignant neoplasms, e.g., endometrial cancer, pancreatic cancer, and ovarian and skin tumors.

Symptoms and Metastasis

▌ *There are no predictable early symptoms!*

Possible signs of disease are:

- General symptoms such as decreased physical capacity, fatigue, and weight loss
- Suddenly altered stool habits
- Blood in the stool, and the possibility of occult bleeding that is not noticed by the patient

▌ *When a patient notices blood in the stool, the symptom must be diagnosed. In the process, one should never be satisfied with a simple diagnosis of hemorrhoids. These occur so frequently that every second CRC patient also has hemorrhoids.*

- Pain
- Ileus as a late symptom or complication (p. 187)

These symptoms are unfortunately only noticed very late, so that 25% of patients already have distant metastases at the time of diagnosis. The principal locations of metastases are liver and lungs.

Early Detection and Diagnosis

With timely diagnosis, 9 out of 10 patients can be cured. For this reason, the following measures for early recognition are recommended, if the patient does not belong to one of the above-mentioned risk groups:

- A test that screens for occult blood in the stool, should be performed annually after the age of 50 years. A positive finding must be further investigated by means of colonoscopy.
- A rectal examination should also be performed annually after the age of 50 because about 20% of cancers are located in the rectum and can be palpated.
- After the age of 50, regular colonoscopies should be performed. If the findings are negative, a control examination in 10 years is recommended.

▌ **Measures for early detection of colorectal cancer:** *From the age of 50, an annual test for occult blood in the stool and a rectal examination as well as regular colonoscopies are recommended.*

If there is a suspicion of CRC, the diagnosis is confirmed endoscopically and histologically (**Fig. 9.16**). If the entire large intestine cannot be visualized in colonoscopy, contrast enema (**Fig. 9.7**) or CT may be necessary. Imaging procedures such as sonography of the liver are used to show the extent to which the tumor has already spread. **Table 9.7** shows the staging classes.

Therapy

Surgical Therapy

The section of the intestine that includes the tumor is removed with at least 5 cm safety margins. Typical resections are:

- Left or right sided hemicolectomy in which half of the large intestine is removed
- Transverse colon resection
- Sigmoidectomy
- Rectum resection

Continuity of the intestine can usually be reestablished by end-to-end anastomosis, and the creation of an artificial intestinal opening—an artificial anus or stoma—is only rarely necessary (**Fig. 9.17a–d**).

Isolated liver or lung metastases can also be surgically removed.

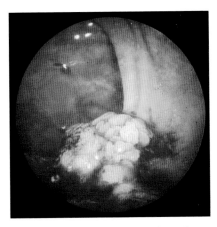

Fig. 9.16 Colonoscopy findings in colorectal cancer. (Baenkler et al. 2001.)

Table 9.7 Modified Dukes classification and UICC stages of CRC and stage-dependent prognosis (UICC = Union for International Cancer Control)

UICC stage	Dukes stage	Definition	5-year survival rate (%)
0	–	Cancer in situ	100
I	A	Tumor limited to mucosal and submucosal layers	up to 95
II	B	Invasion of all wall layers	up to 90
III	C	Invasion of lymph nodes	up to 60
IV	D	Distant metastases	5

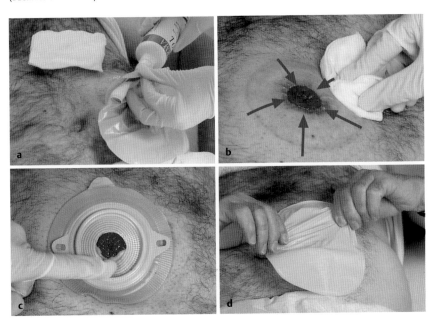

Fig. 9.17a–d Care of an artificial anus. **a** The old bag is removed. **b** Skin and stoma are cleaned. **c** The skin-protective sheet is applied. **d** The new bag is attached. (Kellnhauser 2004.)

Chemotherapy and Radiation Therapy

- Patients with rectal cancer are advised to undergo postoperative adjuvant radiochemotherapy (p. 66).
- In patients with advanced rectal cancer, preoperative, neoadjuvant radiochemotherapy can reduce the size of the tumor so that it becomes operable.
- From UICC stage III, patients with colon cancer profit from additional adjuvant chemotherapy.
- Where there are multiple metastases, palliative chemotherapy can be considered.

■ Ileus

Ileus is also known as intestinal obstruction. This is a life-threatening clinical situation in which passage through the small or large intestine is impeded by a mechanical obstacle or paralysis of the intestine. The differences between mechanical and paralytic ileus are listed in **Table 9.8**.

Table 9.8 Differences between mechanical and paralytic ileus

	Mechanical ileus	Paralytic ileus
Definition	Interruption of passage through intestine by a mechanical obstruction	Intestinal paralysis

Causes	• Intestinal compression, e.g., by:
	  – Adhesions, i.e., postoperative cicatricial contractions
	  – Hernias, i.e., gaps in the abdominal wall through which intestinal sections can emerge
	  – Strangulation
	  – Invagination in which sections of the intestine telescope into each other
	• Obstruction of the lumen by tumors
		• Reflex in inflammations such as pancreatitis and peritonitis
		• Postoperative or posttraumatic intestinal atonia

Symptoms	• Spasmodic pain • Hyperperistalsis (stenotic peristalsis)	• Sensation of pressure • Suspended peristalsis ("silent intestine")
Associated symptoms in both types	• Nausea and vomiting that can also be feculent • Retention of stool and gas • Distended abdomen (meteorism) • Possible volume-deficiency shock since fluid is not sufficiently resorbed • Possible fever	

Diagnosis	• Patient history, e.g., asking about previous surgery
	• Physical examination, especially auscultation of the bowel sounds
	  – Initially loud bowel sounds in mechanical ileus, since the intestine is fighting against blockage (stenotic peristalsis); later, no further bowel sounds
	  – No bowel sounds in paralytic ileus ("silent intestine")
	• Radiographic survey image of the abdomen shows swollen intestinal loops and gas–fluid levels (**Fig. 9.5**)	

Therapeutic principles	Obstruction must be surgically eliminated as quickly as possible	• Causal treatment to the extent possible
		• Conservative measures such as:
		  – Food restriction
		  – Stomach probe
		  – Peristalsis stimulants

■ Irritable Bowel Syndrome

Synonyms

• Irritable colon
• Spastic colon

Definition and Frequency of Occurrence

In irritable bowel syndrome, chronic gastrointestinal complaints cannot be ascribed to an evident organic cause. It manifests from the third decade of life and is one of the most frequent diagnoses in gastroenterology:

• 20% of adults in the industrialized world, with women affected twice as often as men
• 50% of patients with gastrointestinal complaints

Diagnosis

The following diagnostic criteria indicate an irritable bowel syndrome (according to the ROM criteria):

• Chronic or relapsing abdominal pain for at least 3 months during a time span of 6 months with at least two of the following characteristics:
– Bowel movements improve the symptoms
– Changed stool frequency with the beginning of symptoms
– Changed stool consistency with the beginning of symptoms (hard, soft, watery)
– Additional symptoms can be present

The following differential diagnoses must be ruled out:
• Tumors (p. 185 and p. 189)
• Chronic inflammatory intestinal diseases (p. 183)
• Gluten-sensitive enteropathy (p. 182)
• Lactose intolerance (p. 183)
• Infectious diseases (p. 271)
• Abdominal pain resulting from decreased intestinal perfusion
• Gynecological diseases, e.g., endometriosis

The basic diagnosis includes:

- Determination of inflammatory parameters in the blood
- Examination of stool for pathological microorganisms and occult blood
- Abdominal sonography
- Sigmoidoscopy or colonoscopy

Therapy

Effective therapy is very difficult. The physician must take patients and their complaints seriously but educate them about the harmlessness of the finding. Some patients benefit from:

- Changes in diet such as increasing foods rich in fiber, and omitting coffee and foods that cause bloating
- Regular exercise
- Relaxation techniques

Diseases with Various Localizations

■ Polyps

Protrusions of the mucosa into the lumen of the digestive canal are called polyps. If the tumors are benign, with their origin in the glandular epithelium, they are also called adenomas (p. 34). Colorectal polyps are of particular clinical significance.

Colorectal Polyps

Colorectal polyps are found with particular frequency in countries with a high standard of living. The chief factors in their onset are food habits and genetic factors. Frequency increases with age; in the United States, approximately 15%–20% of all adults and 30% of people over 50 years of age have intestinal polyps.

Clinical Picture, Diagnosis and Therapy

Colorectal polyps usually remain asymptomatic and are only noticed during examinations for early identification of cancer (p. 185).

Since they are associated with a 1%–50% risk of becoming cancerous, depending on the size and type of the adenoma (**Fig. 9.18a–c**), they must be completely removed, endoscopically, and then worked up histologically (**Fig. 9.19a–c**). It is advisable to have a control colonoscopy after 3 to 5 years.

Special Forms

In patients with familial adenomatous polyposis (FAP), polyps are scattered throughout the large intestine. As pointed out above, FAP is inherited by autosomal dominant transmission and is an obligate precancerosis, i.e., affected individuals will definitely develop cancer. For this reason, after the age

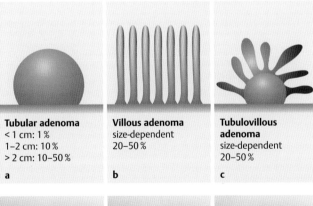

Tubular adenoma
< 1 cm: 1 %
1–2 cm: 10 %
> 2 cm: 10–50 %

a

Villous adenoma
size-dependent
20–50 %

b

Tubulovillous adenoma
size-dependent
20–50 %

c

Fig. 9.18a–c Risk of malignant degeneration of colorectal polyps, depending on the type and size of the adenoma. **a** Tubular adenoma. **b** Villous adenoma. **c** Tubulovillous adenoma.

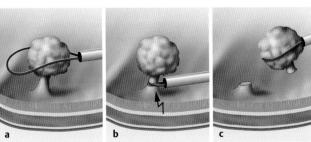

a   b   c

Fig. 9.19a–c Endoscopic removal of a polyp (polypectomy) with a diathermy loop.

of 12 years, they must have regular colonoscopies and after puberty they must undergo colectomy.

▪ Diverticula

Diverticula are bulges in the wall of the digestive canal.
- In true diverticula, the entire wall bulges outward.
- In pseudodiverticula, the mucosa penetrates gaps in the muscle layer.

Diverticula can exist in any section of the digestive tract; esophageal and colonic diverticula are particularly frequent.

Esophageal Diverticula

Esophageal diverticula are usually pseudodiverticula that occur at the three physiologically narrow points of the esophagus. The most frequent are cervical diverticula, also called the Zenker diverticulum, at the entrance to the esophagus (**Fig. 9.6**).

Symptoms

Large diverticula lead to:
- Difficulty in swallowing
- Sensation of pressure
- Regurgitation of undigested food, sometimes with aspiration
- Bad breath

Diagnosis and Therapy

Diagnostic indicators are:
- Patient history and clinical picture
- Esophagoscopy
- Visualization of the esophagus with contrast agent (**Fig. 9.6**)

With intense symptoms, endoscopic or surgical diverticulum resection is indicated.

Diverticulosis and Diverticulitis

Diverticula of the colon are a "disease of civilization," caused by a diet poor in fiber. About 50% of Americans by age 60 and nearly all by age 80 are afflicted by diverticulosis that is usually localized in the sigmoid colon and less frequently, in the cecum. In 80% of patients the diverticulosis is asymptom-

atic and found coincidentally during colonoscopy; 20% of patients develop symptomatic diverticulitis.

Symptoms and Complications

Whereas diverticulosis is asymptomatic, diverticulitis is associated with:
- Pain
- Irregular stool habits in sigmoid diverticulitis
- Possible rise in temperature

Possible complications are:
- Perforation
- Stenosis that can lead to ileus
- Bleeding
- Fistulas

Diagnosis and Therapy

Because of the danger of perforation, no invasive diagnostic procedures should be performed in acute diverticulitis.
- Patient history and clinical picture
- High values for inflammatory parameters in the blood
- Sonography and CT as the most reliable diagnostic methods

Therapy is summarized in **Table 9.9**.

▪ Hernias

Synonyms for hernia are intestinal or soft-tissue rupture (**Fig. 9.20a, b**). In abdominal hernia, the most common type, the peritoneum protrudes through a defect in the abdominal wall, the pelvic floor, or the diaphragm. This creates a sac or bulge contain-

Table 9.9 Therapy of diverticulosis and diverticulitis

Clinical picture	Therapy
Diverticulosis	Regulation of stool through fiber-rich diet, sufficient fluid intake, exercise
Mild diverticulitis	Outpatient therapy: • Diet • Broad-spectrum antibiotics • Spasmolytics
Severe diverticulitis	Inpatient therapy: • Food restriction • Broad-spectrum antibiotics • Spasmolytics
Complications	Surgery

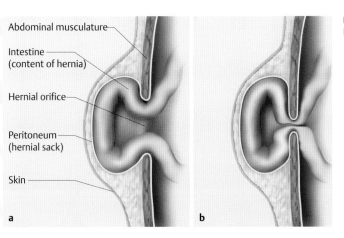

Abdominal musculature

Intestine
(content of hernia)

Hernial orifice

Peritoneum
(hernial sack)

Skin

a   b

Fig. 9.20a, b a Hernia. **b** Incarcerated hernia.

ing the organ or tissue that has broken through the containing wall (**Fig. 9.20a**).

In 95% of cases, the hernia is external, where the hernial sac bulges outward, especially in:

- Inguinal hernias
- Femoral hernias
- Umbilical hernias
- Herniated scars

Internal hernias such as hiatus hernia are not visible outside the body.

Causes

Congenital hernias occur when the abdominal wall does not close completely during fetal development, for example, pediatric umbilical hernias and some inguinal hernias.

Acquired hernias through anatomically weaker areas, such as the protrusion of the spermatic cord in inguinal hernia, are more frequent. Herniation is promoted by increase in intra-abdominal pressure, such as in straining at stool, in pregnancy, or as the result of ascites.

Inguinal Hernia

At 75%, inguinal hernia is the most frequent type of visceral protrusion. In 9 out of 10 cases, it affects men. In the area of the hernial orifice there is a protrusion that can be palpated or even seen, depending on the size of the hernial sac. Normally this sac can be pushed back into the abdominal cavity, but it will protrude again when intra-abdominal pressure is increased.

Incarceration, in which the viscera are pinched in the hernial orifice, is a danger (**Fig. 9.20b**). This results in ileus and life-threatening interruption of the circulation in the organ. Because of this dangerous complication, all inguinal hernias are an indication for surgery. The operation can be open or laparoscopic.

Hiatal Hernia

A hiatal hernia is a rupture of the diaphragm in which the stomach penetrates partially or completely into the thorax through a stretched esophageal hiatus (**Fig. 9.21a, b**).

- Usually, the result is an *axial sliding hernia*, in which the cardia and fundus of the stomach are found above the diaphragm occasionally or permanently (**Fig. 9.21a**). Since the lower closure of the esophagus is missing, axial hernias can cause reflux disease and reflux esophagitis (p. 177). If this does not respond to conservative measures, fundoplication is indicated. This can be performed laparoscopically. In this procedure, a cuff of the gastric fundus is wrapped around the distal esophagus in order to increase pressure on the lower esophageal sphincter.
- In *paraesophageal hernia,* the gastric fundus pushes through the hernial orifice next to the esophagus (**Fig. 9.21b**). On rare occasions, other abdominal organs are also displaced into the thorax. This type of hernia is always surgically treated because of the danger of incarceration.

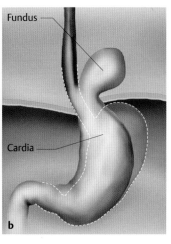

Cardia
Diaphragm
Fundus
a

Fundus
Cardia
b

Fig. 9.21a, b Hiatal hernias. **a** Axial sliding hernia. **b** Paraesophageal hernia.

Diseases of the Liver

■ Viral Hepatitis

Infectious inflammation of liver tissue is caused by:
• Hepatitis viruses A–E
• Rarely, other viruses such as Epstein–Barr virus (p. 277)

Hepatitis viruses A–E are distinguished from each other mainly by the mode of infection, incubation time, and course. **Table 9.10** sets out this information for the frequently occurring hepatitis A, B, and C.

Symptoms

In the acute phase, all forms of hepatitis can exhibit the same signs of illness at different intensities. In addition to icterus (p. 44) ("jaundice"), the patient can exhibit fatigue, tiredness, nausea, feelings of pressure in the right upper abdomen, and pain in muscles and joints. An asymptomatic course is also possible.

Diagnosis

• Patient history and physical examination in which, among other things, an enlarged liver and spleen can be observed, a sign known as hepatosplenomegaly
• Laboratory values, in particular:
  – Elevated liver enzymes as a consequence of tissue damage
  – Signs of reduced synthetic activity in the liver, such as decreased albumin and reduced clotting
  – Viral antigens and virus antibodies that are proof of the disease

Therapy

There is no causal therapy. Symptomatic treatment consists of general measures such as:
• Limited physical exertion; if appropriate, bed rest
• Avoidance of substances toxic to the liver, such as alcohol and certain medications, such as paracetamol

Interferon therapy stimulates the immune system, thus contributing to elimination of the viruses. Hepatitis C and chronic hepatitis B are also treated with antiviral substances such as nucleoside and nucleotide analogs.

■ Liver Cirrhosis

Liver cirrhosis is a chronic process that destroys the structure of hepatic lobes and vessels and replaces them with nonfunctional connective tissue. The transformation to scar tissue is irreversible.

There are no definite epidemiological data. It is estimated that there are 250 new cases per 100 000 persons per year and men are affected twice as frequently as women.

Causes

Liver cirrhosis is the end stage of various liver diseases. In the Western industrialized countries, about 50% of cases can be traced to chronic alcoholism, where the toxic limit of alcohol differs from one individual to the next. The rule of thumb is that those at risk are:
• Men who regularly drink more than 40 g pure alcohol per day

Table 9.10 Comparison of hepatitis A, B and C

	Hepatitis A	Hepatitis B	Hepatitis C
Transmission	• Smear infection • Contaminated water • Contaminated food, e.g., seafood	• Blood and blood products • Sexual intercourse • Birth	• Blood and blood products • Sexual intercourse • Birth
Incubation time	2–6 weeks	1–6 months	0.5–6 months
Danger of infection	As long as viruses are detectable in the stool, i.e., about 2 weeks before and 2 weeks after start of illness	As long as viral DNA can be identified in the blood	As long as viral DNA can be identified in the blood

Spontaneous course	• About 100% cure
	• About 0.2% fulminating course with acute liver failure
		• About 90% cure
		• About 10% chronic course with:
		  – Liver cirrhosis
		  – Liver cell cancer
		• About 1% fulminating course with acute liver failure
			• About 15% cure
			• About 85% chronic course with:
			  – Liver cirrhosis
			  – Liver cell cancer
			• Rarely, fulminating course

Immunization	Indicated vaccination, e.g. before traveling to certain countries	Standard immunization recommended since 1992 by the World Health Assembly	No vaccine available

Women who regularly drink more than 20 g pure alcohol per day

As an example, 20 g of alcohol is contained in 0.2 L of wine or 0.4 L of beer.

About 30% of cases originate with chronic hepatitis B or C (p. 192). At least 10% are the result of a fatty liver in obesity (p. 222), metabolic syndrome (p. 222) or diabetes mellitus (p. 215), i.e., of nonalcoholic steatohepatitis (NASH).

Examples of Less Frequent Causes

Long-term cholestasis (blockage of bile ducts) that leads to biliary cirrhosis

Long-term right heart failure (p. 87) that leads to congestion cirrhosis

Wilson disease, a disease involving excess accumulation of copper in the tissues

Hemochromatosis, a disease involving excess accumulation of iron in the tissues

Hepatotoxic medications such as methotrexate

Autoimmune diseases

Causes:
- *Alcohol 50%*
- *Chronic hepatitis B or C 30%*
- *NASH > 10%*
- *Other causes < 10%*

Clinical Picture

Liver cirrhosis is associated with unspecific *general symptoms*, for example:

- Fatigue and decreased physical capacity
- Feeling of pressure and fullness in the upper abdomen
- Meteorism
- Nausea
- Loss of weight

Skin changes are benign but diagnostically significant. Typical *hepatic skin signs* are (**Fig. 9.22a–d**):
- Icterus (p. 44)
- Itching
- Spider nevi (**Fig. 9.22a**)
- Palmar and plantar erythema, i.e., reddening of the palms and soles (**Fig. 9.22b**)
- Atrophic tongue (**Fig. 9.22c**)
- White nails (**Fig. 9.22d**)
- Rhagades in the corners of the mouth
- Dupuytren contracture with flexion contracture of the fingers due to contracture of the palmar aponeurosis

Since estrogens are only partially inactivated in the liver, *hormone disorders* arise that in women can lead to disturbance and cessation of the menstrual cycle (secondary amenorrhea). Because of the resulting imbalance between testosterone and estrogen, with an excess of the female sex hormone, male patients exhibit (**Fig. 9.23**):
- Gynecomastia (enlarged breasts)
- Loss of secondary hair on the abdomen, which grows under the influence of androgens
- Atrophy of the testicles
- Loss of libido and potency

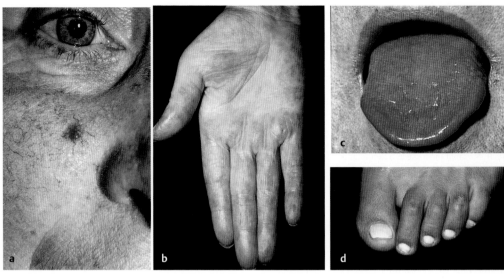

Fig. 9.22a–d Hepatic skin signs. **a** Spider nevus. **b** Palmar erythema. **c** Atrophic tongue. **d** White nails (Baenkler et al. 2001).

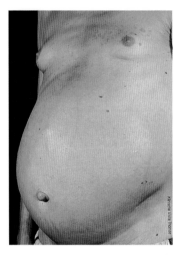

Fig. 9.23 Male patient with ascites, umbilical hernia, gynecomastia, and hairless abdomen as a result of liver cirrhosis.

Liver cirrhosis becomes threatening because of:
- Consequences of disturbed protein biosynthesis
- Consequences of circulation disorders in the liver that lead to high pressure in the portal vein (portal hypertension)
- Hepatic encephalopathy that can result in liver failure coma
- Impaired kidney function
- Primary liver cancer as a late complication (p. 196)

Consequences of Disturbed Protein Biosynthesis

- Tendency to bleed and to clot, since the liver synthesizes both clotting factors and clotting inhibitors (p. 242)
- Susceptibility to infection
- Edema in consequence of decreased oncotic pressure (p. 47)
- Ascites as a result of the decreased oncotic pressure and portal hypertension (p. 49; **Fig. 9.23**)

Consequences of Portal Hypertension

Because vessel structure is destroyed, flow resistance in the liver and pressure in the portal vein are increased. The result is portal hypertension with values of over 12 mmHg. The blood seeks bypasses that offer the least resistance. Externally visible signs are *caput medusae*, the appearance of distended and engorged paraumbilical veins (**Fig. 9.24**) and hemorrhoids resulting from distended rectal veins.

Complications can be caused by esophageal varices. One third of all patients with liver cirrhosis suffer from bleeding of esophageal varices that, because of poor clotting, are associated with a lethality of up to 30%.

Other consequences of portal hypertension are:
- Ascites, since plasma is pressed out into the abdominal cavity. This is promoted by protein deficiency.
- Enlarged spleen (splenomegaly) that captures chiefly platelets, thus increasing the risk of hemorrhage (thrombocytopenia, p. 252).

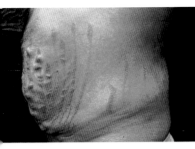

Fig. 9.24 Caput medusae as a sign of portal hypertension. (Greten 2005.)

Hepatic Encephalopathy

Neurological and psychiatric symptoms occur as a result of a decrease in the detoxification function of the liver. For instance, ammonia and other products of protein metabolism have a neurotoxic effect. The course of hepatic encephalopathy has four stages (Table 9.11), which are reversible.

Hepatorenal Syndrome

Limited renal function can arise from the release of vasoactive substances and hypovolemia.

Diagnosis

Patient history and clinical picture
Laboratory values, in particular:
- Elevated liver enzymes that indicate tissue death
- Signs of reduced synthesis in the liver, e.g., decreased values for clotting factors and decreased serum albumin content
- Indications of secondary disease such as thrombopenia with enlarged spleen and elevated ammonia content in hepatic encephalopathy
- Sonography
- CT and MRI if necessary
- Liver biopsy

Therapeutic Principles

Causal Treatment

- Treatment of the underlying disease and elimination of additional hepatotoxic noxae
- Liver transplantation is the standard procedure in severe liver cirrhosis.

Table 9.11 Stages of hepatic encephalopathy

Stage	Symptoms	Survival (%)
I	• Beginning of sleepiness • Confusion • Mood swings • Blurred speech	70
II	• More intense sleepiness • Apathy • Changed handwriting • Flapping tremor	60
III	• Somnolence (patient is asleep but can be aroused) • Agitation • Aggressiveness • Alterations in EEG	40
IV	• Coma • No reaction to pain stimuli • Reflexes such as corneal reflex extinguished • Fetor hepaticus	20

Symptomatic therapy

- Prophylaxis or treatment of deficiencies with balanced increase of calories, nutrients and vitamins
- Prophylaxis or treatment of complications, e.g.:
  - Diet rich in calories and protein
  - Reduction of protein solely in decompensated hepatic encephalopathy, since proteins are transformed into ammonia
  - Fluid and sodium restriction and spironolactone (aldosterone antagonist) and diuretics to treat ascites; paracentesis if necessary
  - Beta blockers to decrease portal vein pressure and avoid consequences
  - Treatment of bleeding esophageal varices with endoscopic hemostasis

Prognosis

Liver cirrhosis is classified into Child stages A–C, depending on severity of the disease. The prognosis is poor for decompensation with ascites, spontaneous bacterial peritonitis, or renal failure. When alcoholic cirrhosis is recognized early, a successful outcome can be achieved by complete abstinence from alcohol. The one-year survival rate is 35% in the worst case. The MELD score (Model for Endstage Liver Disease) is used for assessment of the urgency of a liver transplant.

Acute Liver Failure

Acute liver failure is a relatively rare, life-threatening disease of a previously healthy liver.

Causes

- In 65% of cases, acute liver failure is the result of a viral hepatitis (p. 192).
- Thirty percent of cases are caused by hepatotoxic substances, e.g., medications such as paracetamol, the toxin of amanita mushrooms, and drugs such as Ecstasy.
- Less usual causes are shock liver (p. 54), and fatty liver in pregnancy.

Symptoms and Complications

The typical triad of symptoms consists of:
- Icterus and a smell of ammonia (fetor hepaticus)
- Clotting disorders
- Hepatic encephalopathy up to and including liver failure coma, especially caused by ammonia that accumulates in protein metabolism and produces a neurotoxic effect (**Table 9.11**)

Other possible complications are cerebral edema, gastrointestinal hemorrhage, acute renal failure, infections, and hypoglycemia as a result of decreased gluconeogenesis.

Diagnosis

- Patient history and clinical picture
- Laboratory values, in particular:
  - Elevated liver enzymes as a consequence of tissue damage
  - Signs of reduced liver function such as elevated bilirubin and ammonia
  - Signs of reduced synthetic function in the liver, especially Quick value below 20% as a result of reduced clotting

Therapeutic Principles

Treatment is provided in an intensive care unit:
- Therapy of underlying disease
- Prophylaxis or treatment of complications
- Liver transplantation, which is required by every second patient

Liver Tumors

Overview

A space-occupying lesion in the liver, other tha cysts, can be one of a number of benign or malignan liver tumors. The most frequently occurring tumor are listed here.

Benign Liver Tumors

Hemangioma

Hemangiomas are the most frequently occurring liver tumors. They are benign vascular tumors tha are also called strawberry marks and are usuall found coincidentally in the course of sonography They are usually congenital and show various tendencies to grow. Surgical removal is considere only if a considerable increase in size is observed o monitoring.

Liver Adenoma

Liver adenomas are benign swellings originating in liver cells. They occur especially in women takin oral contraceptives. Since they can have a diamete of more than 20 cm, complaints of pressure in th upper right abdomen and complications such a rupture or degeneration are possible. Thus, onc a tumor reaches a certain size, surgical removal i indicated.

Focal Nodal Hyperplasia

Focal nodal hyperplasia (FNH) is also found mor frequently in women than in men. It is sometime even found in children. Liver cells and the small est bile ducts proliferate and form knots that var in number and size. Since patients are often fre of symptoms and there is no danger of rupture o degeneration, there is no requirement for therapy.

Malignant Liver Tumors

The liver is the second most commonly involve organ in metastatic disease. Metastases aris through hematogenic metastasis, especially in colon bronchial, and breast cancer. They are distinguishe from other benign and malignant liver tumors suc as primary liver cell cancer by:
- Patient history
- Typical appearance in sonography
- Fine-needle puncture under ultrasound control

Primary Liver Cell Cancer

Primary liver cell cancer is also called hepatocellular cancer. In the West, the incidence is low, but worldwide, primary liver cell cancer counts as one of the most frequently occurring malignant tumors. Men are affected three times as often as women; the principal age of onset is between 50 and 60 years.

Causes

- Liver cirrhosis, mostly as a result of chronic hepatitis B or C or chronic alcohol abuse. Other causes are rare (p. 192).
- Aflatoxins, the toxins of the fungus *Aspergillus flavus*, which grows predominantly on grain, nuts, and spices

Symptoms

Patients note uncharacteristic complaints such as weight loss, appetite loss, fatigue, and feelings of pressure in the right upper abdomen. In addition there can be signs of the underlying liver cirrhosis.

Diagnosis

- Patient history and clinical picture
- Sonography and CT, to determine the extent of the tumor
- Alpha-fetoprotein (AFP) is the tumor marker that permits monitoring of progress.

Therapy

A curative approach to therapy with partial resection and, in certain cases, liver transplantation, is only suitable for a few patients. Most patients die an average of 6 months after diagnosis.

Diseases of the Gallbladder and Bile Ducts

■ Gallstones

The incidence of gallstones increases with advancing age. The average prevalence is:
- In women, 15%
- In men, 7.5%
- In patients with liver cirrhosis and Crohn disease, 25% (pp. 192 and 183)

Definitions

- Cholelithiasis: gallstones
- Cholecystolithiasis: gallstones in the gallbladder
- Choledocholithiasis: gallstones in the cystic duct

Pathological Mechanism

Gallstones are usually formed in the gallbladder. In 80% of cases, the stones consist of cholesterol. Bile consists of 80% water and bile acids, phospholipids, and cholesterol. If the cholesterol content rises, it cannot be kept in solution and precipitates in the form of crystals. The chief risk factors are:
- Genetic disposition
- Hormonal factors such as pregnancy
- Age
- Diet high in cholesterol and low in fiber
- Obesity. The probability of disease doubles at 20% overweight.
- Incomplete emptying of the gallbladder, e.g., in fasting

Twenty percent of gallstones consist of bilirubin or pigment; they occur principally in patients with liver cirrhosis and chronic hemolysis.

Symptoms and Complications

Seventy-five percent of patients with gallstones are asymptomatic. Twenty-five percent have the typical biliary colic that arises when a gallstone moves out of the gallbladder and into the cystic duct or the common bile duct. This causes the patient strong, cramping pain in the right upper abdomen that can radiate to the right shoulder and the back. Nausea and vomiting, circulatory collapse, and a slightly elevated temperature are frequent accompanying symptoms.

The following complications of obstruction by a gallstone are possible:
- Bacterial cholecystitis or cholangitis caused by biliary stasis
- Gallbladder edema or gallbladder empyema (accumulation of pus), when the stone obstructs the cystic duct
- Sepsis resulting from massive cholecystitis, cholangitis, or gallbladder empyema
- Icterus caused by blockage (p. 44), if the stone obstructs the bile duct (**Fig. 9.9**)
- Acute pancreatitis (p. 198) if the stone is wedged in place in the region of the papilla

The stones can also perforate and penetrate neighboring organs, leading to peritonitis, liver abscesses, and gallstone ileus.

Diagnosis

The patient's medical history and clinical picture lead to a diagnostic suspicion that is sonographically confirmed.

Therapy

- Asymptomatic cholecystolithiasis is usually a coincidental finding with no therapeutic consequences.
- Acute biliary colic in choledocholithiasis is treated symptomatically with spasmolytics and analgesics as well as food restriction. The patient is advised to undergo surgery for removal of the gallbladder during a symptom-free period. Cholecystectomy is usually performed laparoscopically.
- Cholecystitis caused by gallstones is first treated with antibiotics before a cholecystectomy is performed.
- In case of complications, immediate treatment is required. For instance, if the stone is lodged near the papilla, it can often be removed by endoscopic retrograde cholangiopancreatography (ERCP) with papillotomy (**Fig. 9.8**). In order to avoid repeated complications, a cholecystectomy is performed in a symptom-free interval. If the stone cannot be removed by ERCP, immediate surgery is indicated.

■ Tumors

Tumors in the gallbladder and bile ducts are predominantly malignant. *Gallbladder cancer* and *bile duct cancer*, with an incidence of 3/100 000, are relatively rare.

Symptoms and Diagnosis

General symptoms, such as weakness, loss of appetite and weight loss, icterus, and pain in the upper right abdomen are only very late indications of the disease.

The diagnosis is confirmed by sonography, CT, and ERCP with sampling of biopsy material.

Therapy and Prognosis

Radical surgery with curative intent is only possible in a very few patients. No effective chemotherapy is known. Palliatively, the bile ducts can be dilated endoscopically and held open with a stent.

The 5-year survival rate is 2%; on average patients die within 6 months of diagnosis.

Diseases of the Pancreas

■ Pancreatitis

Inflammations of the pancreas are classified as acute or chronic, depending on their course. After causes have been eliminated and any complications have been overcome, acute pancreatitis can heal. In contrast, chronic pancreatitis is a progressive inflammation that damages the organ irreversibly, with loss of function.

Acute Pancreatitis

Annually, about 20 out of 100 000 persons develop acute pancreatitis, making it five times as prevalent as the chronic form. The principal age of onset is between 30 and 50 years. It is not possible to say at the outset whether the disease will run a mild course or a severe course with lethal outcome.

> Acute pancreatitis is a disease to be taken seriously, having an average lethality of about 15%.

Pathological Mechanism and Degree of Severity

At 40% each, bile duct diseases, especially choledocholithiasis (p. 197), and alcohol abuse are the most frequent causes of acute pancreatitis. Gallstones can obstruct the papilla of Vater and thus block the excretory duct of the pancreas.

Examples of less frequent causes
- Abdominal trauma or surgery
- Medications such as glucocorticosteroids, antibiotics, or cytostatics
- Viral infections, especially mumps
- Hypertriglyceridemia
- Hypercalcemia, e.g., in hyperparathyroidism (p. 228)

In about 15% of patients, no cause can be found.

Congestion of the pancreatic secretions or direct toxic effect first causes edematous swelling of the pancreas and then cell damage. In consequence, digestive enzymes are already activated in the pancreas, instead of later, in the small intestine, so that the organ begins to digest itself and a series of complications is inevitable.

- *80% edematous pancreatitis*
- *20% necrotizing pancreatitis*

Symptoms

A sudden onset of severe pain in the upper abdomen, often radiating in a belt to the back, is typical. Additional possible symptoms are:
- Nausea and vomiting
- "Rubbery belly" characterized by moderate muscular defense, meteorism, and ascites (p. 49)
- Fever
- Signs of triggers, e.g., icterus in case of gallstones
- Signs of complications

Complications

Complications occur chiefly in necrotizing pancreatitis.

Local complications are:
- Bacterial infection of the necrotizing tissue, leading to sepsis
- Pancreatic pseudocysts, accumulation of fluid encapsulated in connective tissue without an epithelial lining. Pseudocysts, which can grow to more than 20 cm, can rupture, bleed, be infected with bacteria, or compromise neighboring tissue.

Systemic complications are:
- Paralytic ileus (p. 187)
- Erosion of neighboring organs and vessels, causing massive bleeding
- Shock due to displacement of fluid into the intestines, ascites, vomiting, or bleeding (p. 54)
- Acute pulmonary failure (p. 163) and acute renal failure (p. 209) in consequence of shock and release of active enzymes
- Consumption coagulopathy caused by proteolytic enzymes (p. 255)
- Hyperglycemia (p. 215)
- Electrolyte imbalance such as hypocalcemia, which can cause cardiac arrhythmias (p. 104) and spasms

Diagnosis

The patient's history and physical examination can already lead to the suspected diagnosis, which is confirmed by laboratory values and imaging.
- Serum lipase and elastase are elevated.
- Sonography and CT show an enlarged, edematous pancreas. In some cases, necrosis, pseudocysts, ascites, and causal gallstones can be visualized.

Therapy

Patients with pancreatitis must be treated in an intensive care unit. The most important conservative measures are:
- Initial food and fluid restriction to spare the pancreas
- Intravenous volume, electrolyte, and energy substitution
- Pain medication
- Prophylaxis and therapy for the complications

Invasive Procedures

- If the acute pancreatitis is caused by gallstones in the region of the papilla of Vater they must be removed endoscopically as soon as possible (p. 175).
- Abscesses and symptomatic pseudocysts are aspirated or endoscopically drained under sonographic or CT control.
- If the conservative measures fail, surgery is indicated. Necrotic material is removed and the abdominal cavity is irrigated and drained. So that lavage can be continued on the following days, the abdomen is temporarily closed with plastic netting.

Chronic Pancreatitis

Chronic pancreatitis is a progressive inflammation that can progress in attacks or gradually, causing irreversible damage to the organ. In the course of the disease, first exocrine and then endocrine function is lost.

Causes

In about 80% of patients, chronic pancreatitis is caused by chronic alcoholism. In rare cases, the disease is caused by medications or genetic defects that trigger aggressive enzymes to become active in the pancreas itself. In 15% of cases, no cause is evident.

Clinical Picture

Patients almost always complain of relapsing upper abdominal pain that can last for days and radiate into the back in the form of a belt. Nausea, vomiting, and icterus are possible.

When more than 90% of the pancreatic tissue has been destroyed, there is:
- Maldigestion with loss of weight, diarrhea, distension, and signs of deficiency as a result of disturbance of exocrine function (p. 173)
- Diabetes mellitus as a consequence of endocrine failure (p. 215)

Possible complications are:
- Pancreatic pseudocysts as in acute pancreatitis
- Stenosis of the bile ducts and duodenum by proliferating connective tissue
- Thromboses of splenic veins and portal vein
- Pancreatic cancer (p. 200)

Diagnosis

- Medical history and symptoms
- Tests for serum lipase and elastase, which are elevated during attacks
- Pancreatic function tests, e.g., pancreas elastase concentration in the stool, which is depressed when exocrine function is disturbed
- Sonography, radiography of the abdomen, CT, and ERCP (p. 175), with which pancreatic calcification and other morphological changes in the organs can be visualized

Therapy

Patients must avoid alcohol in order to retard loss of pancreatic function. Inflammatory attacks are treated like acute pancreatitis. Symptomatic measures are:
- Pain therapy
- Therapy of exocrine pancreatic insufficiency by oral enzyme substitution at every meal and a balanced diet
- Therapy of endocrine pancreatic insufficiency by administration of insulin
- Therapy for complications, such as aspiration of pseudocysts.

◼ Pancreatic Tumors

In addition to cancer of the pancreas, this chapter discusses hormone-producing pancreatic tumors.

Pancreatic Cancer

The incidence of pancreatic cancer, which is continuously increasing in industrialized countries, is currently about 15/100 000. This makes pancreatic cancer the third most frequently occurring tumor of the digestive tract after colon cancer and stomach cancer. The principal age of onset is the seventh decade; men are more frequently affected than women.

Up to 90% of the cancers are located in the head of the pancreas. Usually they are adenocarcinomas, originating in the epithelium of the pancreatic ducts. Since they remain asymptomatic for a long time, cancer of the pancreas is diagnosed (too) late and has a poor prognosis. The average 5-year survival rate is about 2%.

Causes

The cause is unknown but genetic predisposition plays a role. Risk factors are nicotine use and alcohol consumption.

Symptoms

◼ *There are no early symptoms.*

Possible first signs are:
- Loss of appetite, nausea, and weight loss
- Pain radiating to the back
- Relapsing thromboses are a paraneoplastic syndrome (p. 34).
- Icterus: Since most of the tumors arise in the head of the pancreas, they can compromise the papilla of Vater or the bile ducts and thus lead to congestion of bile and posthepatic icterus (p. 44).

Diagnosis

The tumor itself is rarely palpated during physical examination. More frequently, the congested gallbladder can be palpated (Courvoisier sign).

The dimensions of the space-occupying lesion can be determined by sonography, endosonography, MRI, and CT. The diagnosis is confirmed histologically by material obtained during surgery.

Therapy and Prognosis

The 20% of patients who do not yet have distant metastases at the time of diagnosis can be treated surgically. For many years, the main procedure was the Whipple operation. In this procedure, the head of the pancreas, the duodenum, the lower part of the stomach, the gallbladder, and lymph nodes are removed. The partial duodenopancreatectomy described is one of the most extensive abdominal operations and has a surgical lethality of up to 20%. In recent years, Traverso-Longmire partial duodenopancreatectomy, in which the stomach is completely spared, has gained acceptance. The average 5-year survival rate of all surgically treated patients is 5%.

In 80% of patients, the tumor is already so far advanced that only palliative measures can be considered, for example:

- Palliative chemotherapy to retard tumor growth
- Palliative radiation, which can have a good effect on tumor pain
- Other measures to relieve pain
- Implantation of a stent in the bile ducts to permit the flow of bile

Patients receiving palliative treatment die an average of 6 months after diagnosis.

Hormone-Producing Pancreatic Tumors

The following endocrine tumors usually originate in the pancreas but sometimes in other organs of the digestive system. Overall, they are rare.

- *Insulinoma:* Insulinoma is the most frequently occurring pancreatic tumor. It is usually benign and is detected as a result of marked hypoglycemia (insulin effect, p. 214).
- *Glucagonoma:* Glucagonomas are extremely rare, usually malignant. They cause hyperglycemia (glucagon effect, p. 214).
- *Gastrinoma:* This usually malignant tumor is also called the Zollinger–Ellison syndrome. Since gastrin stimulates the secretion of gastric juice, a gastrinoma leads in particular to relapsing gastric and duodenal ulcers (p. 180).
- *Vipoma:* This usually malignant tumor is also known as the Verner–Morrison syndrome. It produces vasoactive intestinal polypeptide (VIP) and causes watery diarrhea with the corresponding consequences (p. 173).

These neoplasms can occur in isolation or in association with other hormonally active tumors as *multiple endocrine neoplasms* (MEN).

Other Gastrointestinal Diseases

- Mucoviscidosis (p. 161)
- Infectious diarrheal diseases (p. 271)

10   Nephrology

Anatomical and Physiological Principles

■   Anatomy

Figure 10.1 shows the macroscopic anatomy of the kidney and the urinary tract.

In each kidney, there are about 1 million *nephrons* (**Fig. 10.2**). A nephron is the smallest functional unit of the kidney. It is composed of the renal corpuscle, located in the renal cortex, and the renal tubule, which extends as far as the renal medulla.

• *Renal corpuscle:* The renal corpuscle consists of a capillary tuft (glomerulus) surrounded by the Bowman's capsule. The primary urine is filtered from

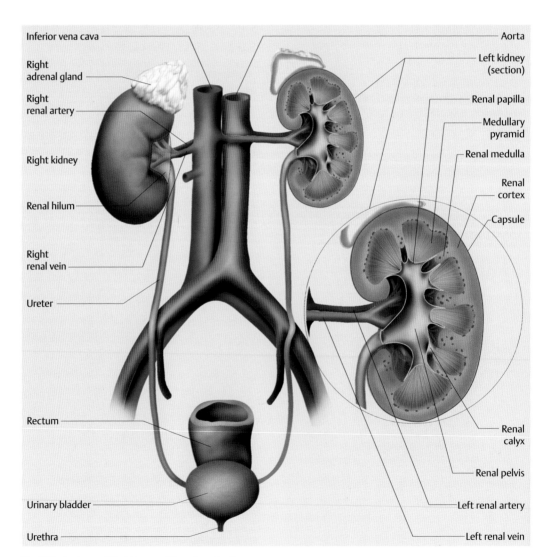

Fig. 10.1 Anatomy of the kidney and the urinary tract.

the glomerular capillary into the capsule. From the 500 mL of blood that perfuses the kidneys every minute, about 120 mL of primary urine is filtered out (this process is measured as the glomerular filtration rate). Every day, about 180 L of primary urine is produced and enters the tubule system.

- *Tubular apparatus:* In the tubules, about 99% of the 180 L primary urine is reabsorbed. This reabsorption of substances that are valuable to the body, such as glucose, amino acids, and electrolytes, is regulated by the adrenal cortex hormone aldosterone and the antidiuretic hormone (ADH) of the posterior lobe of the hypophysis. Some dissolved substances that are waste products are secreted back into the urine through the walls of the tubules and into what is now designated as the secondary urine. Every day about 1.5 L of secondary urine moves through the collecting tubules and the renal calices into the renal pelvis to be poured into the ureters.

- *Kidney perfusion: 500 mL/min*
- *Glomerular filtration rate: 120 mL/min*
- *Primary urine: 180 L/day*
- *Secondary urine: 1.5 L/day*

Functions of the Kidney

Excretory Function

- By means of reabsorption along the tubule, the kidneys regulate:
  - Water balance
  - Electrolyte balance
  - Acid–base balance
- Remaining water-soluble metabolites such as creatinine, urea, uric acid, and ammonia, as well as drugs, are excreted via the kidneys.

Incretory Function

The following hormones are synthesized by the kidneys and secreted into the blood:
- *Erythropoietin* promotes the development of erythrocytes in the bone marrow (p. 242).
- *D hormone (cholecalciferol)* regulates the calcium level (p. 224).
- *Renin*, which is secreted by the juxtaglomerular apparatus (**Fig. 10.2**) of the kidneys when blood pressure falls, elevates the blood pressure via angiotensin and aldosterone (renin–angiotensin–aldosterone system, p. 85).

Fig. 10.2 Structure of a nephron.

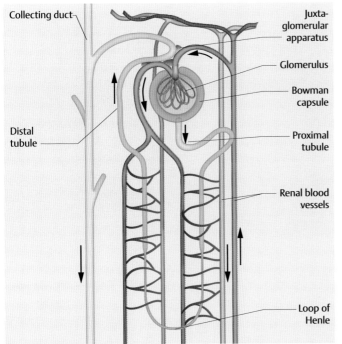

Cardinal Nephrological Symptoms

Many kidney diseases are associated with the following signs of illness:
- Disorders in urine production (diuresis)
- Disorders of urine excretion (micturition)
- Visible changes in the urine
- Flank pain
- Edema (p. 47) and nephrotic syndrome
- Arterial hypertension (p. 117)

◾ Disorders of Diuresis

Problems with urine production can be defined as oliguria, anuria, polyuria, or nocturia (**Table 10.1**).

◾ Disorders of Micturition

Problems with excretory function can be defined as pollakiuria, dysuria, alguria, urine retention, or urinary incontinence (**Table 10.2**).

◾ Visible Changes in the Urine

- *Macrohematuria* refers to the visible red color of urine as a result of the presence of more than 1 mL of blood per liter of urine. Smaller amounts can be found only through laboratory tests and are termed microhematuria. Causes of hematuria include kidney stones, tumors, and inflammations.
- *Pyuria* refers to urine that contains pus. Pyuria results in cloudy urine and occurs in severe infections of the urinary tract.
- *Foamy urine*, urine that foams as it is being released, contains protein (proteinuria).

Table 10.1 Disorders of diuresis

Disorder	Definition	Possible causes	Page
Oliguria	Amount of urine <500 mL/day	• Volume deficiency	
		• Shock	54
Anuria	Amount of urine < 200 mL/day	• Acute renal failure (stage II)	209
		• Advanced stage of chronic renal failure	209
Polyuria	Amount of urine >3000 mL/day	• Diabetes mellitus	215
		• Acute renal failure (stage III)	209
		• Diabetes insipidus	233
		• Alcohol consumption (alcohol inhibits ADH)	
Nocturia	Increased nighttime urination	• Heart failure	87
		• Difficulty in urinating, e.g., enlarged prostate	

Table 10.2 Micturition disorders

Disorder	Definition	Possible causes	Page
Pollakiuria	Frequent urge to urinate although the bladder is not full enough to warrant it	Cystitis	211
Dysuria	A concept with twofold meaning: • Difficulty in urination • Pain and burning during urination	Urinary obstruction, e.g., enlarged prostate	
Alguria	Pain during urination	• Cystitis • Urethritis • Tumor in bladder or urethra	211
Urine retention	Inability to urinate in spite of a full bladder	Enlarged prostate	
Urinary incontinence	Unintended flow of urine	• Weakness of the pelvic floor • Neurogenic disorder	

Flank Pain

- Uni- or bilateral pain, mostly dull, at the level of the kidneys, is typical of acute inflammation of the renal pelvis (pyelonephritis), but can also be present in other kidney diseases.
- Colicky, usually extremely strong, pain in the side, which may radiate to the testicles or labia, indicates the presence of lithiasis.

Nephrotic Syndrome

Definition

Nephrotic syndrome is clinically defined by:
- Pronounced proteinuria (> 3.5 g/day) and hypoproteinemia
- Hyperlipoproteinemia with elevated cholesterol and triglycerides (p. 220)
- Edema (p. 47)

Causes

Normally, the membrane of the glomerulus is not permeable to proteins, since they are too large. However, numerous factors can damage the physiological permeability barrier:
- Glomerulonephritis (p. 209)
- Medications and toxins, e.g., antiphlogistics, gold preparations, and heroin
- Collagenosis (p. 261)
- Vasculitis (p. 265)
- Various other diseases, e.g., diabetes mellitus (p. 215), severe heart failure (p. 87), blood diseases such as lymphoma (p. 250), amyloidosis (p. 209), pregnancy nephropathy (gestosis or toxemia of pregnancy)

Clinical Picture

- Consequences of protein loss and the associated depressed oncotic pressure in the plasma include pronounced edema of the eyelids and the lower extremities and, later, ascites, pleural effusion, and generalized water retention with penile and scrotal edema. Generalized edema is called anasarca.
- Renal loss of AT-III (a coagulation inhibitor) causes an increased tendency to thromboses (p. 242), and heparin is not effective in these cases.
- Loss of immunoglobulins leads to increased susceptibility to infection.
- In advanced disease, there may also be symptoms of renal failure (p. 209).

Nephrological Diagnosis

Laboratory Findings

Urine Studies

Obtaining Urine

- The easiest procedure is to evaluate a urine sample from spontaneous morning urination. In order to avoid contamination from the urinary tract, midstream urine is used: The first portion of urine rinses the urinary tract and is discarded in the toilet. The second portion of urine is caught in a sterile container and the remaining contents of the bladder are emptied into the toilet.
- To ensure elimination of contamination by bacteria in the urinary tract or the vagina, urine can be collected by one-time catheterization or, more rarely, by sterile, suprapubic bladder puncture.
- For some conditions, the patient must collect urine over a period of 24 hours (24-hour urine specimen).

Testing Procedures

- *Test strip:* A test strip that is dipped into the urine provides information concerning erythrocytes, leukocytes, protein and glucose.
- *Urine sediment:* The urine is centrifuged and the solid components are examined with the microscope.
- *Urine culture:* This examination determines the bacterial count in the urine.

Findings

- *Hematuria* is the presence of more than 4 erythrocytes per mL of urine. A distinction is made between macrohematuria, which can be detected by the unaided eye, and microhematuria, which can only be recognized microscopically. Some causes are glomerulonephritis (p. 209) or bleeding in the urinary tract as a result of inflammation, a stone, or a tumor.
- *Leukocyturia* is the presence of more than 4 leukocytes per mL of urine, e.g., in urinary tract infections.
- The excretion of more than 150 mg protein per day results in *proteinuria*. Proteinuria can occur, e.g., in diabetes mellitus (p. 215) or glomerulonephritis.
- With blood sugar values over 180 mg/dL, glucose is present in the primary urine in such high

concentrations that not all of it can be reabsorbed, so that it is excreted with the urine. *Glycosuria* is present in uncontrolled diabetes mellitus.

- The excretion in the urine of more than 10^5 bacteria per mL constitutes *bacteriuria* in the context of a urinary tract infection.
- Tiny cylinders arise in the renal tubule; these are *casts* of the tubulus lumen. They can be made up of erythrocytes, leukocytes, proteins, and components of tubule cells.

Blood Tests

In reduced kidney function, the serum concentration of substances usually excreted by the kidneys rises. Creatinine and urea serve as markers. Their normal values are given in **Table 10.3**.

- *Creatinine* is a decomposition product of muscle metabolism. Creatinine does not become elevated until kidney function is reduced by 50%. Physiologically high values are measured in individuals with pronounced muscle development. The values are low in cachectic patients and individuals with low muscle mass.
- *Urea* is the end product of protein metabolism in the liver. The serum concentration is dependent on protein intake and breakdown as well as on kidney function. An elevated serum urea concentration is not expected until kidney function has been reduced by more than 60%.

Table 10.3 Normal serum creatinine and serum urea values

Substance	Normal value
Creatinine	<1 mg/dL (83 mmol/L)
Urea	10–50 mg/dL (1.6–8.3 nmol/L)

Clearance Measurements

This procedure permits early detection of a decrease in the kidneys' excretory function. Clearance designates the volume of plasma that is cleared of the test substance per unit time. The easiest and most frequently used test is for clearance of endogenous creatinine, which gives values very similar to the glomerular filtration rate (GFR).

The following values are required:
- Urine creatinine concentration ($Crea_{Urine}$)

- Amount of urine collected in 24 hours (urine 24-hour volume, UTV)
- Serum creatinine concentration ($Crea_{Serum}$)

The GFR is calculated with the formula:

$$GFR\ (ml/min) = \frac{Crea_{Urine}}{Crea_{Serum}} \times \frac{UTV\ (ml)}{1440\ (min)}$$

Parameters in the simpler calculation using the MDRD formula (Modification of Diet in Renal Disease) include the serum creatinine concentration and age. Determination of urine creatinine and collection of urine is not required for this.

> GFR is estimated by means of endogenous creatinine clearance or the MDRD (Modification of Diet in Renal Disease) formula.

■ Imaging

Sonography

Ultrasound examination of the kidneys and lower urinary tract gives information about:
- Number, shape, and size of the kidneys
- Structure of the kidneys and indication of tumors, stones, cysts, and hydronephrosis
- Perfusion of the kidneys, by means of color duplex sonography
- Bladder filling

Radiographic Diagnosis

- In an *abdominal survey radiograph* the kidneys are recognizable as shadows. Calciferous stones in the renal pelvis or the ureters can also be seen. This procedure has been largely replaced in nephrological diagnosis by sonography.
- For an *intravenous urogram* (also known as an intravenous pyelogram), the patient receives an intravenous injection of a contrast agent that is excreted by the kidneys. Radiographs are taken at specific times. At first they show the renal pelvis filled with contrast–urine, and after about 20 minutes the filled urinary bladder. This examination provides information about the position and function of the kidneys as well as about the flow of urine. If the passage of urine is impeded by malformations, stones, or tumors, excretion of the contrast agent is delayed and the urinary tracts above the obstacle can still be seen for hours.
- *Computer tomography and more rarely nuclear magnetic resonance imaging* have taken the place of

i.v. urography and can visualize anatomical anomalies such as tumors and metastases. With the use of a contrast agent, the urine flow can be studied.
- *Angiography* permits evaluation of the renal vessels.

◼ Endoscopic Procedures

- *Cystoscopy* (examination of the bladder) is the most frequent endoscopic examination in nephrology and urology. This procedure visualizes the ureteral orifices, space-occupying lesions, and changes in the bladder mucosa.
- Special endoscopes also permit evaluation of the ureters and the renal pelvis. This procedure is called *ureteropyeloscopy.*

Replacement of Kidney Function

◼ Dialysis

In terminal chronic and acute renal failure, kidney function replacement therapy is indicated. A distinction is made between extracorporeal procedures to clean the blood—*hemodialysis* and *hemofiltration*—on the one hand and *peritoneal dialysis* on the other.

The objective of these procedures is to replace the excretory function of the kidneys.

Special blood cleansing procedures such as *hemoperfusion* or *plasma separation* are less frequently used. They serve to remove certain substances from the bloodstream, such as absorbed poisons, antibodies, circulating immune complexes, and inflammation mediators.

Hemodialysis

In hemodialysis, the blood is pumped through a filter, where blood and dialysate ("wash solution") flow on opposite sides of a tubular semipermeable membrane (**Fig. 10.3**). Substances that are normally excreted in the urine pass through the semipermeable surface of the tubes, in response to the concentration difference, and into the dialysate, while cleaned blood returns to the body.

Patients requiring chronic dialysis are provided with a surgically inserted arteriovenous shunt in the forearm as a port for the blood to leave the body and return. If there is no shunt, a central venous catheter with a double lumen can be used for acute dialysis.

As a rule, three dialysis treatments lasting from 3 to 8 hours each are performed per week in a dialysis center.

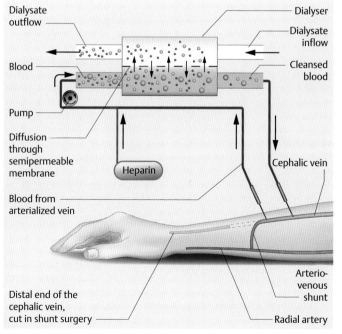

Fig. 10.3 Schematic of the procedure of hemodialysis.

Possible complications are:
- Shunt thromboses and infections
- Bleeding
- Circulatory stress with arterial hypertension and cardiac arrhythmias during the treatment

Hemofiltration

In acute renal failure, *continuous venovenous hemofiltration* (CVVH) is often used. In this procedure, there is no dialysate and no diffusive transport of substances. The drop in hydrostatic pressure is produced by a pump; plasma is filtered through the semipermeable membrane and molecules below a certain size present in the plasma are carried along with it. The loss of plasma water is balanced by substrate solutions according to the balance desired. This procedure exerts less stress on the circulation than hemodialysis and is particularly suited to withdrawing fluid in patients with unstable circulation suffering from acute renal failure.

Peritoneal Dialysis

Peritoneal dialysis procedures include:
- Continuous ambulatory peritoneal dialysis (CAPD)
- Nightly intermittent peritoneal dialysis (NIPD)

In this procedure, the well-perfused peritoneum, about 1 m² in area, is used as a natural semipermeable membrane (**Fig. 10.4**). Dialysate (2–2.5 L) is introduced into the abdominal cavity, under strictly sterile conditions, through an implanted indwelling catheter and is replaced after 4–6 hours with fresh dialysate. The exchange is carried out four to five times a day. Between exchanges, the catheter is clamped off and the patient can move about freely.

Not every patient is able to use this method independently. If the procedure is not carried out with sterile precautions, there is a danger of peritonitis.

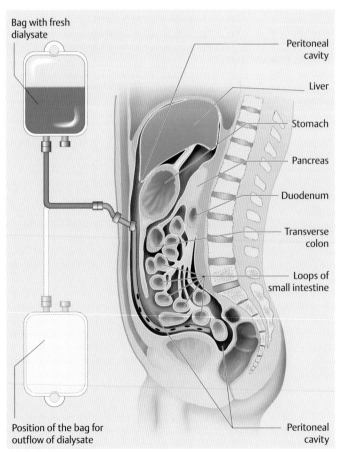

Fig. 10.4 Schematic of the procedure of peritoneal dialysis.

Bag with fresh dialysate

Peritoneal cavity

Liver

Stomach

Pancreas

Duodenum

Transverse colon

Loops of small intestine

Position of the bag for outflow of dialysate

Peritoneal cavity

■ Kidney Transplantation

Kidney transplantation (KTX), a "natural" procedure for the replacement of lost kidney function, provides the patient with a higher quality of life than any form of dialysis treatment. Patients with chronic renal failure who are under 60 years of age and have no serious accompanying diseases can be considered as transplant recipients. Donor organs come from relatives (living donors) or deceased donors with compatible immunological traits.

The organ is implanted in the iliac fossa heterotopically (in an abnormal place) and anastomosed with the iliac vessels. The ureter of the transplant is implanted into the urinary bladder of the recipient. Lifelong immunosuppressant treatment is required in order to avoid rejections.

Acute Renal Failure

Acute renal failure (ARF) is defined as acute-onset, usually reversible, disruption of the kidneys' excretory function with:

- Oliguria, i.e., excretion below 500 mL per day
- Anuria, i.e., excretion below 200 mL per day
- Increased retention of creatinine and urea

Up to 5% of all hospitalized patients suffer from ARF.

Causes

Depending on the localization of the triggering disease, a distinction is made between prerenal, renal, and postrenal ARF. There is a smooth transition between the categories, especially between the first two conditions.

- Prerenal causes, responsible for 70%–80% of all ARF, are the result of ischemia, e.g., shock or hypovolemia.
- Renal causes are toxic kidney damage, for instance by medications and radiographic contrast agent, or kidney diseases caused by inflammatory or vascular kidney disease, e.g., vasculitis or renal artery obstruction.
- Postrenal kidney failure is caused by obstruction of the urinary tract, e.g., stones or tumors.

Symptoms and Course

Acute renal failure usually develops in four stages (**Table 10.4**) but an atypical course is also possible.

Table 10.4 Stages of acute renal failure

Stage	Description
I	Kidney damage: Symptoms of underlying disease
II	Oliguria or anuria: Fluid overload, hyperkalemia, acidosis, uremia
III	Polyuria: Loss of water and electrolytes
IV	Restoration of kidney function with normal function after about 3 weeks

Therapy

Causal treatment is the most important. In addition, the following symptomatic measures can be considered:

- Proper fluid and electrolyte balance, daily weight check
- Treatment of electrolyte disorders and acidosis
- Adjustment of medication to the diminished excretory function
- Administration of diuretics
- Kidney replacement therapy in anuria or uncontrollable volume overload, severe electrolyte disorders, and acidosis

Prognosis

Depending on the underlying disease and accompanying complications, ARF is associated with a mortality of up to 50%.

Chronic Kidney Disease

In Western Europe, 10/100000 persons develop chronic kidney disease (CKD) per year, with irreversibly diminished excretory and incretory kidney function. In the United States, the incidence is even higher with 60/100000 persons affected. According to the latest figures, about 19 million adults in the US are suffering from some stage of chronic kidney disease.

Causes

The most frequent causes are:

- Diabetic nephropathy (p. 215)
- Hypertensive nephropathy (p. 117)
- Chronic glomerulonephritis (see below)
- Other causes, e.g.:
  - Chronic pyelonephritis (page 211)
  - Analgesic nephropathy (see below)

– Collagenoses such as systemic lupus erythematosus (page 261)
– In rare cases, amyloidosis (see below)

In some cases, the cause is not clear.

Glomerulonephritis

Glomerulonephritis (GN) is a general term including inflammatory, immunopathogenic diseases that attack both kidneys and affect glomerular structures and the entire nephron with varying symptoms.

Glomerulonephritis can occur idiopathically, as part of a systemic disease, for example, in collagenoses and vasculitis or in consequence of an infection.

Clinically, GN can manifest in different ways, for example, asymptomatically, as part of a nephrotic syndrome (p. 205), with acute, rapidly progressing or chronic course. Typical consequences of glomerular disease are proteinuria, hematuria, depressed glomerular filtration rate, and hypertension.

Rapidly progressing GN is a nephrological emergency and without therapy leads to rapid loss of kidney function with development of end-stage renal failure within days to weeks.

Analgesic Nephropathy

Chronic misuse of analgesics, especially paracetamol and nonsteroidal antiphlogistics, leads to chronic tubulointerstitial nephritis and to papillary necrosis caused by perfusion disorders. The result is progressive renal failure if the damaging medication is not promptly discontinued.

Amyloidosis

In amyloidosis, proteins accumulate extracellularly in various organs and lead to enlargement and decreasing function. The disease can be primary, i.e., without demonstrable accompanying disease, or secondary, as part of a systemic disease, for example:
• Plasmocytoma (p. 251)
• Chronic infectious diseases
• Chronic inflammation such as rheumatoid arthritis (p. 256)

Congenital familial amyloidosis is rare. The principal location for manifestation is in the kidneys. Nephrotic syndrome (p. 205) progressing to the point where dialysis is required is typical for kidneys affected with amyloidosis. Possible cardiac involvement leads to heart failure.

The diagnosis is confirmed by organ biopsy. Causal treatment is not available.

Table 10.5 Stages of chronic kidney disease according to the National Kidney Foundation, USA 2002 (GFR = glomerular filtration rate)

Stage	Name	GFR (mL/min/1.73m²)
I	Kidney damage with normal or ↑ GFR	>90
II	Kidney damage with mild ↓ GFR	60–89
III	Kidney damage with moderate ↓ GFR	30–59
IV	Kidney damage with severe ↓ GFR	15–29
V	Kidney failure	<15

Stages

Different underlying diseases lead to impairment of kidney function at different rates. Depending on the function remaining in the kidneys, five clinical stages are defined (**Table 10.5**).

Clinical Picture in Advanced Chronic Kidney Disease

Loss of Excretory Function

• Volume overload with the danger of pulmonary edema
• Electrolyte imbalance, particularly hyperkalemia with the risk of cardiac arrhythmias
• Toxic organ damage through retention of substances that should be excreted in the urine ("uremic poisons"), e.g.:
  – Pale yellow skin color and dry skin with pruritus (itching)
  – Thrombocytopathy with tendency to hemorrhage
  – Gastroenteropathy with loss of appetite, nausea, vomiting, and diarrhea
  – Pleuritis and pleural effusion
  – Pericarditis and pericardial effusion
  – Peripheral polyneuropathy
  – Encephalopathy

Loss of Incretory Function

When the failing kidneys cease to produce hormones, the following result:
• Renal anemia through lack of erythropoietin
• Renal osteopathy through lack of vitamin D and secondary hyperparathyroidism (p. 228)

Renal osteopathy manifests in terminal renal failure!

Renal hypertension can be related, among other factors, to:
- Hyperhydration
- Renal prostaglandin deficiency
- Excessive activation of the RAAS by the remaining intact nephrons

Diagnosis

- Patient history
- Sonography of the kidneys
- If appropriate, kidney biopsy
- Laboratory studies
  - Elevated urea or creatinine values in the blood, electrolyte imbalance, metabolic acidosis, and anemia
  - Urine findings related to the underlying disease
- Regular weight monitoring and measurement of urine volume
- Resulting damage

Therapy

In addition to therapy for the underlying disease, symptomatic therapy is particularly important, for example:
- Systematic improvement of blood pressure and blood sugar
- Low-protein diet in advanced renal failure
- Avoidance of nephrotoxic medications, especially analgesics and radiographic contrast agents
- Correction of water, electrolyte, and acid–base balance
- Treatment of renal anemia with erythropoietin
- Prophylaxis and treatment of renal osteopathy with phosphate reduction, vitamin D, and calcium substitution
- Kidney replacement therapy in terminal renal failure (p. 207)
- If appropriate, kidney transplantation (KTX; p. 209)

Case Study: A 52-year-old patient presents with dyspnea on exertion that has been present for a few weeks, loss of appetite, decreased performance, and headaches. His medical history includes untreated high blood pressure. Years previously, microhematuria was found.

Clinical examination shows pale, sallow skin, dry and scaly; a blood pressure of 210/110 mmHg; on auscultation, crackles over the lung bases. The chest radiograph shows a left-sided enlargement of the heart and beginning pulmonary congestion. Sonographically, both kidneys are reduced in size and increased in density, so-called shrunken kidneys. Values for creatinine and urea in the blood are elevated

(creatinine 6 mg/dL, urea 80 mg/dL), anemia is present (Hb 9 g/dL), serum calcium is reduced, and there is metabolic acidosis with respiratory compensation.

No kidney biopsy is performed since shrunken kidneys already correspond to end-stage organ damage.

Treatment consists of systematic lowering of the blood pressure, low-protein diet, and diuretic therapy. This treatment resulted in decrease of complaints and in relative well-being. The patient is seen at 4- to 6-week intervals as an outpatient. Two years later, the patient has a serum creatinine of 9 mg/dL. An arteriovenous shunt is implanted in the forearm and after 8 months, with terminal kidney failure, the patient requires dialysis.

Urinary Tract Infections

Prevalence and Classification

After upper respiratory tract infections, urinary tract infections are the most frequent infections of ambulatory and hospitalized patients. The frequency is a function of age and sex. Four to five percent of all women exhibit bacteriuria; as they grow older, the rate rises to more than 30%. In men, urinary tract infections before the age of 50 years are rare. After this age, they increase as a result of prostate disease.

Depending on localization of the infection, the following classification has been made:
- *Urethritis:* inflammation of the urethra
- *Cystitis:* inflammation of the urinary bladder
- *Pyelonephritis:* inflammation of the renal pelvis
- Special urinary tract infections, e.g., urogenital tuberculosis (p. 268)

Causes and Predisposing Factors

Most urinary tract infections arise from ascending microorganisms, especially bacteria. The most frequent pathogens of simple urinary tract infections are *Escherichia coli* (85%) and *Proteus mirabilis* (15%). When the course is complicated, other bacteria are found, such as *Klebsiella, Enterobacter, Enterococcus,* and *Staphylococcus.* Immunocompromised patients are also vulnerable to fungal infections.

Various risk factors can promote the onset of a urinary tract infection:
- Impediments to urinary flow, e.g., kidney and ureteric stones (p. 212), tumors (p. 213), or neurogenic disorders of bladder emptying, and, in men, an enlarged prostate
- Pregnancy, since the urethra is distended by the action of progesterone

- Metabolic diseases, e.g., poorly controlled diabetes mellitus with the high sugar content of the urine providing a positive environment for pathogens (p. 215).
- Foreign materials such as an indwelling catheter in the urinary bladder promote colonization by bacteria.
- Compromised immune system
- Misuse of analgesics leads to kidney damage and is almost always complicated by urinary tract infections.
- Chilling
- Sexual activity

Symptoms

Urinary tract infections can be symptomatic or asymptomatic. The complaints depend on the anatomical structure affected:
- *Urethritis* is associated with dysuria and pollakiuria and discharge, e.g., in gonorrhea (p. 282).
- In *cystitis,* in addition to dysuria and pollakiuria, there is suprapubic pain and possibly bloody urine.
- *Pyelonephritis* is expressed by dysuria, a severe feeling of illness with fatigue, fever, shivers and rigor, as well as flank pain. In the chronic form, these symptoms are relapsing.

Diagnosis

- Urine findings showing leukocytes, nitrite formed by bacteria, and bacteria or fungi at a concentration higher than 10^5 organisms/mL in the urine culture.
- In addition, in pyelonephritis, elevated values for inflammatory parameters are noted, e.g., accelerated ESR, elevated CRP, and leukocytosis. In about 20% of cases, pathogens are detected in blood cultures (urosepsis). In rare cases, there is kidney dysfunction with elevated values for creatinine and urea concentration.
- Further diagnostic procedures with sonography and, where necessary, contrast-enhanced CT, are indicated in relapsing urinary tract infections, in order to reveal predisposing risk factors.

Therapy

Symptomatic urinary tract infections are treated with antibiotics appropriate to the pathogen. Diuresis is increased by increased fluid intake. In infectious urethritis, the sexual partner must also be treated. Where bacteriuria occurs repeatedly, predisposing factors should be sought and eliminated.

Asymptomatic bacteriuria only requires treatment when there are special accompanying conditions, for example, for pregnant women and children, for patients with urinary tract obstruction or restricted kidney function, for diabetics, and for immunocompromised patients.

Kidney Stones

Synonyms for kidney stone disease are calculosis, nephrolithiasis and urolithiasis.

About 5% of the population suffers from calculi made up of urinary components. They can be found in the renal pelvis or the urinary tract.

Causes

The following are predisposing factors:
- Low volume of urine with correspondingly higher concentration, e.g., with low fluid intake or hot climate
- High calcium or oxalate concentration in the urine, e.g., in hyperparathyroidism (p. 228) and immobilization; oxalate in food such as spinach, rhubarb, citrus fruits and black tea
- High uric acid concentration in the urine, as in gout (p. 222)
- Alkaline urine that promotes the precipitation of calcium salts. Urinary tract infections lead to alkaline urine.
- Acidic urine that promotes the precipitation of uric acid crystals
- Lack of stone-formation inhibitors, such as magnesium
- Urinary tract obstruction

Calculi are classified according to their composition:
- In 80% of cases, the stones consist of calcium phosphate or calcium oxalate.
- About 15% are uric acid stones that can be formed in gout (p. 222).

Clinical Picture

Symptoms depend on the size and location of the calculus.
- If the stone is located in the renal pelvis, it can remain unnoticed or cause a feeling of pressure or dragging pain in the region of the kidneys. Some patients notice blood in their urine.
- Stones remaining lodged in the ureter as they pass cause *ureteric colic.* The patient complains of

severe pain that can radiate to the back, the lower abdomen, or the groin. Accompanying symptoms are nausea and vomiting and sometimes reflex ileus (intestinal obstruction, p. 187).

Calculi promote urinary tract infections that can develop into urosepsis (p. 211).

Diagnosis

- Medical history and clinical data
- Sonography
- Abdominal survey radiography, but this cannot visualize uric acid stones
- Where necessary, intravenous urogram or contrast-enhanced CT to detect uric acid stones (p. 205)
- Urinalysis
- Analysis of passed or removed calculi
- Search for causes

Therapy and Prophylaxis

Acute ureteric colic is treated with analgesics and spasmolytics. Frequently, stones pass spontaneously if the patient increases fluid intake and exercise. Otherwise, urological treatment is required.
- The method of choice for stones in the renal pelvis or high in the ureters is extracorporeal shock wave lithotripsy (ESWL). In this procedure, stones are located sonographically and shattered with shock waves. The fragments are excreted with the urine.
- Ureteral stones can be removed endoscopically during ureterorenoscopy. If the attempt to grasp the stone with forceps fails, the stone can be broken up by means of intracorporeal shock wave lithotripsy (ISWL).
- Surgical removal of a stone is necessary only in rare cases.

Without prophylaxis, up to 70% of patients suffer a relapse; with prophylaxis, the relapse rate is lower than 5%. The appropriate measures, for example, high level of fluid intake or systematic treatment of urinary tract infections, can be determined on the basis of the risk factors.

Kidney Cell Cancer

Kidney cell cancer, also known as Grawitz tumor, has shown a rising incidence during the last years with a recent estimate of 10/100 000 persons. Men are affected twice as often as women and the principal age of onset is in the seventh decade of life.

The causes are largely unknown; cigarette smoking and exposure to cadmium are risk factors.

Symptoms and Metastasis

Kidney cell cancer remains unnoticed for a long time. In more than 60% of patients, the tumor is discovered coincidentally during sonography. The following signs often indicate an advanced finding:
- Hematuria
- Pain in the side
- Palpable tumor

Tumors with endocrine activity cause:
- Arterial hypertension with renin secretion
- Polyglobulia with erythropoietin secretion
- Hypercalcemia with secretion of a substance resembling parathyroid hormone (p. 224)

Kidney cell cancer metastasizes early, through the blood. Most distant metastases are to the lungs, liver, bones, and brain.

Diagnosis, Therapy, and Prognosis

After the tumor has been found sonographically, its extent is determined by CT or MRI.

The kidney with the tumor is removed, along with the adrenal gland, lymph nodes, blood vessels, and ureter in a radical nephrectomy. Palliative measures are chemotherapy (p. 68) and immunotherapy (p. 69).

If the tumor is still confined in the renal capsule, the 5-year survival rate is about 80%. If there are distant metastases, it is under 5%.

11   Metabolic Diseases and Endocrinology

Disorders of Carbohydrate Metabolism

◼ Physiological Principles

Basic Concepts of Carbohydrate Metabolism

Blood glucose concentration (blood sugar, BS) in the fasting state is 70–100 mg/dL (normoglycemia). Deviations are called hyperglycemia or hypoglycemia.

▮ *Fasting blood sugar: 70–100 mg/dL (3.9–6.6 mmol/L)*

Glucose is the principal energy source for the human organism. Its degradation is called glycolysis. In order to maintain a constant blood sugar, glucose is stored or made available, depending on need (**Fig. 11.1**).
   If the glucose concentration exceeds the need, storage deposits are created:
- First the rapidly available glycogen storage depots in the liver and muscles are filled. This process is called *glycogenesis.*
- The process of creating fat deposits is called *lipogenesis.*

If the glucose concentration does not fulfill need, the deposits must be mobilized.
- The breakdown of glycogen to glucose is called *glycogenolysis.*
- *Lipolysis* is the breakdown of fats, in which glycerol and free fatty acids are produced.

- In *gluconeogenesis*, glucose is formed from glycerol, amino acids, or lactate.

These processes are hormonally controlled. Important hormones of carbohydrate metabolism are insulin and glucagon (endocrine pancreas, p. 171).

Insulin

Insulin is produced by the B cells of the islets of Langerhans in the pancreas. It is secreted when blood sugar rises.

▮ *BS ↑ → Insulin secretion.*

Insulin binds with the receptors of the cells that can metabolize glucose, for example, muscle cells, and functions as follows (**Fig. 11.2**):
- It promotes the uptake of glucose in the cells.
- In the cells, it stimulates the enzymes that convert glucose into glycogen and fat storage depots.
- It inhibits the enzymes that mobilize the storage depots.

Special Characteristics of the Insulin Receptors

The sensitivity of insulin receptors is variable.
- Use of the muscles increases receptor sensitivity and more glucose can enter the cells where it is needed.
- When too much glucose is supplied, the pancreas secretes more insulin. Under the increased insu-

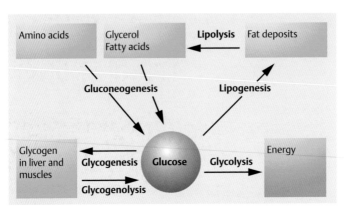

Fig. 11.1 Basic concepts in carbohydrate metabolism.

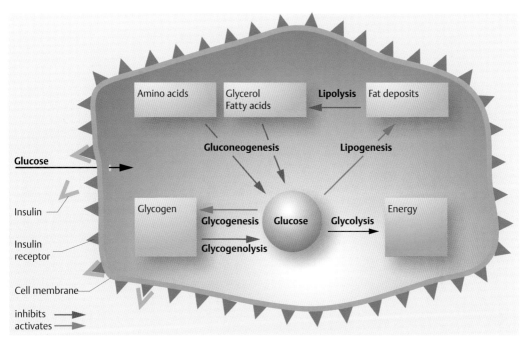

Fig. 11.2 Effect of insulin: the permeability of the cell membrane to glucose increases. In the cell, the glucose is transported to storage.

lin effect, the sensitivity of the insulin receptors decreases (down-regulation). The result is insulin resistance, less glucose enters the cells and the blood sugar rises.

These mechanisms are important for the understanding of the pathomechanism of Type 2 diabetes.

Glucagon

Glucagon is produced by the A cells of the pancreas; it is the antagonist of insulin, secreted in hypoglycemia. Glucagon mediates a sensation of hunger and mobilizes glycogen and fat storage depots to raise the blood sugar level.

■ Diabetes Mellitus

The term diabetes mellitus designates a group of metabolic disorders that lead to chronic hyperglycemia as a result of absolute or relative insulin deficiency. In the United States about 10% of all people aged 20 years or older suffer from diabetes mellitus and have to expect metabolic disorders and long-term damage to blood vessels and the nervous system.

Classification

In 1997, the World Health Organization (WHO) and the American Diabetes Association elaborated the following classification:

- Type 1 Diabetes
- Type 2 Diabetes
- Pregnancy diabetes (gestational diabetes), which occurs in about 3% of pregnant women as a result of decreased sensitivity of the insulin receptors and usually resolves after childbirth
- Other forms of diabetes, e.g.:
  - Genetically determined B cell defects or disorders of insulin activity
  - Pancreatic diseases that have led to destruction of more than 90% of the tissue (p. 198)
  - Endocrine disease such as Cushing syndrome (p. 239) and acromegaly (p. 229)
  - Medications that cause hyperglycemia, e.g., glucocorticosteroids

Type 1 Diabetes

About 5% of all diabetics have Type 1 diabetes, which usually manifests between the ages of 14 and 18 years (**Table 11.1**). Genetic disposition results in an autoimmune process directed against the B cells of the pancreas, creating an absolute insulin deficiency.

Table 11.1 Comparison of Type 1 and Type 2 diabetes

	Type 1	Type 2
Frequency	About 5% of all diabetics	About 95% of all diabetics
Pathogenesis	Autoimmune process → absolute insulin deficiency	• Insulin resistance • Secondary exhaustion of insulin reserve (secondary insulin deficiency)
Age of onset	Usually at 14–18 years	Usually after 40 years
Clinical aspects	• Slim patients • Rapid development of symptoms • Ketoacidotic coma	• 90% obese patients • Slow development of symptoms • Hyperosmolar coma
Therapy	Insulin therapy	Stepwise therapy 1. Diet and exercise 2. Oral antidiabetics 3. Insulin therapy in secondary insulin deficiency

The previously used terms, *insulin-dependent diabetes mellitus* or *juvenile diabetes mellitus* are no longer used.

▌ *Absolute insulin deficiency results in Type 1 diabetes.*

Type 2 Diabetes

About 95% of diabetics have Type 2 diabetes, a component of the metabolic syndrome (**Table 11.1**; p. 222). Where there is a genetic disposition, insulin resistance is created through excessive carbohydrate and glucose consumption and a lack of exercise (see above). When permanently elevated blood sugar values cause the pancreas to produce more and more insulin, it becomes exhausted over the course of time and stops production.

Up to now, Type 2 diabetics have usually been over the age of 40 years at onset of the disease. Lately this form has also been observed in children who are markedly overweight because of their lifestyle. Accordingly, the terms *non–insulin dependent diabetes mellitus* or *age-related diabetes* are no longer used.

▌ *Insulin resistance and possibly exhaustion of the insulin reserves is found in Type 2 diabetes.*

Clinical Picture

Type 1 Diabetes

The typical signs of disease in Type 1 diabetes often have an acute onset, and diagnosis can be made in days or weeks.

• *General symptoms*: Unspecific symptoms are fatigue and decrease in physical capacity.
• *Increased urine production (polyuria)*: In hyperglycemia, the glucose concentration in the primary urine is so high that glucose can no longer be completely reabsorbed; instead, it is excreted with the urine. The literal translation of diabetes mellitus is "honey-sweetened flow." Glucose in the urine binds water osmotically and as a result, patients excrete large amounts of urine. The osmotic diuresis increases the sense of thirst (polydipsia) in spite of increased fluid intake.
• *Loss of weight*: Since, with the lack of insulin, lipolysis and gluconeogenesis from fats and amino acids are not inhibited, there is a marked loss of weight.
• *Metabolic crises*: Sometimes the diagnosis is only made on the basis of a dangerous ketoacidosis or a diabetic coma (see below).

Type 2 Diabetes

Type 2 diabetes develops insidiously and patients remain asymptomatic for a long time. Often the finding is coincidental or is made when a secondary disease develops. Only a few Type 2 patients show the symptoms typical of Type 1 diabetes: polydipsia, loss of weight, and metabolic crises.

Acute Metabolic Crises

▌ *Hyperglycemic and hypoglycemic metabolic crises are life-threatening medical emergencies. Patients, their relatives, and all carers must be able to recognize the symptoms.*

Hyperglycemic Metabolic Crises

Severe hyperglycemia with blood sugar values up to 700 mg/dL are principally the result of:
• Absolute lack of insulin
• Relative lack of insulin with increased insulin demand, for instance in infectious diseases and after surgery
• Severely inappropriate diet

▌ *Hyperglycemia is expressed as fatigue, decreased muscle tone, nausea and vomiting, polyuria and polydipsia, arterial hypotension and tachycardia.*

- As the disease progresses, especially a patient with Type 1 diabetes is at risk for ketoacidotic coma.
- The patient with Type 2 diabetes can develop hyperosmolar coma.

Ketoacidotic Coma

Ketoacidosis is the result of uncontrolled lipolysis. The free fatty acids in the blood are metabolized to acid ketone bodies such as acetone, and these lead to metabolic acidosis. Clinical signs are:

- Accelerated, deep breathing as a result of acidosis (p. 139) and breath smelling of acetone
- Pseudoperitonitis with signs of an acute abdomen (p. 50)
- Symptoms of shock (p. 54)
- Loss of consciousness to the point of coma, which is called diabetic coma

Hyperosmolar Coma

This complication is also called hyperglycemic, hyperosmolar, nonketoacidotic dehydration syndrome, since the symptoms of marked dehydration due to osmotic diuresis are dominant. Ketoacidosis does not develop, since the insulin present is sufficient for partial inhibition of fat mobilization.

Typical signs of hyperosmolar coma are:

- Arterial hypertension up to and including shock
- Clouding of consciousness, where patients seldom become comatose
- Other neurological symptoms such as convulsions and stiff neck

Hypoglycemic Metabolic Crises

Hypoglycemia with blood sugar values below 40 mg/dL can develop under drug treatment of diabetes mellitus. Triggers are:

- Relative or absolute overdose of insulin or oral antidiabetics (see below)
- Increased physical activity
- Consumption of alcohol, since alcohol inhibits gluconeogenesis

The action of glucagon, counterregulation by the sympathetic nervous system, and lack of glucose in the brain determine the symptoms of hypoglycemia, which are summarized in Table 11.2.

A patient can also suffer a hypoglycemic crisis during physiotherapeutic treatment. In that case, a conscious patient is given rapidly absorbable sugar, in the form of a solution of glucose or fruit juice. An unconscious patient is given an intravenous infusion of glucose by an emergency physician.

Table 11.2 Signs of hypoglycemia

Mechanism	*Important symptoms*
Effect of glucagon	• Ravenous hunger
Counterregulation by the sympathetic system	• Restlessness, anxiety • Excessive activity, aggressiveness • Trembling • Cold sweat • Tachycardia • Dilated pupils
Cerebral glucose deficiency	• Inability to concentrate • Headache • Confusion • Motor restlessness • Disorders of speech and vision • Hypertonic muscles • Spasms • Primitive automatisms, e.g., grimacing and lip-smacking • Disturbance of consciousness up to and including coma • Death

Long-Term Damage

Chronic hyperglycemia can damage large and small blood vessels after an average of 10–15 years of illness.

Macroangiopathy

Diabetes mellitus presents a severe vascular risk since it contributes to the development of arteriosclerosis (p. 31). Because the vessels that are altered have a diameter of more than 2 mm, arteriosclerosis is also known as macroangiopathy. The manifestations are summarized in **Table 11.3**.

Microangiopathy

Diabetic microangiopathy affects vessels with a diameter of less than 2 mm in the kidneys, retina, and nerves.

Diabetic Nephropathy

Diabetes mellitus can lead to chronic kidney failure (p. 209). More than 30% of patients requiring dialysis are diabetics.

Diabetic Retinopathy

About 50% of all diabetics experience the first retinal damage after 10 years: Uncontrolled vascular neogenesis, bleeding, and detachment of the retina can cause blindness.

Table 11.3 Complications of diabetes mellitus

Complications	Consequences

Metabolic crises	• Hyperglycemia
	  – Ketoacidotic coma
	  – Hyperosmolar coma
	• Hypoglycemia

Macroangiopathy (arteriosclerosis; p. 31)	• Coronary artery disease (CAD, p. 98); • Myocardial infarction (p. 101) • Cerebral vascular disease (p. 126) • Stroke • Peripheral arterial disease (PAD; p. 123) • Acute arterial occlusion (p. 126) • Aortic dissection (p. 127) • Aortic aneurysm (p. 127)

Microangiopathy	• Diabetic nephropathy
	• Diabetic retinopathy
	• Diabetic neuropathy:
	  – Peripheral polyneuropathy
	  – Autonomic neuropathy

Other	• Susceptibility to infections • Fatty liver and liver cirrhosis (p. 192)

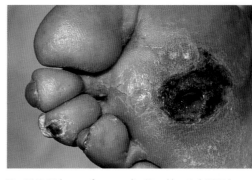

Fig. 11.3 Malum perforans pedis. (Baenkler et al. 2001.)

Diabetic Neuropathy

Involvement of the nerves is caused by microangiopathy of the vessels supplying the nerves, the vasa nervorum. The somatic and vegetative nervous systems are affected.

• *Peripheral sensorimotor polyneuropathy* is often associated with stocking-type sensory disorders, unpleasant sensations (burning feet), or paresis.
• *Autonomic neuropathy* leads to:
  – Disorders of circulatory regulation such as orthostatic dysregulation
  – Digestive problems such as constipation and diarrhea (p. 173)
  – Disorder of compensatory regulation in hypoglycemia
  – Disorders of the urogenital tract such as erectile dysfunction

> *Autonomic neuropathy impairs pain sensation in myocardial ischemia so that "silent infarctions" can occur (p. 101).*

Diabetic Foot

For a diabetic, the most minor foot injuries can develop into widespread ulceration. The sharply defined ulcers on the ball of the foot are called malum perforans pedis (**Fig. 11.3**). Causes of diabetic foot are:

• Poor perfusion in macro- and microangiopathy
• Disorder of the sensation of touch in peripheral polyneuropathy
• Susceptibility to infection, which is typical for diabetics

Diagnosis

• Patient history and clinical picture
• Laboratory parameters:
  – Blood sugar
  – Autoantibodies in Type 1 diabetes
  – Hemoglobin A1c (HbA1c) is the "blood sugar memory" of the previous 6–8 weeks and serves to monitor therapy.
  – Fructosamine is also a blood sugar memory and gives information about the blood sugar levels of the previous 14 days.
  – Glucose and ketone bodies in the urine
• Oral glucose tolerance test (OGTT): In case of doubt, an OGTT is performed. Blood sugar is tested nil by mouth (NBM) and 120 minutes after intake of a standardized amount of glucose.
• Diagnosis of possible complications, by regular monitoring of renal function and the fundus of the eyes
• Screening for additional risk factors that can promote premature arteriosclerosis (p. 31)

Therapy

The objective of diabetes therapy is optimal metabolic function, allowing the patient to be energetic and free of symptoms, as well as delaying damage as long as possible. This requires systematic patient education, which could take place initially during a two-week residence in a specialized facility. The diabetes education team consists of internists with specialties in endocrinology or diabetology as well as trained general practitioners, diabetes consultants, dietetics assistants, psychologists, and physiotherapists.

> *Therapy for Type 1 diabetes is fundamentally different from therapy for Type 2 diabetes because of the difference in pathomechanism.*

- For Type 1 diabetes, insulin therapy is indispensable.
- For Type 2 diabetes, treatment follows a stepwise plan:
  - First, the sensitivity of the insulin receptors must be restored through diet and exercise.
  - If these measures are not sufficient to achieve normoglycemia, oral diabetic medication is instituted.
  - If exhaustion of the endocrine pancreas has resulted in secondary insulin deficiency, insulin therapy is indicated.

Lifestyle Changes

Individuals at risk (see metabolic syndrome, p. 222) can reduce their risk of developing diabetes by half, by means of deliberative improvement of their diet, weight loss, and physical activity. Type 2 diabetics can retard the progress of their disease.

Nutrition

The recommended diet is largely the same as that recommended for healthy persons.

- If the patient is overweight, calorie intake should be reduced and calorie consumption should be increased to achieve weight loss.
- Sugar and fat metabolism can be improved by decreasing the carbohydrate content (glycemic load) in the diet. This improvement comes from avoiding rapidly-absorbed carbohydrates from white flour products, bread, cereals, noodles, rice, and sweets or soft drinks.
- Preferred foods should be high in fiber and water and low in calories, like vegetables, salad, fruit and legumes.
- Unsaturated fats should be preferred to saturated fats. Healthy fats, unsaturated and rich in omega-3 fatty acids are contained, for example, in olive oil, canola oil, avocados, nuts, nut oils and fish.
- A long-lasting feeling of satiety is provided by proteins from fish, lean meat or poultry, legumes, eggs and milk products.

Exercise

Regular physical training is essential to increase the sensitivity of the insulin receptors in the muscles. It decreases the insulin requirement of Type 1 diabetics and the usual insulin resistance of Type 2 diabetics, thus improving metabolic function. Sports decrease the diabetic's risk of developing cardiovascular diseases or dying of them.

The specific recommendation is moderate endurance training of at least 30 minutes for at least 5 days a week and strength training on at least 2 days a week.

> *The insulin dose must be adjusted to physical activity, to avoid hypoglycemia.*

Oral Antidiabetic Medication

If normoglycemia cannot be achieved in the Type 2 diabetic patient through lifestyle changes, oral antidiabetic medications are instituted. Examples are:

- *Metformin* for overweight Type 2 diabetics to achieve appetite control, reduction of glucose absorption, improvement of insulin receptor sensitivity, and inhibition of gluconeogenesis
- *Incretins*, to elevate insulin secretion from the pancreas and inhibit glucagon release, to reduce appetite and slow stomach emptying
- *Sulfonyl urea compounds*, to elevate insulin secretion from the pancreas and increase the insulin receptor sensitivity and to improve glucose uptake by the liver
- *Acarboses*, to delay the breakdown and absorption of carbohydrates in the intestines

Insulin

Indications for insulin therapy are:

- Type 1 diabetes
- Type 2 diabetes when lifestyle changes and oral antidiabetic medications are insufficient
- Pregnancy diabetes
- Hyperglycemic metabolic crises

Treatment consists largely of human insulin prepared with gene technology, which is usually injected subcutaneously. An insulin pen can be used for injection. Application in the form of a nasal spray is currently in trials. The insulin types summarized in **Table 11.4** can be combined according to three therapeutic principles.

Conventional Insulin Therapy

In conventional insulin therapy, a combination of short-acting and long-acting insulins is used. Two-thirds of the daily dose is injected in the morning and one-third in the evening, before meals. In practical application, conventional insulin therapy leads to a rigid diurnal rhythm and a defined nutrition program.

Table 11.4 Start and duration of effect for different insulins (simplified)

Insulin	Start of effect	Maximal effect	Duration of effect
Short-acting insulins	After 15–20 min	After 1–2 h	4–6 h
Long-acting insulins	After 1–4 h	After 4–12 h	9–24 h

Intensive Insulin Therapy

Intensive insulin therapy is also known as the basal-bolus concept.
- *Basis*: Up to 50% of the daily dose is given in the evening in the form of long-acting insulin.
- *Bolus*: The remaining quantity of insulin is administered in the form of normal insulin. The timing and dose are determined by the meal times.

The basal-bolus concept makes for a freer life but requires good patient education.

Insulin Pump Therapy

Insulin pump therapy is an alternative to intensive insulin therapy. A portable pump imitates pancreatic function by continuously injecting normal insulin subcutaneously through a thin plastic catheter. In addition to this base rate, the patient must take a bolus at mealtimes.

Disorders of Lipid Metabolism

Increased lipids in the blood (hyperlipidemia), together with cigarette smoking, elevated blood pressure, overweight and diabetes mellitus is one of the classic vascular risk factors that accelerate the development of arteriosclerosis (p. 31).

▧ Physiological Principles

The most important lipids in the plasma are:
- Cholesterol
- Triglycerides
- Phospholipids

Because lipids are not soluble in water, they can only be transported after they have been surrounded by proteins. The resulting complexes are called lipoproteins. At least three classes of lipoproteins are distinguished on the basis of their densities:
- Very low-density lipoproteins (VLDL)
- Low-density lipoproteins (LDL)
- High-density lipoproteins (HDL)

VLDL

Absorbable lipids are broken down in the intestinal mucosa and are carried to the liver by the blood. There they are mixed with the fats formed by the liver and are combined with proteins to make lipoproteins. The liver excretes "light" lipoproteins (VLDL) rich in triglycerides, into the blood.

LDL

In the blood, the triglyceride components of VLDL are split off to form LDL. These are very rich in cholesterol and are recognized by special LDL cell receptors and taken up into almost all cells of the human body.

There, their cholesterol becomes available for inclusion in cell membranes and as starting substances for the synthesis of steroid hormones.

LDL receptors are highly significant for regulation of the blood cholesterol level. They can exhibit genetically determined defects and thus lead, for example, to familial hypercholesterolemia (see below).

> The LDL cholesterol level in particular is an important risk factor for the development of arteriosclerosis.

HDL

HDL is also formed in the liver and partially in the small intestine. These lipoproteins are able to take up cholesterol from the periphery and transport it to the liver, which transforms it to bile acid and excretes it with the bile.

> HDL cholesterol protects the blood vessels in this way.

▧ Hyperlipidemia

Classification

Three categories of hyperlipidemia are differentiated on the basis of cholesterol and triglyceride concentration in the plasma.
- Hypercholesterolemia > 200 mg/dL (5.2 mmol/L)
- Hypertriglyceridemia > 150 mg/dL (1.7 mmol/L)
- Mixed hyperlipidemia

Table 11.5 Recommendations of the National Cholesterol Education Program (NCEP), 2001 (modifications of 2004 are shown in parentheses)

Risk group	Cardiovascular 10-year risk	Target values LDL cholesterol
Primary prevention: Low risk with 0–1 risk factor	<10%	<160 mg/dL
Primary prevention: Moderate risk with >1 risk factor	<20%	<130 mg/dL (<100 mg/dL)
Secondary prevention: High risk with • CAD and other manifestations of arteriosclerosis • Diabetes mellitus	>20%	<100 mg/dL (<70 mg/dL)

Disorders of lipid metabolism can be divided into three groups, depending on the cause:
- Reactive physiological forms arise from inappropriate lifestyle, e.g., high alcohol consumption or a diet rich in calories, fats, and sugar.
- Primary disorders of lipid metabolism, such as defects in specific metabolic steps or receptors, are genetically determined.
- Secondary symptomatic hyperlipidemias are caused by diseases and medications, e.g., metabolic syndrome, diabetes mellitus, hypothyroidism, renal insufficiency, alcoholism, glucocorticosteroid treatment.

Symptoms and Clinical Significance

Hypercholesterolemia

More than 50% of individuals over 40 years old in the Western world have hypercholesterolemia. Often this is only noticed in a test for blood lipids, for instance during a medical checkup. Otherwise, hypercholesterolemia is suggested by cardiovascular complications.
- The risk of a myocardial infarction or cardiovascular death rises proportionally with the LDL cholesterol level.
- An HDL cholesterol level under 35 mg/dL also increases the risk of arteriosclerosis.

Hypertriglyceridemia

- In familial hypertriglyceridemia with excessively high triglyceride levels above 2000 mg/dL, there is a risk of severe pancreatitis (p. 198). Occasionally there are xanthomas, i.e., benign skin changes in the form of yellowish lumps, in which lipids are stored. When these occur on the eyelids, they are called xanthelasmas.
- Elevated triglycerides can be part of a metabolic syndrome and reflect the associated cardiovascular risk.

Therapeutic Principles

Therapeutic Goal

The plan of therapy for patients with disorders of lipid metabolism consists of working toward blood lipid target values determined by the individual cardiovascular risks. The target values for LDL cholesterol have been defined by national and international associations on the basis of the underlying risk profiles (**Table 11.5**). A distinction is made between:
- Primary prevention of arteriosclerosis in patients without or with additional risk factors
- Secondary prevention in already-existing arteriosclerosis. In this context, diabetes mellitus is considered as an equivalent of coronary artery disease.

Therapeutic Measures

Therapeutic, nonpharmacological measures are:
- Improvement of eating habits and lifestyle (see p. 219)
- Elimination of additional risk factors

If dietetic attempts are insufficient and the underlying risk profile is significant (**Table 11.5**), lipid-reducing medications are indicated:
- Statins or cholesterol synthesis inhibitors are the most effective cholesterol-lowering medications; they act to protect the vessels and reduce the risk of myocardial infarction and death.
- Sometimes a combination with additional substances, such as fibrates or cholesterol absorption inhibitors, is necessary. Fibrates reduce triglycerides preferentially.

In rare cases of severe familial hyperlipidemia or pancreatitis resulting from hypertriglyceridemia, plasma exchange can become necessary.

Disorders of Purine Metabolism

■ Physiological Principles

Purines are important building blocks of nucleic acids and thus of DNA. They are released during natural cell replacement and also taken in with food.

Purine breakdown generates uric acid; 80% of this is excreted by the kidneys and 20% through the intestines.

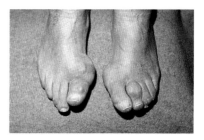

Fig. 11.4 Pronounced podagra bilaterally and gout tophi on the great toes and the left second toe. (Greten 2005.)

■ Hyperuricemia and Gout

Hyperuricemia is an elevated uric acid level in the blood. When crystals of uric acid are deposited in the joints and kidneys and trigger an inflammatory reaction there, gout can result. This usually occurs together with other metabolic disorders, as metabolic syndrome (p. 222). Men are affected significantly more often than women. In the industrialized world, 15%–20% of all men exhibit hyperuricemia and fewer than 1% suffer from gout.

Causes

- *Primary hyperuricemia and gout*: About 95% of gout patients have a genetically determined disorder of purine metabolism.
- *Secondary hyperuricemia*: Much more rarely, the elevated uric acid level is caused by increased cell division, e.g., in leukemia or tumors, or by decreased excretion of uric acid by the kidneys.

Clinical Picture

The course of hyperuricemia is asymptomatic for a long time.

The first *acute gout attack* is often triggered by a lavish meal and consumption of alcohol. At first, only one joint exhibits the typical signs of inflammation. Usually, this joint is the metatarsal-phalangeal joint at the base of the great toe (podagra, **Fig. 11.4**), more rarely a finger joint. The affected joint is very painful, so that even a light touch or the weight of blankets cannot be tolerated.

Without treatment, *chronic gout* develops over the course of about 10 years, with joint deformation and deposit of uric acid crystals in bones and soft tissue, for example, visible gout tophi (**Fig. 11.4**). The chronic form has become rare.

Since crystals of uric acid are precipitated in the kidneys, *gout nephropathy* can set in at any time,

with inflammation, kidney stones, and increasingly limited kidney function.

Diagnosis

- Patient history and clinical picture
- Hyperuricemia and inflammatory parameters in the blood

Therapy

- As long as the serum level of uric acid is under 9 mg/dL, asymptomatic hyperuricemia is treated with diet, e.g., avoidance of offal and limited consumption of alcohol. Medication is necessary only at higher levels of uric acid.
- An acute attack of gout is treated with colchicine and nonsteroidal antiphlogistics.
- When the acute attack of gout resolves, long-term dietetic and pharmaceutical therapy is introduced. Preparations are prescribed that inhibit production of uric acid or increase excretion of uric acid.

Overweight, Obesity, and Metabolic Syndrome

Overweight and Obesity

Obesity is a genetically determined syndrome reinforced by excessive food intake with insufficient physical activity. The number of overweight people is continually increasing. According to the CDC 2010, more than 34% of the adults in the United States are overweight, and the number of overweight children and youth is increasing seriously. More than 33% of the adults can be classified as obese.

According to WHO, body weight is classified on the basis of the body mass index (BMI) (**Table 11.6**).

Table 11.6 Classification of body weight

Classification	BMI (kg/m²)	Cardiovascular risk
Underweight	<18.5	Low, but with increased risk of other diseases
Normal weight	18.5–25	Normal
Overweight	25–30	Slightly elevated
Grade I obesity	30–35	Moderately increased
Grade II obesity	35–40	Strongly increased
Grade III obesity	>40	Very strongly increased

$$BMI = \frac{Weight\ [kg]}{(Height\ [m])^2}\ kg/m^2$$

Obesity leads to a significant decrease in quality of life and is an important partial cause of arterial hypertension as well as lipid and sugar metabolism disorders. In particular truncal obesity, the apple-shaped figure with increased waist circumference, is a significant risk factor for cardiovascular disease. It correlates with metabolic syndrome. BMI does not give sufficient information about fat distribution, so that guidelines additionally recommend the waist measurement as a direct measure for truncal obesity.

> A BMI of > 25 kg/m² is associated with an increased morbidity and mortality risk.

Metabolic Syndrome

Metabolic syndrome is the co-occurrence of:
- Truncal obesity
- Disorder in lipid metabolism (p. 220)
- Type 2 diabetes (p. 215)
- Arterial hypertension (p. 117)
- Hyperuricemia and gout (p. 222)

Excessive eating leads to increased blood lipids of qualitatively unfavorable composition. More than half of all obese persons have arterial hypertension, since with increased body weight, activity of the sympathetic nervous system is always increased and the renin–angiotensin system is stimulated (p. 85). With increasing mass of body fat, the response to insulin is decreased and insulin resistance rises. The risk of developing Type 2 diabetes is tripled in obesity.

Individual cardiovascular risk factors are not merely additive in metabolic syndrome but to some

Table 11.7 Clinical criteria for metabolic syndrome according to IDF 2010 (International Diabetes Federation)

Risk factor	Positive in
Abdominal obesity	Waist measurement at level of navel: • Men >94 cm • Women >80 cm
Triglycerides	>150 mg/dL (>1.7 mmol/L)
HDL-cholesterol	• Men <40 mg/dL (<1.04 mmol/L) • Women <50 mg/dL (<1.29 mmol/L)
Blood pressure	≥130/85 mmHg
Fasting blood sugar	≥100 mg/dL (>5.6 mmol/L)

extent they reinforce each other. For instance, metabolic syndrome increases the risk of coronary artery disease (p. 98) and other cardiovascular diseases by a factor of 3. The life expectancy of a 40-year-old obese woman is shortened by 7 years and of a 40-year-old man by 5.8 years.

Clinical diagnostic criteria of metabolic syndrome are listed in **Table 11.7**; three out of five points must be met in order for the diagnosis to be made.

Therapy

The principal objective of treatment is sustainable weight reduction, but this succeeds in only about 15% of obese patients.
- *Nutrition therapy* consists of modified eating behavior with selection of healthy foods and reduction of energy intake (p. 219). Losing 5%–10% of the starting weight requires an energy reduction of 2100–3300 kJ/day (500–800 kcal/day) over a period of many months. The accompanying dietetic consultation with physicians, dieticians, food scientists, or trained nursing per-

sonnel or accomplished training in groups is suitable for motivating patients to apply principles of nutrition therapy consistently and regularly.

- Increased *physical activity* accelerates the loss of weight and stabilizes long-term success of treatment. Decrease in muscle mass caused by diet is slowed down and cardiovascular risk factors such as hypertension and lipid and sugar metabolism disorders are also positively affected. In order to achieve optimal effects and the greatest possible reduction of fat, regular aerobic endurance training should be instituted after a physician's approval and with medical supervision. The target is a stress of 60%–70% of maximal heart rate for a period of 40–60 minutes or two 20–30 minute sessions per day. Suitable forms of exercise for obese patients are bicycling, walking, hiking, Nordic walking, and water exercises, which are easier on the joints but associated with high energy consumption because of the many muscles used. Adding strength training at least twice a week produces a long-term increase in basal metabolism.
- Systematic *therapy and reduction of existing cardiovascular risk factors* is always a component of treatment for obesity.
- *Surgical procedures* are considered in cases of extreme obesity, with careful determination of indication. The most widely used procedures at present are stomach restriction procedures, e.g., *gastric banding*, in which a band is placed around the stomach laparoscopically and fastened under the skin. In this position, it can be adjusted to limit the size of the stomach and thus induce an early feeling of satiety.

> Good physical fitness is a much more important factor than body weight for decreasing morbidity and mortality. So, better "plump and fit" than "slim and flabby".

Case Study: The 61-year-old, obese Mrs. D. F. (164 cm, 89 kg, BMI 33 kg/m²) consults her primary physician because of pollakiuria and polyuria. She reports that she already has had this type of complaint earlier and that up to now, "bladder tea" has always helped.

Examination of the urine shows glucosuria, a trace of albumin as well as leukocyturia and bacteria (*E. coli*). Further diagnostic studies show elevated blood sugar between 200 and 300 mg/dL. The HbA1c value is elevated at 12%. There is a hypertriglyceridemia at 286 mg/dL and arterial hypertension with resting blood pressure at 185/90 mmHg.

Because of the urinary tract infection, a diagnosis is made of metabolic syndrome, with obesity, Type 2 diabetes mellitus, hyperlipidemia and arterial hypertension.

Disorders of Bone Metabolism

◼ Physiological Principles

Bone Structure

Bone consists of the ground substance, bone cells, and minerals (**Table 11.8**).
- The ground substance is chiefly collagen, a protein that gives the bone its elastic properties.
- The bone cells are influenced by mechanical stress and hormones.
  - Osteoblasts build up bone.
  - Osteoclasts break down bone.
  - Osteocytes, together with the other two cell types, regulate mineral metabolism.
- Minerals embedded in the ground substance stabilize the bone. The most important component is hydroxyapatite, a complex compound that contains chiefly calcium and phosphate. Mineralization depends largely on hormonal factors and mechanical stress.

> Bone compression promotes mineralization; immobilization leads to breakdown of bone.

Calcium and Phosphate

Calcium

Calcium constitutes about 2% of body weight. Ninety-nine percent of this amount is located in bone and 1% is dissolved in body fluids. Forty percent of total serum calcium is bound to proteins and 60% is present as free calcium ions. The concentration of free calcium ions is decisive for electrophysiological processes in the heart and neuromuscular system.

Table 11.8 Composition of bone

Proportion (%)	Component	

30	Organic components	• Ground substance (matrix, 98%)
		  – Collagen (95%)
		  – Other proteins (5%)
		• Cells (2%)
		  – Osteocytes
		  – Osteoblasts
		  – Osteoclasts

70	Inorganic components (minerals)	• Hydroxyapatite (95%) • Other minerals (5%)

Calcium is absorbed with food in the intestines and is excreted by the kidneys. It can be incorporated into the bones as needed or mobilized from the bones.

Phosphate and Solubility Product

Phosphate balance is closely related to calcium balance. The product of the two substances is called the solubility product.

- If the solubility product exceeds a certain value, calcium phosphate is precipitated out of the solution. Calcium phosphate salts are stored in the bones and, in extreme cases, in other organ systems as well.
- If a patient receives a phosphate infusion, this combines with free calcium so that the solubility product is exceeded and calcium phosphate is precipitated. This lowers the calcium concentration in the serum (hypocalcemia).
- The opposite is true when a lack of phosphate causes hypercalcemia.

> *Phosphate ↑ → Hypocalcemia.*
> *Phosphate ↓ → Hypercalcemia.*

Hormonal Regulation

Calcium Metabolism

Three hormones regulate calcium balance and to some extent phosphate balance:

- *Parathyroid hormone*, produced by the parathyroid glands, which are also called epithelial bodies
- *Calcitonin*, formed by the C cells of the thyroid gland
- *D hormone (cholecalciferol)*, whose precursors are formed in skin and liver under the influence of UV radiation. The actual active substance is only produced in the kidneys. When UV light is lacking, insufficient D hormone is produced. Since the deficit must be corrected by means of nutrition, this substance is also called vitamin D.

Main target organs of this hormone are the intestines, the kidneys, and the bones (**Table 11.9**).

> *Numerous electrophysiological processes depend on the serum calcium concentration. It is therefore the objective of hormonal regulation to maintain the serum calcium level, if necessary at the expense of the bones.*

Other Hormones that Affect Bone Metabolism

- *Growth hormone* (somatotropic hormone, STH) controls skeletal growth.
- *Thyroid hormones* promote mineralization.
- *Estrogen and androgen* retain calcium in the bone tissue.
- *Glucocorticosteroids* decrease calcium absorption in the intestine and increase calcium excretion by the kidneys. The resulting hypocalcemia increases the amount of parathyroid hormone released (secondary hyperparathyroidism, p. 228).

■ Osteoporosis

In the fourth decade of life, the human skeleton has the greatest bone mass before a gradual, age-dependent bone breakdown begins at the age of 40 years. By the age of 80, women lose up to 40% of cortical bone and up to 60% of the spongiosa. Men lose only about two-thirds of these amounts.

This physiological old-age atrophy is distinguished from osteoporosis in which the bone mass is decreased more severely than indicated above. Pathological bone loss affects the organic and mineral components equally and promotes the occurrence of fractures without adequate trauma (pathological fractures or spontaneous fractures; **Fig. 11.5a, b**).

In the US, according to projections made by the National Osteoporosis Foundation in 2002, the number of individuals with osteoporoses by 2010 would

Table 11.9 Regulation of calcium and phosphate balance (PTH = parathyroid hormone, Ca^{2+} = calcium ions, HPO_4^{2-} = phosphate ions)

Hormone	Stimulus for release	Effect on target organs		
		Bones	Kidneys	Intestine
PTH	Ca^{2+} ↓ HPO_4^{2-} ↑	Demineralization	• Ca^{2+} excretion ↓ • HPO_4^{2-} excretion ↑ • D hormone ↑	Ca^{2+} absorption ↑ (indirectly via D hormone)
Calcitonin	Ca^{2+} ↑	Mineralization	Ca^{2+} excretion ↑	
D Hormone	Ca^{2+} ↓ HPO_4^{2-} ↓ PTH	Mineralization	• Ca^{2+} excretion ↓ • HPO_4^{2-} excretion ↓	Ca^{2+} absorption ↑

be 52 million, comprising 35 million women and 17 million men. Prevalence increases with age, resulting in increasing numbers of fractures, such as vertebral fractures. For the US, the estimated numbers of such fractures are in the hundreds of thousands.

Forms and Causes

Ninety-five percent of the affected individuals suffer from primary osteoporosis without a known underlying disease. Three forms of the disease are distinguished:

- Idiopathic osteoporosis in young people
- Type I osteoporosis, also known as postmenopausal osteoporosis, which leads to a loss of bone concentrated in the spongiosa
- Type II osteoporosis, also called senile osteoporosis, which affects spongiosa and compacta

At 80%, Type I osteoporosis is the most frequently occurring form. Predisposing factors are summarized in **Table 11.10**.

Considerably less frequent is secondary osteoporosis, which can be ascribed to an underlying disease (**Table 11.11**).

Clinical Picture

In contrast to old-age atrophy, osteoporosis involves vertebral deformation without trauma. Kyphosis of the thoracic spine and lordosis of the lumbar spine are intensified; clinical signs are formation of a gibbus (hump) and loss of body height (**Fig. 11.6a–c**).

Patients complain of spinal pain that at first occurs only under stress and finally persists continuously.

In addition to spontaneous fractures of the vertebrae, frequently occurring fractures are pathological fractures of the femoral neck, the subcapital humerus, and the distal radius.

Table 11.10 Risk factors for development of primary osteoporosis

Unalterable factors	Alterable factors
• Age	• Estrogen deficiency
• Sex	• Lack of exercise
• Genetic disposition	• Nutritional factors, e.g.:
	– BMI under 20 kg/m²
	– Calcium deficiency
	– Vitamin D deficiency
	• Cigarette smoking
	• Alcoholism

Table 11.11 Causes of secondary osteoporosis

Causes	Important examples	Page
Endocrine disorders	• Type 1 diabetes, also moderately in Type 2 diabetes	215
	• Osteomalacia	
	• Hyperparathyroidism	228
	• Hypothyroidism	228
	• Hyperthyroidism	236
	• Cushing syndrome	235
	• Hypogonadism	239
Rheumatologic diseases	• Rheumatoid arthritis	256
	• Bechterew disease	260
Malabsorption diseases	• Gluten-sensitive enteropathy	229
	• Lactose intolerance	230
	• Crohn disease	232
Kidney diseases	• Chronic kidney failure	209
Malignant diseases	• Multiple myeloma	251
	• Hormone therapy in oncological treatment	69
Medications	• Long-term therapy with glucocorticosteroids	77
	• Long-term therapy with heparins	73
	• Phenytoin (antiepileptic)	

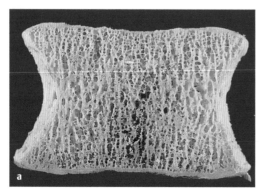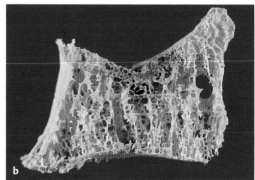

Fig. 11.5a, b   a Normal lumbar vertebra. **b** Osteoporotic lumbar vertebra (Niethard 2005).

Diagnosis

- Patient history and clinical picture
- Radiography is applied to confirm fractures. Early radiological diagnosis is problematic because increased transparency to radiation of the bones does not set in until more than 30% of the bone mass has been broken down. In the late stage, the typical vertebral deformations can be seen.
- Measurement of bone density, called osteodensitometry, using DXA (dual X-ray absorptiometry) permits conclusions about the risk of fracture.
- Laboratory studies to rule out secondary osteoporosis or other bone diseases.

Therapy

Therapy of Primary Osteoporosis

The basic therapy takes risk factors into account (**Table 11.10**) and includes, in particular:

- Diet rich in calcium and vitamin D
- Exercise therapy, e.g., in osteoporosis groups: Coordination training, muscle strengthening, encouragement and maintenance of mobility
- Fall prevention
- Use of therapeutic appliances if applicable (corset, hip protector, walker, rollator)
- Avoidance of underweight
- Cessation of smoking

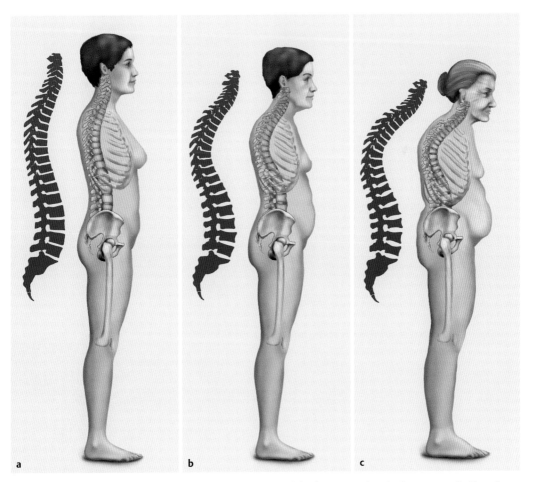

a   **b**   **c**

Fig. 11.6a–c Spinal changes in osteoporosis. Compression fractures of the thoracic vertebrae lead to a progressive thoracic spine kyphosis and decrease in body height. Under certain circumstances, the thorax can rest on the pelvic crest and the abdominal intestines can cause the abdominal wall to protrude. Wedge-shaped vertebrae form in the thoracic spine and the start of concave deformation ("cod-fish vertebrae") can be seen in the lumbar spine. **a** 55 years. **b** 65 years. **c** 75 years.

In addition, there is pharmacotherapy:
- Calcium and vitamin D (but these do not suffice alone)
- Medications that inhibit bone breakdown, e.g., bisphosphonates, parathyroid hormone analoga
- If necessary, pain therapy (analgesics)

Therapy of Secondary Osteoporosis

First of all, the underlying disease must be treated. Supplementary measures correspond to those described for therapy of primary osteoporosis.

Case Study: Mrs. S., 67 years old, trips while out on a walk and suffers a right distal radius fracture. This is conservatively treated.

Two years later, the patient knocks against an open cabinet door and suffers a rib fracture.

At 70, the patient is diagnosed with arteritis temporalis (p. 266) and is treated with glucocorticosteroids for a period of 12 months. At the age of 73, Mrs. S suffers acutely occurring back pain, which she describes as the strongest pain imaginable and the strongest she has ever experienced. Her primary physician prescribes analgesics. One year later, she again suffers equally strong pain. At this point, for the first time, a radiological study of the spine is made. It shows breaks in vertebrae at the level of the thoracic spine and one vertebral break in the lumbar spine. The result of a bone density measurement corresponds to osteoporosis.

Since the disease is already advanced and has manifested in the form of several fractures, the patient now receives osteoporosis-specific therapy for the first time. After 9 months, the medication is no longer prescribed.

At the age of 77, a fall from a standing position results in a medial femoral neck fracture. As a result of a complicated recovery and failure of attempts at rehabilitation the patient becomes dependent on care in a nursing home.

■   Osteomalacia

In osteomalacia, bone tissue is insufficiently mineralized. The comparable disease in children is rickets with insufficient mineralization of the epiphysis.

Causes

The principal cause is a vitamin D deficiency as a result of insufficient ingestion with food and low UV exposure. Less frequent causes are:
- Malassimilation with disturbed vitamin D uptake (p. 173)
- Renal or hepatic insufficiency with decreased synthesis of hormone D (renal osteopathy; p. 209)

- Phosphate deficiency with reactive mobilization of calcium from the bones, since the solubility product decreases (p. 224)

Symptoms

Development of symptoms is insidious. The consequences of insufficient mineralization are:
- Bone pain
- Bone deformities such as kyphosis formation in the spine and bow legs
- Pathological fractures

As a result of hypocalcemia, muscle weakness develops and in some cases, tetany. There can be signs of the underlying disease.

Diagnosis

- Indications in the patient's history regarding symptoms and where applicable, existing underlying disease
- Clinical picture
- Increased transparency to radiation and deformations on the radiograph
- Hypocalcemia and serum vitamin D deficiency

Therapy

Vitamin D substitution with monitoring of serum calcium. Where applicable, the underlying disease must be treated.

■   Hyperparathyroidism

Hyperparathyroidism exists when the parathyroid glands release too much parathyroid hormone (PTH).

Forms and Causes

- *Primary hyperparathyroidism:* In primary hyperparathyroidism, hormone production usually emanates from an adenoma in the parathyroid glands. Sometimes there is also a general enlargement of the parathyroid glands (hyperplasia).
- *Secondary hyperparathyroidism:* In the secondary form, the parathyroid gland reacts to a lowered calcium level with increased release of PTH, e.g., in:
  - Malassimilation syndrome with decreased calcium absorption (p. 173)
  - Chronic kidney failure with D hormone deficiency (p. 209)

About 50% of patients exhibit symptoms due to the action of PTH (**Table 11.9**).

- Calcium phosphate precipitates in the kidneys and calculi are formed (nephrolithiasis p. 212). Moreover, the ability to concentrate the urine is impaired, which increases diuresis.
- Demineralization of the bone tissue results in osteopenia with spine and joint pain.
- Gastrointestinal complaints include loss of appetite, nausea, weight loss, and constipation. Some patients develop gastroduodenal ulcer disease (p. 180) or pancreatitis (p. 198).

In addition, some patients exhibit neuromuscular and psychiatric symptoms, for example, rapid tiring, muscle weakness, and depressive mood. At any time a life-threatening *hypercalcemic crisis* can develop. This is associated with:

- Vomiting
- Increased diuresis
- Signs of dehydration
- Adynamia and clouded consciousness up to and including coma

Diagnosis

- Patient history and clinical picture
- PTH and serum calcium are elevated, whereas phosphate is decreased in primary hyperparathyroidism.
- Proof of adenoma by sonography or CT

Therapy

Primary Hyperparathyroidism

Surgical removal of the enlarged parathyroid glands in:

- Symptomatic patients
- Patients with changes in bone density
- Patients with changes in kidney function

Secondary Hyperparathyroidism

- Therapy of the underlying disease
- Supplementation with vitamin D and, if appropriate, calcium

Diseases of the Pituitary Gland

■ Physiological Principles

Hormonal Regulatory Cycle

Hierarchy of Hormone Regulation

The hypothalamus and the pituitary gland (hypophysis) are the superordinate centers of the endocrine system. The hypothalamus is located in the diencephalon and secretes releasing hormones. These hormones cause the pituitary gland to release glandotropic hormones that stimulate the peripheral hormone-secreting glands (**Fig. 11.7**).

Feedback Mechanism

Hormone production is regulated by negative feedback. Thus sufficient concentrations of the peripheral hormones or their metabolic effects cause the hypothalamus and pituitary gland to decrease or stop the release of superordinate hormones. The same is true for medication with hormone preparations.

In contrast, underfunctioning of a peripheral hormone-secreting gland causes increased secretion of releasing hormones and glandotropic hormones.

Pituitary Hormones

The pituitary gland is an important control organ in the endocrine system. It can be divided anatomically and functionally into the anterior lobe and the posterior lobe.

Hormones of the Anterior Pituitary Lobe

The glandotropic hormones are produced by the anterior lobe of the pituitary gland (APL). They are:

- Thyroid-stimulating hormone (TSH), which activates the thyroid gland
- Adrenocorticotropic hormone (ACTH), which stimulates the adrenal cortex to produce glucocorticosteroids
- Follicle-stimulating hormone (FSH) and luteinizing hormone (LH), which stimulate release of sex hormones by the ovaries or the testes

Other hormones of the anterior lobe have a direct effect on target organs:

- Growth hormone (somatotropin, STH)
- Prolactin promotes milk production in nursing women.

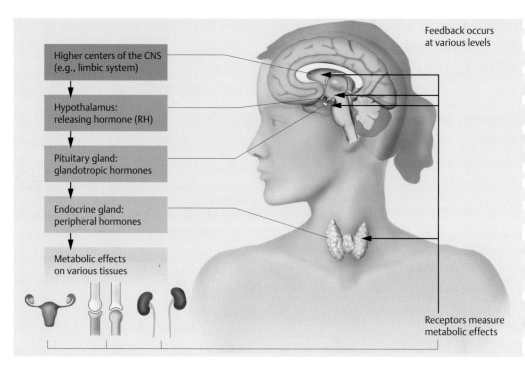

Fig. 11.7 Hierarchy of hormone regulation.

- Melanocyte-stimulating hormone (MSH) regulates the production of melanin in the melanocytes.

Hormones of the Posterior Pituitary Lobe

The posterior pituitary lobe (PPL) releases two hormones:
- Antidiuretic hormone (ADH), which inhibits urine production (diuresis) in the kidneys
- Oxytocin, which causes contraction of the smooth muscles in the uterus and the excretory ducts of the milk glands and thus leads to lactation

These two hormones are produced in neurons of the hypothalamus and released by the axons into the pituitary circulation. They are then stored and released by the pituitary gland.

■   Pituitary Tumors

Overview

The incidence of pituitary tumors is difficult to define because many of them are asymptomatic. Up to 15% of all brain tumors are neoplasms of the pituitary gland.

These are usually benign tumors. More than 90% are adenomas, which are classified as endocrine-active and endocrine-inactive tumors (**Table 11.12**).

Symptoms

Tumor-specific endocrine symptoms of large space-occupying lesions can include the following signs of disease:
- Headache
- Visual disorders due to compression of the optic nerve
- APL and PPL insufficiency due to compression of the hormone-producing cells

Prolactinoma

A prolactinoma is a prolactin-producing tumor of the APL. This is the most frequently occurring endocrine-active pituitary tumor, usually manifesting in the third or fourth decade of life. It occurs five times as often in women as in men.

Table 11.12 Overview of pituitary tumors

Group	Frequency (%)	Tumor	Consequences, clinical picture	Page
Endocrine-active	60	Producing prolactin	Prolactinoma	230
		Producing STH	Acromegaly	230
		Producing ACTH	Cushing disease	239
		Producing TSH (rare)	Hyperthyroidism	235
		Producing FSH or LH (rare)	Premature puberty (pubertas praecox)	
Endocrine-inactive	40	• Craniopharyngioma • Cysts • Metastases, etc.	Possible consequences of all endocrine-inactive tumors • Headache • Visual disorders • APL insufficiency • PPL insufficiency: diabetes insipidus	232 233

Symptoms

- Prolactin suppresses the secretion of FSH and LH, so that menstrual periods and ovulation are absent in women (secondary amenorrhea). Also possible are loss of libido, flow of breast milk (galactorrhea), and secondary osteoporosis (p. 225).
- Men suffer from loss of libido and impotence and sometimes enlarged breasts (gynecomastia).
- In both sexes there is a possibility of headache, visual disturbances through compression of the optic nerve, and APL and PPL insufficiency through compression of the hormone-producing cells.

Diagnosis

- Patient history and clinical picture
- Elevated serum prolactin level
- Determination of the remaining pituitary hormones
- Visualization of the tumor by CT or MRI
- Ophthalmological examination

Therapy

Under drug therapy with dopamine agonists the tumor shrinks in 95% of patients and the prolactin level is normalized. In the remaining patients, surgical removal of the prolactinoma is indicated.

Pituitary Gigantism and Acromegaly

Definition and Symptoms

Underlying both clinical pictures is an adenoma of the APL that produces growth hormone.
- If the tumor appears before the epiphyses of the bones have closed, the result is pituitary gigantism with a body height of over 2 meters.
- After the growth in height is complete, an excess of STH leads to acromegaly with enlarged hands and feet, coarse facial traits, and enlarged organs (**Fig. 11.8a–c**).
- Every second patient suffers from arterial hypertension.
- As a result of pathological glucose tolerance, about 15% of affected patients develop diabetes mellitus (p. 215).
- If the tumor is large, there may be headaches, visual disorders, and APL and PPL insufficiency.

Diagnosis

- Patient history and clinical picture
- Hormone analysis with monitoring of STH and the other pituitary hormone levels
- Visualization of the tumor by CT or MRI
- Ophthalmological examination

Therapy

The therapy of choice is microsurgical removal of the adenoma. In exceptional cases, radiation therapy or inhibition of hormone secretion with dopamine agonists and somatostatin analogs may be considered. Somatostatin is the antagonist of growth hormone.

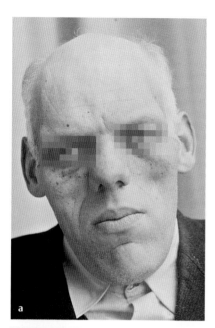

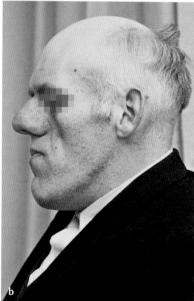

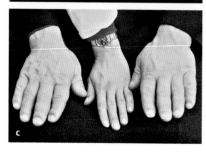

Fig. 11.8a–c A patient with acromegaly. **a** and **b** Coarsened facial traits with enlargement of nose and lower jaw. **c** "Bear paw" hands compared with a normal hand (Gerlach 2000).

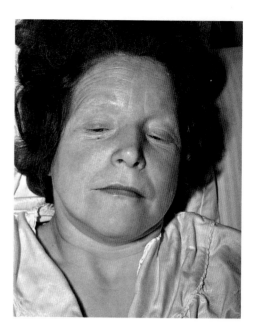

Fig. 11.9 A patient with total APL insufficiency in Sheehan syndrome. The sallow paleness and loss of eyebrows are notable. (Gerlach 2000.)

■ Insufficiency of the Anterior Pituitary Lobe

Definition and Causes

APL insufficiency is a rare clinical picture in which one, several, or all functions of the APL are absent. Causes include:

- Tumors (p. 230)
- Skull–brain trauma
- Consequences of surgery or radiation
- Autoimmune processes
- Ischemic necrosis, e.g., shock or Sheehan syndrome (**Fig. 11.9**). The latter can occur in women during childbirth if the pituitary gland is insufficiently perfused.

Symptoms

APL insufficiency does not manifest until 70% of the tissue has been destroyed. If the illness is caused by a pituitary adenoma, the symptoms develop slowly and in a typical order (**Table 11.13**).

Complications

In situations such as infections, trauma, or surgery, the lack of ACTH and TSH can lead to *pituitary coma*.

The signs are:
- Bradycardia and arterial hypotension
- Hypothermia
- Consequences of hypoglycemia (**Table 11.2**)
- Hypoventilation with hypercapnia and acidosis

Diagnosis and Therapy

Patient history and the clinical picture lead to a suspected diagnosis that is confirmed by numerous endocrinological tests:
- Base values of APL hormones
- APL hormone levels after stimulation with releasing hormones
- Peripheral hormone levels such as thyroid hormones and glucocorticosteroids

In addition to causal treatment, for example, surgical removal of a tumor, lifelong replacement of the peripheral hormones is required.

Table 11.13 Development of symptoms in chronic APL insufficiency

Disappearance of hormones	Resulting symptoms

1. STH	• In children: Pituitary dwarfism
	• In adults:
	  – Adynamia
	  – Decreased muscle mass
	  – Increased fat mass
	  – Metabolic disorders
	  – Secondary osteoporosis

2. FSH, LH	• Secondary amenorrhea in women • Loss of libido and potency • Decrease in secondary hair patterns
3. TSH	Signs of hypothyroidism (p. 236) such as: • Sensitivity to cold • Fatigue, apathy • Bradycardia
4. ACTH	Signs of adrenocortical insufficiency (p. 241) such as: • Adynamia • Weight loss • Arterial hypotension
5. MSH	Sallow paleness due to depigmentation (**Fig. 11.9**)
6. Prolactin	In nursing women: agalactia, i.e., lack of milk production

▪ Insufficiency of the Posterior Lobe of the Pituitary Gland

The decreased production of antidiuretic hormone (ADH), which leads to diabetes insipidus, is clinically significant.

Diabetes Insipidus

Diabetes insipidus is a rare disease in which the kidneys are unable to absorb sufficient water to concentrate the urine. This causes polyuria with urine volumes up to 25 liters per day.

Forms and Causes

- Usually, *central diabetes insipidus* is associated with decreased ADH production by the PPL. Causes may be dominant inheritance, autoimmune processes, tumors, trauma, or surgery, meningitis or encephalitis.
- Much less frequent in occurrence is *renal diabetes insipidus*, in which the kidneys do not respond to ADH.

Symptoms

Since large quantities of unconcentrated, clear urine are excreted, the patient increases fluid intake. If the loss of fluid cannot be balanced through polydipsia, there is a threat of dehydration with circulatory failure, acute renal failure (p. 209), and thromboses (p. 131).

Diagnosis and Therapy

Diagnostic clarification is indicated when amounts of urine and fluid intake exceed 4 liters per day.
- The diagnosis is confirmed if the osmolarity of the urine does not rise after a thirst test.
- CT or MRI is used to screen for an underlying tumor.

If causal treatment is impossible or insufficient, ADH is replaced by synthetic vasopressin analogues. In the renal form, thiazide diuretics and nonsteroidal antiphlogistics can improve the symptoms.

Thyroid Diseases

■ Physiological Principles

Hormonal Regulatory Cycle

- Hypothalamus: thyrotropin-releasing hormone (TRH)
- Anterior lobe of the pituitary gland: thyroid-stimulating hormone (TSH)
- Thyroid gland: triiodothyronine (T_3) and thyroxine (T_4)

Under the influence of TSH, the thyroid gland produces the thyroid hormones triiodothyronine and thyroxine, which contain three and four atoms of iodine, respectively, and are therefore designated as T_3 and T_4.

The thyroid gland releases much more T_4 than T_3 into the bloodstream. T_4 has only slight biological effect and serves primarily as a hormone precursor that is transformed in the liver to the active T_3 by the splitting off of one atom of iodine.

Effect

Thyroid hormones have numerous target organs and effects, resembling those of the catecholamines epinephrine and norepinephrine.

- Increased energy consumption is associated with increased need for oxygen, increased carbohydrate and lipid consumption, and increasing heat production.
- In addition, thyroid hormones promote growth and maturation, especially of the central nervous system and bones.

■ Goiter

An enlarged thyroid gland is known as a goiter or struma (**Fig. 11.10**). The term conveys no information regarding:

- The mode of thyroid enlargement, which can be diffuse or nodular
- Cause
- Quantity of hormone production

Depending on hormone production, three metabolic situations are distinguished:

- Euthyroidism with normal blood hormone levels
- Hypothyroidism with decreased hormone levels
- Hyperthyroidism with elevated hormone levels

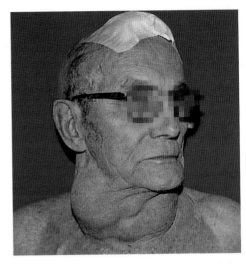

Fig. 11.10 A patient with large nodular goiter. (Gerlach 2000.)

Euthyreotic Goiter

Euthyreotic or bland goiter is a thyroid gland with normal hormone production and an enlargement that is not caused by inflammation or malignancy.

The most important cause of a bland goiter is a lack of iodine, which causes release of growth factors in the thyroid gland. In the United States, where most people use iodized salt, bland goiter caused by iodine deficiency is not often found.

Symptoms

Most patients are symptom-free at first, but later observe an increase in the circumference of the throat and a feeling of pressure and tightness that is intensified when wearing a high collar.

Where the goiter is large, compression of neighboring organs can also result in the following symptoms:

- Difficulty in swallowing
- Dyspnea, possibly with inhalation stridor (p. 144)
- Hoarseness if the recurrent nerve, which innervates the larynx, is damaged
- Superior vena cava congestion due to compression of large veins

In an enlarged thyroid gland, autonomous centers that lead to hyperthyroidism can develop (p. 234). More rarely, cells can degenerate and give rise to thyroid cancer (p. 237).

Diagnosis

The basic diagnosis includes:
- Inspection and palpation
- Sonography to determine the size of the enlargement and possible presence of nodes
- TSH determination

> To assess the supply of thyroid hormones to the body, TSH level is determined first (hormonal regulatory cycle, p. 229):
> TSH ↓ → Hyperthyreosis.
> TSH ↑ Hypothyreosis.

- Scintigraphy, in which a radionuclide is injected intravenously. The uptake of the radionuclide is registered with a special camera, so that the metabolic status can be assessed.

Therapy

Drug Therapy

The volume of the thyroid gland can be reduced by about 40% by administration of iodine or iodine and thyroxine.

Surgical Therapy

If the goiter is large, compressing the neighboring organs, or if the benign/malignant status is unclear, subtotal strumectomy is indicated, sparing a small remnant of the thyroid gland.

Possible surgical complications are paresis of the recurrent nerve with hoarseness and dyspnea as well as damage to the parathyroid glands. The latter can lead to hypocalcemia (**Table 11.9**) and tetany through parathyroid hormone deficiency.

Postoperatively, TSH levels must be determined regularly and, where necessary, hormone replacement therapy must be instituted. For prophylaxis of relapse, iodine is prescribed.

Radioiodine Therapy

In a relapsing goiter or where there is elevated surgical risk, radioiodine therapy is undertaken. The patient swallows radioactive iodine, which is concentrated exclusively in the thyroid gland, where it destroys the tissue. The goiter can be reduced in size by 50% with this procedure. The most common complication is hypothyroidism, which requires hormone replacement.

Prophylaxis

> In some geographical areas, there is insufficient iodine in locally produced food. Such a deficit cannot be balanced by using iodized salt or eating marine fish, and iodine tablets are recommended. The daily dose is 100–200 μg iodine.

■ Hyperthyroidism

Definition and Causes

Hyperthyroidism is caused by excessive functioning of the thyroid gland, which in 90% of cases is caused by functional autonomy of the thyroid gland or Basedow disease.
- In *functional autonomy*, some cells of the thyroid gland have escaped from the hormonal regulatory cycle and produce T_3 and T_4 without stimulation by TSH. The autonomous thyroid gland tissue can be restricted to one or more circumscribed areas or be distributed throughout the whole thyroid gland.
- *Basedow disease* is an autoimmune disease (p. 29) in which autoantibodies against TSH receptors are produced. These stimulate the thyroid gland to hormone production and growth. In addition to signs of hyperthyroidism and of a goiter, immunogenic hyperthyroidism can entail endocrine orbitopathy with protruding eyeballs (exophthalmic goiter, Graves disease; **Fig. 11.11**).

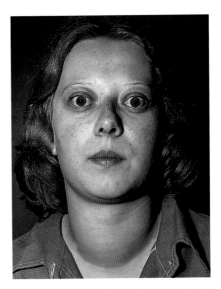

Fig. 11.11 A patient with exophthalmic goiter (Graves disease, Basedow disease): Protruding eyes and goiter are notable. (Kellnhauser 2004.)

Examples of less frequent causes of hyperthyroidism are:

- Thyroid gland cancer (p. 237)
- Thyroiditis, which results in transitory increase of thyroid hormone release
- Elevated exogenous hormone supply (hyperthyreosis factitia)

Symptoms

- Up to 90% of patients have a goiter.
- They suffer from psychomotor restlessness associated with tremors, nervousness, irritability, and insomnia. Even though they are operating at high speed, affected persons feel tired and weak.
- Patients are inclined to break out in a sweat. The skin is warm and moist and the head hair is sparse.
- Noticeable vital signs are tachycardia, sometimes cardiac arrhythmias, and elevated blood pressure.
- Heightened intestinal activity results in higher stool frequency and sometimes in diarrhea.
- Elevated basal metabolism leads to weight loss in spite of ravenous hunger.
- The motor apparatus suffers from myopathy that increases generalized weakness. In addition, some patients develop osteoporosis (p. 225).

Complications

A *thyrotoxic crisis* can be caused by the administration of iodine-containing medications or contrast agents. The symptoms described are intensified and result in:

- Tachycardia with a heart rate of over 150/min and cardiac arrhythmias
- Fever up to 41 °C
- Dehydration due to fever, sweating, vomiting and diarrhea
- Pronounced muscle weakness
- Altered states of consciousness
- Circulatory failure

Diagnosis

Information in the patient history and the clinical picture lead to a suspected diagnosis, confirmed by a depressed TSH level. The thyroid hormones in the blood are elevated. Further diagnostic information can be obtained as follows:

- In Basedow disease, TSH receptor autoantibodies can be demonstrated.
- Sonography shows a thyroid gland increased both in size and in perfusion; possibly nodules can be visualized.
- In hyperthyroidism, scintigraphy shows homogeneous or focal concentrations ("warm" or "hot" nodules).

Therapy

Hyperthyroidism must first be treated with medication. Administration of thyrostatics is aimed at achieving euthyreosis. Long-term therapy with thyrostatics is only justified in individual cases. In general, surgery or radioiodine therapy is indicated for definitive therapy (p. 234).

■ Hypothyroidism

The various forms and causes of insufficient thyroid function are summarized in **Table 11.14**.

Symptoms and Complications

- Patients with hypothyroidism are characterized by decreased physical and mental capacity. They are tired, lacking in drive, slowed-down, and give the impression of lacking interest (**Fig. 11.12a**).
- Patients are sensitive to cold and the skin is dry, cool, doughy, and scaly.
- The doughy appearance is caused by generalized *myxedema* (**Fig. 11.12b, c**) caused by deposition

Table 11.14 Forms and causes of hypothyroidism

Form	Localization of cause	Important examples

Primary hypothyroidism	Thyroid gland	• Congenital hypothyroidism
		• Acquired hypothyroidism:
		  – Hashimoto thyroiditis with an underlying immune process
		  – Iatrogenic, e.g., after surgery, after radiotherapy and from use of thyrostatics

Secondary hypothyroidism	Pituitary gland (rare)	APL insufficiency (p. 232)
Tertiary hypothyroidism	Hypothalamus (rare)	• Tumors • inflammation • Skull–brain trauma and surgery

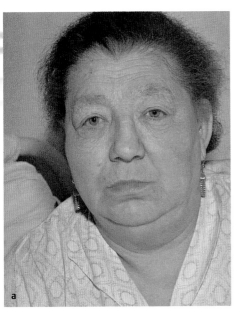

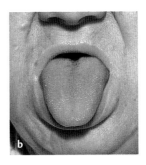

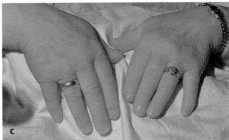

Fig. 11.12a–c A patient with hypothyroidism caused by autoimmune thyroiditis. **a** Pale, doughy skin and dry hair, hard to comb. **b** Enlarged tongue due to myxedema. **c** Doughy swelling of hands due to myxedema (Gerlach 2000).

of mucopolysaccharides in the tissue. Myxedema leads to increase in weight and possibly to organ involvement. Bradycardia and possible signs of heart failure can point to a "myxedema heart."
- Additional symptoms are dry, brittle hair, coarse voice, and constipation.
- Decreased basal metabolism results in hyperlipidemia (p. 220) that promotes premature arteriosclerosis (p. 31).
- Myxedema coma with extreme hypothermia, bradycardia, arterial hypotension, bradypnea, hypoglycemia, and altered states of consciousness seldom occurs today.

Diagnosis

- Patient history and clinical picture
- Elevated TSH level in primary hypothyroidism; the other, rarely occurring, forms are characterized by decreased TSH levels
- Decreased blood level of thyroid hormones
- Decreased radionuclide concentration in the scintigram
- Evidence of antibodies in Hashimoto thyroiditis

Therapy

Hypothyroidism is treated by lifelong replacement of thyroid hormones and regular monitoring of TSH levels.

■ Malignancies of the Thyroid Gland

Malignant tumors of the thyroid gland constitute 0.5% of all cancers, i.e., they are rare. In most cases, the tumor is a carcinoma of the thyroid gland. Far behind come lymphoma, sarcoma, and metastases of other tumors.

The following are risk factors:
- Genetic disposition
- Ionizing radiation. There was a 20-fold increase in carcinomas of the thyroid gland after the nuclear reactor catastrophe at Chernobyl.
- Iodine deficiency

Clinical Picture

- Evidence of a thyroid gland malignancy is a rapidly growing, fixed lump or a goiter that rapidly increases in size in spite of all treatment.
- As the disease progresses, compression and invasion of neighboring organs can cause the following symptoms:
  - Difficulty in swallowing
  - Dyspnea with stridor on inspiration
  - Hoarseness with damage to the recurrent nerve
  - Horner syndrome with narrowed pupils (miosis), drooping upper lid (ptosis), and the appearance of sunken eyeballs (enophthalmos) with damage to the cervical sympathetic trunk

– Superior vena cava congestion due to compression of large veins.
- Lymph node metastases may be palpable at the neck and above the collarbone.
- Distant metastases in lungs and bones can also produce symptoms.

Diagnosis

- Evidence in the patient history of radiation to the neck or a positive family history
- Visual or sensory findings
- Sonography
- "Cold nodes" in the scintigram; the lack of radionuclide concentration may also have other causes, e.g., cysts, and requires further clarification.
- Fine needle puncture
- Staging studies such as CT or MRI, to determine the size of the tumor

Therapy

In a radical thyroidectomy, the entire thyroid gland and regional neck lymph nodes are removed. About 3 weeks postoperatively, radioiodine therapy is begun (p. 235). Undifferentiated tumors not sensitive to radioiodine can be treated with percutaneous irradiation.

In any case, high-dose hormone replacement therapy is required in order to suppress secretion of TSH since TSH stimulates the growth of the tumor cells.

Diseases of the Adrenal Cortex

■ Physiological Principles

The adrenal cortex produces:
- Glucocorticosteroids (also: glucocorticoids), especially cortisol
- Mineral corticosteroids (mineralocorticoids), especially aldosterone
- Androgens

These hormones are steroid hormones, all derived from the starting material cholesterol (p. 220).

Glucocorticoids

Glucocorticoids are named after their effect on carbohydrate metabolism. Their main role is to make glucose and fatty acids available as energy sources by causing their release in greater quantities in stress situations. Their numerous effects are summarized in **Table 11.15**.

Table 11.15 Effect of glucocorticoids

Location of effect	Effect	Mechanisms
Carbohydrate, lipid and amino acid metabolism (alarm reaction)	Glucose availability	• Gluconeogenesis through catabolic action, i.e., protein breakdown in: – Muscles – Bones – Skin – Lymphatic tissue • Redistribution of fat
Coronary circulation (alarm reaction)	Elevated blood pressure	• Enhancement of epinephrine action • Vasoconstriction • Sodium and water retention by the kidneys
Kidneys	Decrease in diuresis	At higher doses, it acts like aldosterone, i.e., causes retention of sodium and water
Immune system	• Anti-inflammatory • Antiallergic • Immunosuppressive	At high doses it inhibits: • Lymphocyte formation • Antibody formation (proteins) • Phagocytosis • Histamine release
Stomach	Increase in production of gastric juice	
Brain	At high doses it causes: • Effects on the hypothalamus • Psychological alterations	

Glucocorticoid secretion by the adrenal gland is controlled by the corticotropin-releasing hormone (CRH) of the hypothalamus and by the adrenocorticotropic hormone (ACTH) of the pituitary gland.

Mineralocorticoids

Mineralocorticoids are named according to their effect on electrolyte balance. The functionally most important mineralocorticoid is aldosterone, which acts in the kidney to cause excretion of potassium and retention of sodium. The sodium retains water and diuresis decreases.

Secretion of aldosterone is regulated by the renin–angiotensin–aldosterone system (p. 85) and the potassium balance.

Androgens

In men, the androgens that are produced in the adrenal cortex play a subordinate role; considerably more androgens are produced in the testes. In women, more than 50% of the total androgens are produced in the adrenal cortex. They are responsible, first of all, for the secondary sex hair pattern and for anabolic effects.

Regulation of androgen production is also controlled by the ACTH of the pituitary gland.

▨ Excessive Adrenocortical Function

Cushing Syndrome

Forms and Causes

Cushing syndrome is caused by increased production of the body's glucocorticoids or by exogenous glucocorticoids. Another name for this disease is therefore *hypercortisolism.*

Exogenous Cushing Syndrome

The most common form is exogenous or iatrogenic Cushing syndrome caused by long-term treatment with glucocorticosteroids or ACTH.

Endogenous Cushing Syndrome

- Central Cushing syndrome: A pituitary adenoma (p. 230) produces uncontrolled ACTH, to which the adrenal cortex reacts with an overshoot of cortisol production.

- Paraneoplastic syndrome (p. 34): Some malignant tumors are able to produce ACTH, e.g., bronchial carcinoma.
- Adrenal Cushing syndrome: Tumors of the adrenal cortex that are not subject to the hormonal regulatory cycle can produce glucocorticosteroids even without ACTH stimulation.

Symptoms

Most symptoms are caused by the metabolic effects of cortisol (**Fig. 11.13a, b; Table 11.15**):
- Hyperglycemia is also called steroid induced diabetes (p. 215).
- Consequences of protein breakdown in skin, muscles and bones are:
  - Parchment skin
  - Hemorrhaging as a result of capillary fragility
  - Connective tissue weakness and tears in the dermis, leading to the typical red stripes (striae rubrae)
  - Disorders of wound healing
  - Muscle atrophy
  - Osteoporosis, also promoted by decreased calcium absorption in the intestine and increased calcium excretion by the kidneys
  - Rarely, aseptic bone necrosis.

> In physiotherapy, the relevant factors are especially osteoporosis, parchment skin and fragile vessels.

- The redistribution of fat deposits results in the full-moon face, bull neck and torso obesity.

Further consequences of hypercortisolism are:
- Secondary arterial hypertension (p. 117)
- Tendency to edema
- Susceptibility to infections
- Gastric ulcers (ulcus ventriculi, p. 180)
- Psychological alterations, such as depression
- Loss of libido and impotence in men, since cortisol inhibits LH secretion by the pituitary gland
- Menstrual disorders in women. If the underlying disease is Cushing disease, ACTH causes increased release of androgens, so that women develop masculine characteristics.

Diagnosis

Patient history and clinical findings are indicative. Diagnosis is based on the following laboratory findings:
- Plasma cortisol levels over the course of the day are elevated and the diurnal rhythm is interrupted.

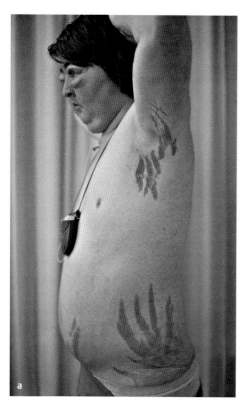 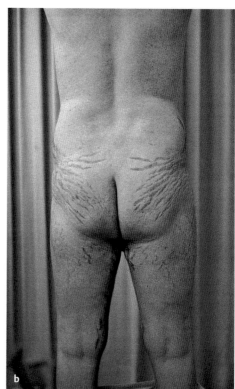

Fig. 11.13a, b Patient with Cushing syndrome. Marked torso obesity and striae rubrae. (Gerlach 2000.)

- Cortisol excretion in the urine is elevated.
- Dexamethasone inhibition test: Dexamethasone is a highly potent synthetic glucocorticosteroid. After administration of dexamethasone a healthy individual produces less cortisol in the adrenal cortex (negative feedback). In Cushing syndrome, the plasma cortisol level does not fall.
- CRH (corticotropin-releasing hormone) stimulation test to screen for the cause: CRH is injected intravenously. ACTH rises in central Cushing syndrome. In adrenal or paraneoplastic Cushing syndrome, pituitary function is intact and, because of negative feedback, there is no increase in ACTH.

The tumor is localized by imaging procedures such as sonography, CT, or MRI.

Therapy

- The therapy of choice for ACTH-producing pituitary tumors is surgical removal.
- In the adrenal form, the affected adrenal gland is removed surgically. At first, after adrenalectomy, steroid hormones must be replaced until the other adrenal gland has taken over the function of both.

- In paraneoplastic Cushing syndrome, the underlying neoplasm must be treated.

Conn Syndrome

Conn syndrome is also called *primary hyperaldosteronism*. It is caused by aldosterone-producing adrenocortical adenoma and more rarely by carcinoma or adrenocortical hyperplasia.

A distinction must be made between Conn syndrome and secondary hyperaldosteronism that develops when renin production by the kidneys is triggered, for example, in kidney disease.

Symptoms

- All affected individuals have secondary arterial hypertension because of decreased diuresis and elevated plasma volume (p. 117).
- Hypokalemia is characterized by headache, fatigue, muscle weakness, lameness, and constipation.

- Hydrogen ions are in equilibrium with potassium ions. As a result, hypokalemia produces alkalosis that can lead to paresthesia and tetany.

Diagnosis

Typical laboratory parameters are:
- Hypokalemia, hypernatremia, and alkalosis
- An elevated aldosterone level with depressed renin level; in secondary hyperaldosteronism, however, renin is elevated.

Space-occupying lesions in the adrenal glands are localized by means of CT or MRI.

Therapy

An adrenocortical adenoma is removed laparoscopically, whereas patients with adrenocortical hyperplasia are treated pharmaceutically with spironolactone, an aldosterone antagonist.

■ Adrenocortical Insufficiency

Definition and Causes

Adrenocortical insufficiency is marked by decreased production of cortisol and aldosterone.
- The *primary form* is caused by the adrenal gland itself. The most common cause is Addison disease, in which autoimmune processes damage the adrenal cortex. Less frequently, infectious diseases such as tuberculosis and cytomegaly in AIDS patients, as well as hemorrhage and metastases of the adrenal cortex, can lead to primary adrenocortical insufficiency.
- In the *secondary form,* the stimulation of the adrenal cortex disappears with the loss of ACTH. Causes are disorders in the hypothalamus or the pituitary gland. Even in long-term treatment with corticosteroids, ACTH secretion by the pituitary gland is suppressed by the feedback mechanism (p. 229).

Symptoms and Complications

If more than 90% of the adrenal cortex is destroyed, the decreased hormone production causes hypoglycemia, increased diuresis and electrolyte shift with the following signs of disease:
- Fatigue and weakness
- Nausea and vomiting
- Diarrhea or constipation
- Weight loss
- Arterial hypotension
- In the primary form, skin and mucosa are hyperpigmented, since the increased ACTH released also stimulates the melanocytes in the skin.

There is a threat of an *Addison crisis.* The symptoms described are intensified and result in:
- Massive decrease in blood pressure up to and including shock
- Fever as a result of dehydration
- Consequences of hypoglycemia (**Table 11.2**)
- Altered states of consciousness or even coma

Diagnosis

Patient history and clinical picture lead to a suspected diagnosis that is confirmed by laboratory studies:
- Hyponatremia and hyperkalemia
- Decreased serum cortisol
- Primary form with elevated serum ACTH, secondary form with depressed serum ACTH
- ACTH test: After intravenous injection of ACTH, in primary adrenocortical insufficiency there is no rise in serum cortisol.
- Autoantibodies in Addison disease

Sonography, CT, and MRI can be used to demonstrate processes in the pituitary or the adrenal glands.

Therapy

Patients with primary adrenocortical insufficiency must replace glucocorticoids and mineralocorticoids orally for the rest of their lives. In the secondary form, the administration of glucocorticoids is sufficient.

12 Hematology

Physiological Principles

■ Composition of Blood

The blood volume of an adult represents 6%–8% of body weight. The blood consists of cellular elements and fluid plasma (**Table 12.1**).
- The proportion of blood volume occupied by red blood cells is called the *hematocrit*.
- Serum is the portion of the *plasma* separated from clotting factors.

■ Erythrocytes

Morphology

Erythrocytes have no nucleus. They have the shape of a round-to-oval biconcave disk with a diameter of about 8 µm and a thickness of about 2 µm. Their red color is provided by hemoglobin, which serves to transport oxygen and carbon dioxide. Hemoglobin consists of four amino acid chains (globin) to each of which a heme molecule is bound. The central iron ion of the heme group can bind an oxygen molecule reversibly. The erythrocyte membrane carries the blood group antigens.

Life Cycle

Like all blood cells, the erythrocytes originate in the pluripotent stem cells of the blood-forming (hematopoietic) bone marrow (**Fig. 12.1**). Iron is one of the components necessary for erythropoiesis. It is provided by food or reclaimed from the breakdown products of erythrocytes. After a life of about 120 days, erythrocytes are broken down in the spleen (hemolysis). The heme released in hemolysis is metabolized to bilirubin and secreted in the bile (p. 44).

■ Leukocytes

Classification

Leukocytes include:
- Granulocytes
- Lymphocytes
- Monocytes (**Fig. 12.1**)

Defensive Function

Leukocytes have a defensive function, which can only be presented here in very simplified form.

Microorganisms invading the organism activate B lymphocytes, which can distinguish between the body's own substance and foreign substances. After contact with antigens, B lymphocytes become either plasma cells or memory cells.
- *Plasma cells* produce specific antibodies called immunoglobulins. The "invader" is marked by the antibodies and other elements of the defense system, e.g., phagocytes, that gather to eliminate it.
- *Memory cells* register the structure of the antibodies and if this antigen appears again, they provide a more rapid and stronger immune response (booster effect).

■ Hemostasis

When a blood vessel is injured, hemostasis is required. This is a complex interplay of:
- Vessel wall
- Platelets (platelets)
- Clotting factors

Table 12.1 Blood composition

Cells (about 42%)	Plasma (about 58%)
• Erythrocytes (red blood cells) • Leukocytes (white blood cells) • Platelets (blood platelets) The normal values are given in **Table 12.2**)	• Water (about 90% of the plasma) • Proteins, e.g., clotting factors, antibodies, etc. (about 8% of the plasma) • Electrolytes • Glucose • Hormones • Metabolic products e.g., creatinine and urea

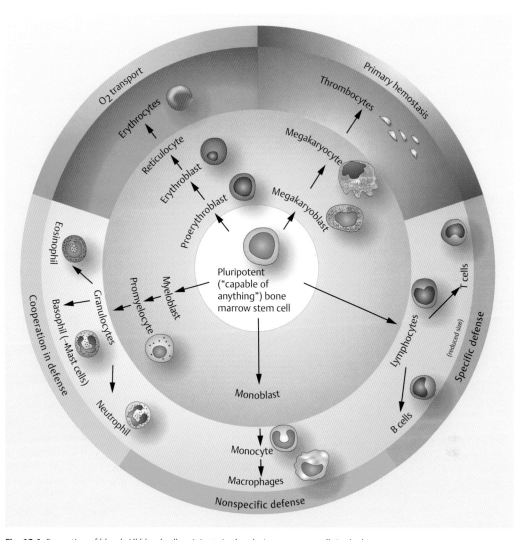

Fig. 12.1 Formation of blood: All blood cells originate in the pluripotent stem cells in the bone marrow.

Primary Hemostasis

When a vessel is injured, platelets adhere to the collagen fibers below the injured intima. The platelets are activated by mediators like the von Willebrand factor, which is released by damaged endothelial cells. These activated platelets release mediators such as thromboxane and serotonin, which cause vasoconstriction and platelet aggregation. The resulting clump of platelets, called a white thrombus, temporarily blocks the leak.

Clotting

The white thrombus produced by primary hemostasis is unstable. It must be covered by a stabilizing network of fibrin (red thrombus). Fibrin is the product of blood clotting, also called secondary hemostasis. **Figure 12.2** shows the cascade of events in the activation of clotting factors produced by the liver. Vitamin K is required for the synthesis of some clotting factors.

Clotting Inhibitors

To avoid an overshoot in the production of fibrin, there are natural inhibitors that act at different points in the clotting cascade (**Fig. 12.2**). Important inhibitors are:

- Protein S
- Protein C
- Antithrombin III (AT III), which inhibits the transformation of prothrombin into thrombin

Fibrinolysis

Tiny amounts of fibrin are constantly being formed in intact vessels and immediately broken down again by the fibrinolytic system. Plasminogen is activated for this purpose. Plasmin is produced, which breaks the fibrin down into fibrin fragments (**Fig. 12.3**).

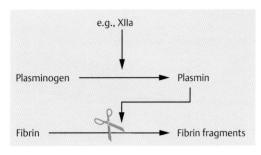

Fig. 12.3 Fibrinolysis

Cardinal Hematological Symptoms

Important hematological symptoms are:

- Unspecific general symptoms that are considered as a whole as "B symptoms"
- Susceptibility to infections (p. 30)
- Lymph node enlargement (p. 53)
- Tendency to hemorrhage (p. 46)
- Tendency to excessively produce clots (p. 131)

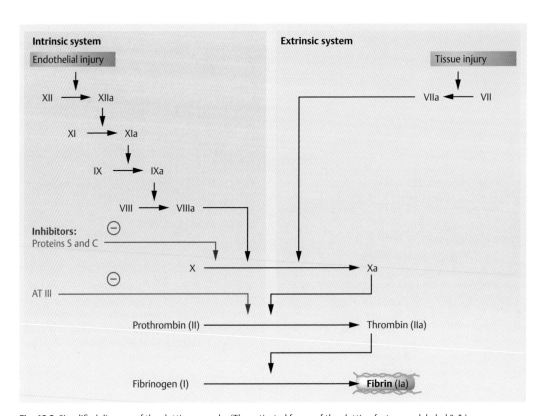

Fig. 12.2 Simplified diagram of the clotting cascade. (The activated forms of the clotting factors are labeled "a".)

B Symptoms

The B symptoms with an unfavorable prognosis include:
- Fever
- Night sweats
- Loss of more than 10% of body weight within 6 months

Hematological Diagnosis

■ Blood Count

The blood count (BC) determines the number of erythrocytes, leukocytes, and platelets (**Table 12.2**). The values for hemoglobin and hematocrit are closely related to the erythrocyte count. Additional parameters are:
- The average volume of an erythrocyte, also called median corpuscular volume (MCV)
- The average hemoglobin concentration, also called median corpuscular hemoglobin (MCH)

For some issues, leukocytes must be classified into subgroups and stage of maturity.

■ Clotting Status

The individual steps of hemostasis are monitored by means of various laboratory values (**Table 12.3**).
- The *platelet count* is included in the blood count.
- To measure the *bleeding time*, which is normally less than 6 minutes, the patient is pricked with a lancet and the time to the end of bleeding is measured.

- The *Quick value*, also called the *thromboplastin or prothrombin time*, is a check of the extrinsic clotting system. The normal value is 70%–100%.
- The Quick value depends on the reagents used, so that results from different laboratories are difficult to compare. For this reason, it is more usual to give the *international normalized ratio* (INR). The normal value is 1.0.
- The *partial thromboplastin time* (PTT) is a check of the intrinsic clotting system. The normal value is 30–40 seconds.
- In certain problems, it is possible to determine the activity of various clotting factors, AT III, and fibrin breakdown products (D-dimers).

Table 12.3 Clotting status (INR = international normalized ratio, PTT = partial thromboplastin time)

Process examined	Laboratory parameters	Normal value
Hemostasis	Platelet count	140–345 × 10⁹/L
	Bleeding time	<6 min
Extrinsic clotting	Quick value	70%–100%
	INR	1.0
Intrinsic clotting	PTT	30–40 s

■ Bone Marrow Studies

Bone Marrow Aspiration

Bone marrow aspiration is carried out on the posterior pelvic crest and in rare cases on the sternum to obtain bone marrow. Aspiration cytology is particularly useful for diagnosis of:

Table 12.2 Normal values for blood count (p. 245)

Parameter	Women	Men
Erythrocytes	3.9–5.3 × 10¹²/L	4.3–5.7 × 10¹²/L
Hematocrit (Hct)	37%–48%	40%–52%
Hemoglobin (Hb)	7.4–9.9 mmol/L (12–16 g/dL)	8.3–10.5 mmol/L (13.5–17 g/dL)
Leukocytes	3.8–10.5 × 10⁹/L	
Platelets	140–345 × 10⁹/L	
Mean corpuscular volume (MCV)	85–98 fL	
Mean corpuscular hemoglobin (MCH)	28–34 pg/cell	

Bone Marrow Biopsy

A bone marrow biopsy must be taken from the pelvic crest for histological examination. It is indicated if bone marrow aspiration was unsuccessful and no cells could be aspirated. This technique is used when there is suspicion of:

- Osteomyelosclerosis, in which the bone marrow that produces the blood is fibrosed and ceases to function
- Myeloproliferative diseases, in which the bone marrow produces an increased number of cells of one cell line
- Granulomatous bone diseases such as sarcoidosis (p. 162) and tuberculosis (p. 268)

Anemia

Overview

Definition

Anemia is present when the hemoglobin concentration (Hb), the hematocrit (Hct), or the erythrocyte count is decreased below normal. Hb and Hct are the most sensitive parameters for detecting anemia (**Table 12.4**).

Causes

Anemia can develop if too few erythrocytes are produced, too many erythrocytes are broken down, or erythrocytes are lost.

Anemia caused by *production disorders* arise when:

- Function of the erythropoietic stem cells in the bone marrow is impaired or inhibited, e.g., in toxic damage to the bone marrow or in diseases that affect the bone marrow, such as leukemia or other hematological diseases (p. 247).
- Hemoglobin formation is impaired, as in iron deficiency (see below).
- Maturation of erythrocyte nuclei is impaired, as in vitamin B_{12} or folic acid deficiency (see below).
- There is an erythropoietin deficiency in consequence of a kidney disease (renal anemia, p. 209).

Table 12.4 Laboratory diagnosis in anemia

Parameters		Decreased	Increased
Blood count	Hemoglobin (Hb)	• Men <8.1 mmol/L (13.0 g/dL) • Women <7.4 mmol/L (12.0 g/dL)	–
	Hematocrit (Hct)	• Men <40% • Women <37%	–
	Reticulocytes (young erythrocytes)	Formation disorder	Elevated erythropoiesis, e.g., in: • Hemolytic anemia • Successful anemia treatment
	Mean corpuscular volume (MCV)	Microcytic anemia, e.g., in iron deficiency anemia	Megaloblastic anemia, e.g., in pernicious anemia
	Mean corpuscular hemoglobin (MCH)	Hypochromic anemia, e.g., in iron deficiency anemia	Hyperchromic anemia, e.g., in pernicious anemia
Iron status	Serum iron	• Iron deficiency anemia • Tumor anemia	• Hemolytic anemia • Pernicious anemia
	Ferritin (iron-storage protein)	Iron deficiency anemia	Tumor anemia
	Transferrin (iron-transport protein)	Tumor anemia	Iron deficiency anemia

Hemolytic anemia results from *increased erythro-cyte breakdown*. The cause is structurally changed erythrocytes with a shortened lifespan.
- These forms can be congenital, for example, in spherocytosis with membrane defects, sickle cell anemia, or thalassemia with hemoglobin changes.
- Numerous acquired forms are due to factors that damage erythrocytes, such as antibodies, medications, physical and chemical agents, or infectious diseases like malaria (p. 285).

Hemorrhagic anemia results from blood loss.

Iron Deficiency Anemia

> *At 80% incidence, iron deficiency is the most frequent cause of anemia.*

Causes include:
- Insufficient iron in the diet
- Malabsorption of iron, e.g., after gastric resection, in malassimilation syndrome (p. 173)
- Increased demand for iron in growing children and women during menstruation, pregnancy, and lactation
- Iron loss through chronic bleeding, e.g., from the gastrointestinal tract or other organs, as a result of menstrual bleeding, surgical or trauma-induced bleeding, frequent blood draws or blood donation, and where there is a tendency to hemorrhage

Pernicious Anemia

Vitamin B$_{12}$ deficiency can result, for example, from type A gastritis, caused by autoimmune processes (p. 179). Autoantibodies attack the parietal cells of the gastric corpus which, in addition to hydrochloric acid, produce *intrinsic factor*. If this substance is missing, vitamin B$_{12}$ cannot be absorbed by the small intestine. As a consequence of vitamin B$_{12}$ deficiency, formation of blood is limited and the result is pernicious anemia.

Symptoms

Anemia causes pale mucosa and general symptoms such as fatigue, tiredness, decreased physical capacity, and in some cases tachycardia and dyspnea on exertion because of the decreased number of oxygen carriers in the blood.

In addition to the symptoms of the underlying disease, certain consequences are typical for a few forms of anemia:

- In manifest iron deficiency, skin and mucosal symptoms such as disturbances in nail growth, rhagades (small cracks) in the corners of the mouth, burning sensation in the tongue and swallowing disorders, as well as headache, lack of concentration, and inner unrest
- Vitamin B$_{12}$ deficiency is expressed by neurological symptoms such as polyneuropathy, spinal ataxia, and gastrointestinal complaints.
- Folic acid deficiency in pregnancy can cause defects in the embryonic neural tube, leading to spina bifida.

Diagnosis

Patient history and clinical findings lead to a suspected diagnosis that is confirmed by the blood count. One of the factors investigated to clarify the cause of the anemia is the iron status (**Table 12.4**).

Therapy

Treatment depends on the underlying disease. Deficiency of iron, folic acid, vitamin B$_{12}$, or erythropoietin is treated by supplementation. In pronounced cases of anemia, a transfusion of erythrocytes may be required.

Leukemia

Leukemias are malignant diseases of the blood-producing system that can attack all organs, in addition to bone marrow and blood. Untreated, leukemia has a mortality of 70%–100%. In the year 2010, over 43 000 new cases of leukemia were diagnosed in the United States. Around 250 000 people in the United States are currently living with or in remission from leukemia.

Pathogenesis and Causes

In leukemia, there is uncontrolled and uninhibited production of one type of white blood cell as a result of a stem cell defect (**Fig. 12.4**). These cells do not mature at all or mature insufficiently to perform their function. They impair normal blood production so that the number of effective leukocytes as well as erythrocytes and platelets decreases.

The causes of this process have not yet been completely understood, but certain factors have been identified that are associated with an elevated risk of contracting the disease. Risk factors are:

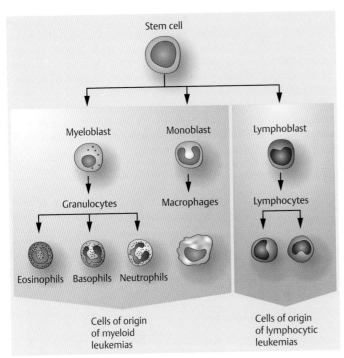

Fig. 12.4 Diagram of leukocyte origin: cells of origin for myeloid and lymphocytic leukemias.

Stem cell

Myeloblast   Monoblast   Lymphoblast

Granulocytes   Macrophages   Lymphocytes

Eosinophils Basophils Neutrophils

Cells of origin of myeloid leukemias

Cells of origin of lymphocytic leukemias

- Ionizing radiation, i.e., radioactivity and X-rays, which at high doses can trigger genetic changes in the blood-forming cells
- Chemical substances, e.g., insecticides, herbicides, organic solvents, and others
- Certain medications, e.g., cytostatics and immunosuppressants that impair bone marrow function
- Genetic disposition; for instance, Down syndrome carries an 18-fold risk for leukemia

Classification

Leukemias are classified according to their course into acute and chronic forms, and according to the origin of the affected blood cells into lymphocytic and myeloid leukemias (**Fig. 12.4**). The resulting categories are:
- Chronic lymphocytic leukemia (CLL)
- Chronic myeloid leukemia (CML)
- Acute lymphocytic leukemia (ALL)
- Acute myeloid leukemia (AML)

This distinction has clinical relevance since both symptoms and course of the disease as well as treatment strategy and prognosis are different for the different forms.

Chronic leukemias have an insidious course and often remain unnoticed over a long period. The leu-kemia cells appear in mature form, for example, as lymphocytes in chronic lymphocytic leukemia or as leukocytes in chronic myeloid leukemia.

Acute leukemias are rapidly progressing diseases characterized by the appearance in the peripheral blood of immature blood cells, so-called *blasts*. The typical childhood leukemia is acute lymphocytic leukemia in which the lymphocyte precursors in the bone marrow undergo malignant changes. Acute myeloid leukemia occurs more frequently in adults. It is characterized by degradation of leukocyte precursor cells in the bone marrow. Various types of these leukemias are distinguished, depending on the type of cell affected, for example, myeloblastic or monoblastic leukemia.

Symptoms

The disease begins with general signs of illness, such as loss of appetite, unexplained weight loss, elevated body temperature, and night sweats. The following symptoms can be ascribed to disrupted blood formation:
- Anemia as a consequence of decreased erythrocyte production causes paleness, decreased physical capacity, tiredness and fatigue.
- The reduced platelet count inclines patients to nosebleeds, bleeding gums, petechiae and hema-

tomas and bleedings that are difficult to control after trivial injuries (p. 46).

Since the pathologically increased white blood cells are nonfunctioning, susceptibility to infections increases.

If the disease is advanced, the organs may be infiltrated. The following are possible:

Swollen lymph nodes

Enlargement of liver and spleen, called hepatosplenomegaly

Joint and bone pain

CNS involvement with headache, vomiting, cranial nerve palsy, and seizures

Diagnosis

Patient history, thorough physical examination, and laboratory tests:

Blood count and bone marrow studies provide information as to which blood cell group is affected. Typically a chromosome analysis can provide evidence of the so-called Philadelphia chromosome in the leukemia cells in CML, sometimes even in ALL.

Imaging techniques such as radiography, sonography, CT, and MRI are used for staging, which determines the extent of organ and lymph node involvement.

Therapy and Prognosis

The principal component of leukemia treatment is chemotherapy. Depending on the clinical picture and the course of the individual disease, it can be supplemented or replaced by other forms of therapy, such as radiation therapy, administration of hormonelike substances, or bone marrow transplantation.

Acute Leukemia

After the diagnosis is established, there is intensive and aggressive therapy in specialized hematological centers.

In the first phase of treatment, the *induction treatment*, in-patient combined chemotherapy is administered in order to destroy the majority of leukemia cells and thus achieve a full remission, the most complete elimination possible of all manifestations. In ALL patients, irradiation of the skull may be required to destroy leukemia cells in the meninges.

> Since chemotherapy destroys all leukocytes, the patient is highly susceptible to infections and must therefore be in protective isolation (reverse barrier nursing).

In addition there may be consolidation cycles and maintenance therapy, which can be administered on an outpatient basis, with regular monitoring. The objective is to turn remission into cure, i.e., to prevent relapses caused by remaining leukemia cells.

> Induction treatment → Complete remission.
> Maintenance therapy → Cure.

Treatment lasts about 2–3 years. A patient who remains in remission for 5 years is considered cured. Up to 80% of all children and 40% of all adults with ALL can be cured. AML is often associated with relapses. Therefore, every attempt is made to achieve early allogenic bone marrow transplantation (BMT) or stem cell transplantation (SCT).

Chronic Leukemia

- CML is associated with a chromosome defect (Philadelphia chromosome). It is treatable with the tyrosine kinase inhibitor Imatinib, among other drugs. A definitive cure is only possible with BMT or SCT.
- CLL is a disease of old age. It is not curable but it progresses very slowly and does not always require treatment. Chemotherapy or immune-modulating therapy is only indicated for symptomatic patients or a complicated course.

Bone Marrow and Stem Cell Transplantation

For many leukemia patients, chiefly with AML or CML, transplantation of bone marrow or stem cells is the only possibility for a cure. BMT and SCT are performed in centers where the facilities and the personnel are specialized in this treatment.

Requirements

To receive BMT or SCT, the patient must have achieved remission through a previous course of chemotherapy and must be free of infection. Other factors, such as age and general condition of the patient, affect the decision to undertake a transplantation, which is a stressful and risky treatment.

Course

- Preparation for the transplantation is *conditioning*, in which all the patient's leukemia cells and stem cells are destroyed to the fullest extent possible by high-dose chemotherapy and, where applicable, by whole-body irradiation.
- After conditioning, the stem cells are transferred intravenously. They settle in the bone marrow and produce all the blood cell lines throughout the patient's lifetime. In BMT these cells are obtained from the bone marrow and in SCT from the circulating blood after special pretreatment.
- It takes 1 year for the body's own defense system to become completely intact again. Patients are specially trained to minimize the risk of infection.

Donors

In principle, either autologous or foreign donors are possible.

Autologous Transplantation

In this procedure, patients receive their own bone marrow or stem cells back after they have been cleared of leukemia cells as completely as possible.

Allogenous Transplantation

The patient receives bone marrow or stem cells from a family member or an unrelated donor. The donor must have tissue characteristics compatible with those of the recipient (histocompatibility) to minimize rejection reactions of the donated bone marrow against the recipient's body. Between siblings, the chances of finding a compatible donor are about 25%. In the United States, compatible unrelated donors are located through regional and national registries.

It should be noted that patients with a bone marrow transplant have the donor's blood group after the treatment.

Complications and Aftercare

- Typical cytostatic side-effects occur during conditioning therapy (p. 68).
- During the bone marrow suppression, patients are still at risk for about 3–6 weeks of infections and a septic course. Patients must remain in isolation units and receive antibiotics and antimycotics. During this time, the foreign bone marrow grows and blood production becomes normal again.

- Rejection reactions are particularly possible in allogenous transplantation. In such a reaction, the transplant attacks the host and the dreaded *graft versus host disease* (GVHD) sets in. This disease primarily attacks skin, liver, and the intestines and, where the course of the disease is severe, requires immunosuppressive therapy. When the defense reaction attacks leukemia cells remaining in the body, this desirable effect is called *graft versus tumor effect*.
- Late consequences of BMT or SCT are usually the result of the high-dose chemotherapy, e.g., infertility in women and men.

Malignant Lymphoma

Lymphomas are malignant diseases of the lymphatic system caused by degraded lymphatic cells and manifesting at various lymph node stations and organs. On the basis of histological criteria, Hodgkin lymphoma (Hodgkin disease) is distinguished from B- and T-cell diseases, which are grouped together as non–Hodgkin lymphomas.

■ Hodgkin Disease

The disease, which is also known as lymphogranulomatosis, is local at first and then develops into a systemic disease attacking extralymphatic organs as well. The origin is a degraded B lymphocyte line the Hodgkin–Reed–Sternberg cells. The etiology is unknown; the role of HIV or Epstein–Barr virus infection (mononucleosis, p. 277), is discussed as a cofactor. It is probable that genetic disposition is a factor.

The age-adjusted incidence of Hodgkin lymphoma in the United States is 2.8 cases per 100 000 individuals. Men are affected somewhat more frequently than women. There are two peaks in age distribution of the disease: the first peak is at the age of 30 years and the second is at the age of 60 in Europe and the United States.

Symptoms and Staging

- Hodgkin lymphoma is usually localized in a lymph node group, at first expressed by swollen lymph nodes that often begin in the head and neck region, more rarely in the chest or armpits. The swollen lymph nodes are not painful.
- In the course of the disease, several lymph node stations and possibly even extralymphatic organs.

such as skin, liver, lungs, bone marrow, bones, pleura, and spleen are affected (**Table 12.5**).

- B symptoms (p. 245) can set in. They are signs of an unfavorable prognosis: fever, night sweats, weight loss of more than 10% of body weight in the last 6 months.

Diagnosis and Therapy

Histological confirmation of the diagnosis is a requirement for therapy. For this purpose, an affected lymph node is surgically removed and examined. Knowledge of the extent of spread as well as of the histological subgroup at the time of diagnosis is important for prognosis and therapy. The manifestations are determined by:

- Medical history in which the patient is queried about B symptoms
- Physical examination for palpably enlarged lymph nodes
- Laboratory studies
- Bone marrow and liver biopsy
- Imaging

Treatment with curative intent takes place in specialist centers after first-line therapy protocols using polychemotherapy and additional irradiation. Side-effects and consequences of chemotherapy and irradiation have already been discussed on page 66.

Prognosis

Cure rates of 50%–90% can be achieved, depending on the stage of the disease. About 50% of patients experience complete remission. However, the overall favorable prognosis is associated with late consequences of radiation therapy and chemotherapy.

■ Non–Hodgkin Lymphomas

Overview

Frequency and Causes

The majority of persons afflicted with non–Hodgkin lymphoma (NHL) are older people and AIDS patients (p. 283). Annually up to 19.8 in 100 000 people contract NHL. The tendency is increasing.

NHL arises from B or T lymphocytes with malignant transformation and, as in Hodgkin disease, can affect other tissues and organs in addition to the lymphatic organs. The most frequently affected organs are the gastrointestinal tract, bones, skin, and the brain.

The following factors have etiological significance:

- Immune deficiencies, e.g., as late complications of immunosuppressive or cytostatic therapy, in HIV infection, and in autoimmune diseases
- Irradiation, radioactive substances
- Infections, e.g., with Epstein–Barr virus in Burkitt lymphoma and *Helicobacter* infection in MALT lymphoma of the stomach
- Genetic alterations

Classification

The NHL group comprises numerous diseases that can be histologically and clinically distinguished. Examples are listed in **Table 12.6**. They overlap in part with other hematological diseases such as leukemias (CLL; p. 247).

Table 12.5 Simplified staging for Hodgkin disease (Ann Arbor Classification; LN = lymph node)

Stage	Definition
Stage 1	A single LN region affected
Stage II	2 or more LN regions on one side of the diaphragm affected
Stage III	2 or more LN regions on both sides of the diaphragm affected
Stage IV	One or more extralymphatic organs affected extensively with or without LN being affected
Additive A Additive B	No general symptoms B symptoms

Table 12.6 Simplified Classification of the NHL (WHO 2001)

B cell line (80%–85%)	T cell line (15%–20%)
Precursor B cell neoplasms, e.g., precursor cell B lymphoblastic lymphoma	Precursor T cell neoplasms, e.g., precursor cell T lymphoblastic lymphoma
Mature B cell neoplasias, e.g.: • Plasmacytoma (see below): • CLL (p. 247) • Hair cell leukemia • Immunocytoma • MALT gastric lymphoma • Mantle cell lymphoma • Diffuse large-cell B cell lymphoma • Burkitt lymphoma	Mature T cell neoplasias, e.g.: • Fungoid mycosis • Nonspecific T cell lymphoma

Diagnosis and Therapy

Diagnosis of NHL is comparable to that of Hodgkin disease. Therapy depends on the underlying neoplasia and usually consists of polychemotherapy.

Plasmacytoma

Plasmacytoma (multiple myeloma) is a neoplastic plasma cell disease caused by numerous factors. It occurs principally in older people. A plasma cell line exhibiting malignant proliferation produces excessive identical but inactive immunoglobulins.

Consequences

- Malignant plasma cells infiltrate the bone marrow and cause osteolysis (**Fig. 12.5a, b**). Bone pain is a typical resulting symptom. Pathological fractures are also possible.
- Since normal blood production is impaired, anemia and increased susceptibility to infection set in over the course of the disease.
- The immunoglobulins coat the platelets and impair their function (thrombocytopathy; p. 253).
- The massively increased production of immunoglobulins overloads the kidneys and can lead to kidney failure.

In physiotherapy, the principal concern must be with increased risk of fracture.

Diagnosis and Therapy

Diagnostic indicators are laboratory studies, skeletal radiographs, and histological examination of bone marrow.

The disease progresses chronically. Usually a curative approach is not available.

- Tumor-modifying chemotherapy is adapted to the individual case.
- For patients under 60 years of age, allogenous stem cell transplantation can be considered (p. 247).
- Solitary plasmacytomas can be irradiated.
- Pathological fractures are treated surgically.

Disorders of Hemostasis and Clotting

▪ Thrombocytopenia

Definition and Causes

Thrombocytopenia is characterized by a platelet count below 140×10^9/L (140 000/µL). Thrombocytopenia, the most frequent cause of a tendency to hemorrhage, is mainly caused by a disorder of formation in the bone marrow or by increased breakdown.

Decreased Platelet Formation

The formation of platelets in the bone marrow can be impaired by congenital or acquired factors:

- Damage to the bone marrow through medications such as cytostatics, chemicals such as benzene, and ionizing radiation as in radiotherapy

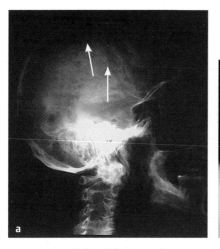
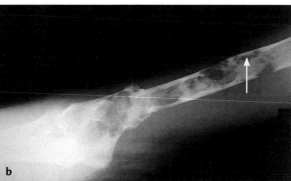

Fig. 12.5a, b Radiological findings in plasmacytoma. **a** Small spot osteolysis in the skull cap. **b** Extensive osteolysis in the humerus (Baenkler 2001).

- Bone marrow infiltration in malignant diseases, e.g., leukemia (p. 247) and malignant lymphomas (p. 250)
- Osteomyelosclerosis, in which the blood-forming bone marrow fibroses and loses its functionality

Increased Turnover

Increased breakdown of platelets is often caused by autoimmune processes:
- Idiopathic thrombocytopenic purpura (ITP), which can arise as postinfectious ITP or as a chronic ITP (Werlhof disease)
- Secondary immunothrombocytopenia in known underlying diseases such as systemic lupus erythematosus (p. 261)
- Drug-induced immunothrombocytopenia, e.g., induced by heparins

Further causes leading to increased turnover of platelets are:
- Increased consumption in consumptive coagulopathy (p. 255)
- Enlarged spleen (hypersplenism) resulting in increased capture of blood cells
- Artificial heart valves that damage platelets mechanically

Clinical Picture

As long as the count of functional platelets remains above 30×10^9/L (30 000/µL) and the clotting system is intact, there is no danger of hemorrhage. Petechial bleeding with punctiform hemorrhages (p. 46) is characteristic for thrombocytopenia (p. 46).

> Platelets $< 30 \times 10^9$/L (30 000/µL)
> → Danger of hemorrhage

Diagnosis

- Patient history and clinical picture
- Blood count
- Bleeding time extended beyond 6 minutes
- Screening for causes, e.g., autoantibody screening

Therapy

The basic procedure is causal treatment. Replacement of platelets is only undertaken after rigorous establishment of indication and in the case of hemorrhage.

Idiopathic Thrombocytopenic Purpura

At first, the ITP is observed without taking any action. Glucocorticosteroids are not administered until the platelet count falls below 30×10^9/L (30 000/µL). Possibly immunosuppressants and surgical removal of the spleen (splenectomy) may become necessary.

■ Thrombocytopathy

Definition and Causes

Functional disorders of the platelets are called thrombocytopathies. Congenital thrombocytopathies are rare. Some causes of acquired functional disorders are:
- Therapy with platelet aggregation inhibitors such as acetylsalicylic acid (p. 73)
- Plasmacytoma (p. 251), in which the platelets are coated with immunoglobulins
- "Uremic poisons" in chronic kidney failure (p. 209)

Clinical Picture

Spontaneous bleeding does not usually occur in thrombocytopathy. The disorder is not manifest until hemostasis becomes problematic in cases of injury or surgery.

Diagnosis and Therapy

- Patient history and clinical picture
- Extended bleeding time
- Search for causes

Diagnosis is followed by causal treatment.

■ Hemophilia

Importance and Forms

This familial disease is the second most frequent congenital coagulopathy, after von Willebrand syndrome (p. 254); one male in 10 000 is affected. Since inheritance of hemophilia is X-linked recessive, usually only boys and men have the disease (p. 13). In 30% of affected individuals, there is no mention of the disease in the family history and it must be attributed to a new mutation.

Two forms are distinguished, depending on which clotting factor is absent.
- In 85% of cases, the disease is hemophilia A, in which Factor VIII is inactive or absent. The vari-

Table 12.7 Degree of severity of hemophilia A

Degree of severity	Factor VIII activity	Consequences
Normal	>75%	None
Subhemophilia	16%–50%	Usually asymptomatic
Mild hemophilia	5%–15%	Hematomas after significant trauma and postoperative bleeding
Moderate hemophilia	1%–5%	Hematomas after even slight trauma
Severe hemophilia	<1%	Spontaneous bleeding and hemarthroses

ous degrees of severity of hemophilia A are summarized in **Table 12.7**.

- Fifteen percent of patients have hemophilia B (Christmas disease), in which Factor IX is inactive or absent.

Consequences

Depending on the degree of severity, one of the following may result:

- Spontaneous bleeding or hemorrhage after minor trauma, leading to extensive hematomas (p. 46)
- Dreaded CNS bleeding or bleeding in the mouth and throat
- Bleeding in the muscles, especially the psoas muscle, leading to modification of the muscle and contractures
- Hemorrhages in the joints, called hemarthroses, which can lead to permanent limitations
- Mucosal hemorrhages
- Postoperative hemorrhages

Diagnosis

The following parameters are indicative for diagnosis:

- Partial thromboplastin time
- Factor VIII or Factor IX activity

Therapy

The purpose of therapy is to allow the patient to lead as normal a life as possible. The most important objective is prophylaxis of hemorrhage. For this purpose, patients learn how they can replace Factor VIII or Factor IX intravenously themselves, as needed. In mild cases, administration of desmopressin can be enough to release the clotting factors stored in the endothelium.

Timely initiated physiotherapy is aimed at avoiding loss of function through joint and muscle hemorrhage. Damaged joints require surgical joint replacement.

All physiotherapeutic measures must take into account the increased risk of bleeding.

Complications of Therapy

- Up to 30% of patients develop antibodies against Factor VIII. Attempts are made in specialized centers to counter this antibody hemophilia with high doses of Factor VIII. Sometimes the antibodies must be removed from the blood by plasmapheresis.
- The risk of hepatitis or HIV infection through Factor VIII preparations or blood transfusions is low in the meantime.

■ Von Willebrand Syndrome

In von Willebrand syndrome (vWS), the von Willebrand factor, which plays a decisive role in hemostasis, and clotting Factor VIII are defective or absent. About 1% of the population has this clotting disorder, which is thus the most frequently occurring coagulopathy. vWS is usually congenital (**Table 12.8**) but it can also be acquired, for example, in malignant lymphomas or autoimmune processes.

Both men and women can be affected by the von Willebrand syndrome.

Clinical Picture

Most affected patients have little or no tendency to spontaneous bleeding; that which does occur primarily affects the mucosa.

Hemostasis and clotting are impaired, so that a hemorrhage can lead to a combination of petechial and hemophilic bleeding types (p. 46).

Diagnosis

- (Family) history and clinical picture
- Extended bleeding time

Table 12.8 Forms of congenital vWS (vWF = von Willebrand factor, F VIII = Factor VIII)

Type (frequency)	Defect	Heredity
Type 1 (80%)	• vWF decreased • F VIII decreased	Autosomal dominant
Type 2 (15%)	• vWF defective • F VIII normal	Autosomal dominant
Type 3 (5%)	• vWF absent • F VIII strongly decreased	Autosomal recessive

- Evidence of decreased or defective von Willebrand factor and decreased Factor VIII

Therapy

In patients with vWS, acetylsalicylic acid and other platelet aggregation inhibitors are contraindicated. Additional therapeutic consequences usually occur only in surgery and with injuries:
- Thorough hemostasis
- Where appropriate, administration of desmopressin, which causes release of the clotting factors stored in the endothelium
- Where appropriate, replacement of Factor VIII and von Willebrand factor

■ Disseminated Intravasal Clotting and Consumptive Coagulopathy

Pathological Mechanism

Various factors can trigger disseminated (generalized) intravasal clotting and lead to microthrombi:
- Prothrombin activators can enter the bloodstream in:
  - Obstetrical complications such as amniotic embolism
  - Surgery on organs with a high clotting potential, especially lungs, pancreas and prostate
  - Disintegration of tumors

- Shock (p. 54)
- Messenger substances activate clotting, for instance in sepsis, e.g., meningococcal sepsis (Waterhouse–Friedrichsen syndrome).

In the course of the disease, platelets and clotting factors are consumed by the clotting process, resulting in a tendency to bleeding that is called consumptive coagulopathy. In addition, clotting causes fibrinolysis that further intensifies the hemorrhagic diathesis.

Clinical Picture

Microthrombi can lead to organ infarctions and the consumptive coagulopathy, in particular, causes:
- Extensive skin bleeding
- Gastrointestinal bleeding
- Renal bleeding
- Cerebral hemorrhage

The bleeding produces hypovolemic shock with the corresponding complications (p. 54).

Diagnosis and Therapy

Patient history and clinical picture lead to a suspected diagnosis that is confirmed by clotting status:
- Thrombocytopenia
- Low Quick value
- Decreased fibrinogen and AT III
- Evidence of D-dimers (breakdown products of fibrin)

The patient is treated in an intensive care unit:
- Causal treatment
- Symptomatic therapy depending on the stage, with heparins, AT III, fresh frozen plasma with the contained clotting factors as well as platelet concentrates
- Treatment of complications

13   Rheumatology

The spectrum of rheumatic disorders includes numerous diseases that can affect blood vessels and internal organs as well as the motor apparatus. These are *systemic diseases* whose exact causes are usually not known. Often genetic disposition and autoimmune processes play a role (p. 29).

Rheumatology is a subspecialty of internal medicine, concerned with conservative therapy, and a subspecialty of orthopedics, concentrating on surgery.

Rheumatoid Arthritis

Rheumatoid arthritis (RA), which is also known as chronic polyarthritis, is a systemic connective-tissue disease. Its underlying cause is an autoimmune process of unknown origin. RA manifests mainly in the joints, but 10% of patients also have a clinically relevant organ involvement. In the course of the disease, the patient may become disabled and unable to work.

The prevalence of the disease is about 1%; women are affected more than three times as often as men. A first peak of incidence falls between the ages of 20 and 30 years and a second one between 50 and 65.

Pathological Mechanism

Where there is a genetic disposition, autoantibodies of the IgM type are formed against the body's own IgG. The IgM antibodies are detected in the serum of many patients as "rheumatoid factors." It is still unclear what triggers this autoimmune reaction. Virus infections are one factor under discussion.

The resulting immune complex triggers an inflammatory reaction in which the complement system is activated and inflammation mediators and cartilage-attacking enzymes are released. The inflammatory reaction is aimed at the synovial membrane, which thickens as a result of synovitis, so-called pannus formation. Pannus and cartilage-attacking enzymes destroy the joints up to and including complete loss of function.

■ *IgM against IgG → Inflammation → Synovitis.*

Clinical Picture

RA usually begins insidiously with a general feeling of unwellness, decreased performance, and unspecific muscle and joint complaints. Typical symptoms develop in the course of the first two years of the illness.

Joint Symptoms

Polyarthritis is characterized by:
- Effects concentrated in the hand, base of the fingers, middle finger joints, and base joints of the toes (**Fig. 13.1**)
- Symmetrical pattern that may be absent at first
- Swelling (**Fig. 13.2**)
- Elevated temperatures without reddening
- Painful restrictions of motion
- Stiffness, especially in the morning

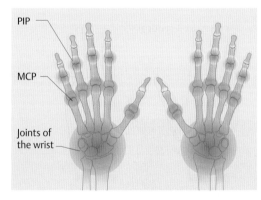

Fig. 13.1 Incidence pattern of rheumatoid arthritis. Symmetrical involvement of hand, metacarpophalangeal (MCP) and proximal interphalangeal (PIP) joints.

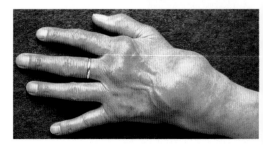

Fig. 13.2 Rheumatoid arthritis. Distinct synovitis of the hand and metacarpophalangeal joints with massive swelling. (Greten 2005.)

In the course of the disease, (sub-)luxations and deformities can develop (**Fig. 13.3**).

- Swan's neck deformity: The middle joint of the finger is overstretched and the distal joint is bent.
- Keyhole deformity: Since the extensor tendons of the fingers deviate in a palmar direction, the middle joint of the finger is bent and the distal joint is overstretched.
- "Ninety-nine" deformity: The joint at the base of the thumb exhibits a bending contracture of about 90° and the distal joint is overextended by 90°.
- Ulnar deviation: Fingers and hand are bent toward the small finger.
- Hallux valgus (inward deviation of the great toe) and subluxation of the heads of the basal phalanges II–V of the foot in a dorsal direction

Additional Signs in the Motor Apparatus

- Involvement of the cervical spine, where atlantoaxial subluxation as a result of degeneration of the transverse ligament is a threat, since the spinal canal is narrowed
- Osteoporosis, which can often be detected a few months after the start of the disease
- Tendovaginitis
- Bursitis
- Carpal tunnel syndrome
- Baker cyst

Changes in Skin and Organs

- Twenty percent of patients have rheumatic nodules (**Fig. 13.4**). These are harmless subcutaneous bumps that are found predominantly on the extensor side of the joint. The most frequent localization is the elbow joint, followed by the finger joints, the Achilles tendon, and the sacrum.
- Ten percent of patients have significant organ manifestations in heart, lungs, liver, kidneys, vessels, and eyes (**Table 13.1**).

Special Forms

Felty Syndrome

This is a severe form of RA with spleen and lymph node enlargement and decreased neutrophil granulocyte counts. A consequence of granulocytopenia is a massively increased susceptibility to infection.

Juvenile Rheumatoid Arthritis and Still Syndrome

One child in 1000 develops juvenile rheumatoid arthritis (JRA), which appears between the ages of 1 and 15 years. Depending on the age and sex of the child, the number and pattern of the affected joints, evidence of the rheumatoid factor, and eye or organ involvement, five different subtypes are distinguished.

The prognosis for JRA is considerably better than for the adult form. Thus, in 80% of children, the

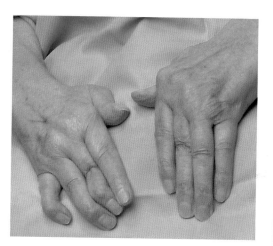

Fig. 13.3 Joint deformities in the late stage of rheumatoid arthritis. Distinct "ninety-nine" deformity of thumb and swan's neck deformity of the right second and third digit. (Riede 2004.)

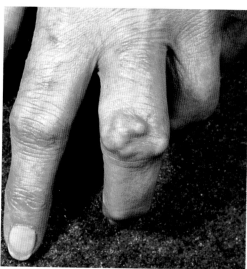

Fig. 13.4 Rheumatoid arthritis. Rheumatic nodules over the extensor side of the proximal interphalangeal joint of the second finger. (Greten 2005.)

Table 13.1 Organ manifestations in RA

Organ	Possible consequences	Page
Vessels	• Premature arteriosclerosis	31
	• Vasculitis causes, among other complaints:	
	– Polyneuropathy through inflammation of the vasa nervorum	
	– Skin ulcers on the lower leg	
	– Necrosis of fingertips	
Heart	• CAD	98
	• Pericarditis	115
	• Myocarditis	113
	• Usually asymptomatic valve involvement	111
Lung	• Frequently asymptomatic pleuritis	167
	• Pulmonary fibrosis	160
	• Pulmonary nodes	
Liver	• Elevated liver enzymes	
Kidneys	• Consequences of amyloidosis	209
Eyes	• Secondary Sjögren syndrome with reduced secretion of tears	265
	• Scleritis	

Table 13.2 ACR criteria: If at least four criteria are satisfied, a diagnosis of RA can be made

Criterion	Comment
• Morning stiffness in joints lasting at least 1 hour	These criteria must be present for a period of at least 6 weeks
• Arthritis in at least three joints	
• Arthritis of hand, base of fingers or middle finger joints	
• Symmetrical arthritis, i.e., simultaneous involvement of the same joint areas on both sides	
• Rheumatoid nodules	
• Detection of rheumatoid factor	
• Typical radiological changes	

• HLA-DR4: Leukocytes can be typed according to various membrane characteristics that are designated as human leukocyte antigens (HLA). Seventy percent of patients with RA have human leukocyte antigens of class DR4, which occur in healthy individuals with a frequency of only 25%.
• Nonspecific laboratory parameters of inflammation, chronic disease anemia, antinuclear antibodies (ANA), and circulating immune complexes

inflammatory process is self-limiting and the disease resolves spontaneously after 1–2 years, without permanent damage.

An exception is Still syndrome, the systemic form of JRA with pronounced organ involvement. With this form, about 60% of affected children suffer permanent impairment.

Diagnosis

The American College of Rheumatology (ACR) established diagnostic criteria in 1987 that take laboratory parameters and radiological findings into account, in addition to the clinical picture.

> Of the seven criteria summarized in **Table 13.2**, at least four must be satisfied to confirm the diagnosis.

Laboratory Parameters

• Rheumatoid factor: IgM autoantibodies against IgG can be found in 70% of patients and 5% of the healthy population. The prognostic value of the rheumatoid factor is greater than the diagnostic value. Patients with high concentrations often exhibit a severe course and a tendency to vasculitis.

> Thirty percent of patients are seronegative, i.e., no rheumatoid factor can be detected.

Radiological Findings

• In the first months of illness, there are no specific radiological changes. **Table 13.3** summarizes the radiological changes over the course of the disease.
• MRI can visualize synovial hyperplasia, cartilage, and joint damage.

Table 13.3 Radiological stages of RA according to Steinbrocker

Stage	Radiological findings
I	• Possible osteoporosis near joints
II	• In addition, beginning of cartilage and bone destruction
III	• In addition, beginning of subluxations and misalignments
IV	• Joint disorders and deformations
	• Joint luxations
	• Ankyloses (stiffening of joints)

Therapy

Antirheumatic treatment is used to decrease pain, inhibit inflammation, and prevent or retard loss of function and joint destruction.

Systemic Therapy

There are three large groups of medications for systemic therapy:

- Nonsteroidal antirheumatics (NSARs), which alleviate pain but do not affect the pathological mechanism
- Glucocorticosteroids (p. 77)
- Disease-modifying antirheumatic drugs (DMARDs)

DMARDs have an immunomodulating effect. It is recommended to begin therapy in the first 3 months of the disease. An effect can be expected after about 3 months of treatment. If there is no effect, the dose can be adjusted, the DMARD can be changed, or combination therapy can be considered. The following are important DMARDs:

- Methotrexate
- Sulfasalazine
- Cyclosporine (ciclosporin)
- Chloroquine and hydroxychloroquine
- Azathioprine
- Gold preparations

If therapy fails, other substances are available, for example, etanercept or infliximab, which inhibit specific inflammatory mediators. These drugs entail high costs and there is no long-term experience with them.

Local Therapy

- Intra-articular injection of glucocorticosteroids
- Radiosynoviorthesis, in which a radionuclide is injected into the joint, leading to scarring of the synovial structure
- Surgical procedures such as:
  - Synovectomy, i.e., removal of the synovium
  - Corrective surgery
  - Arthrodesis, i.e., joint bracing
  - Joint replacement

Physical Therapy

▮ *Every RA patient needs regular physiotherapy.*

The objective of the treatment is rapid restoration of mobility in the affected joint in order to prevent capsule shrinkage and muscle atrophy. Possible measures are:

- Active and passive movement therapy
- Application of cold in an acute episode, otherwise application of heat
- Massage
- Balneotherapy
- Electrotherapy
- Assistive technology, sometimes provided by the ergotherapist

Concomitant Therapy

- Psychosomatic care
- Industrial medicine and social care
- Support by groups such as the Arthritis Foundation (ww.arthritis.org) providing patient education

Prognosis

There are mild but also rapidly progressing systemic forms. One in three patients with this disease becomes an invalid. Elevated mortality is primarily due to cardiovascular events (**Table 13.1**).

Spondylarthropathies

The categorization of spondylarthropathy includes five clinical pictures:

- Bechterew disease (p. 260)
- Reactive arthritis and Reiter syndrome (p. 260)
- Psoriatic arthritis (p. 261)
- Enteropathic arthritis with sacroiliitis, e.g., in Crohn disease and ulcerative colitis (p. 183)
- Undifferentiated spondylarthritis

These are chronic inflammatory diseases that have clinical, biochemical, and radiological characteristics in common.

Clinical Common Features

One clinical sign is back pain due to sacroiliitis and spine involvement with the following characteristics:

- Start before the age of 40
- Insidious development
- Persistence for more than three months
- Stiffness in the morning, which improves through movement
- Additional joint manifestations, such as asymmetrical oligoarthritis, frequently affecting the knee joint
- Inflammatory enthesopathies, i.e., involvement of tendon attachments and ligaments
- Extra-articular manifestations, such as Crohn disease, ulcerative colitis, psoriatic disease, inflammatory involvement of the eyes and other extra-articular manifestations

Biochemical Common Features

- HLA-B27 in almost all patients
- Lack of rheumatoid factors

| *Since rheumatoid factors are characteristically absent, the diseases are also called seronegative spondylarthritis.*

Radiological Common Features

In an X-ray image, sacroiliitis can only be seen on average 8 years after the onset of the disease. An MRI of the iliosacral joints permits earlier diagnosis.

▦ Bechterew Disease

Bechterew disease is also known as ankylopoietic spondylarthritis (AS). Three men are diagnosed with AS for every one woman; the overall prevalence is <1%. Many rheumatologists believe the number of patients, especially women, with AS is underdiagnosed. Eighty percent of cases manifest between the ages of 15 and 35 years. Genetic disposition and familial concentration have been recognized. Ninety-five percent of patients are HLA-B27-positive. *Klebsiella* or *Chlamydia* infections of the urogenital tract or gastrointestinal tract have been considered as triggers.

Clinical Picture

Bechterew disease has a chronically progressive course. Characteristic signs of disease are:
- Sacroiliitis with night and morning pain in sacrum and buttocks as well as pain on percussion and shifting of the iliosacral joints
- Spondylitis with pain in the thoracolumbar junction
- Impaired movement progressing from caudal to cranial along the intervertebral joints, culminating in complete stiffening of the spinal column
- Increasing restriction of movement of the costovertebral joints and thus restrictive ventilation disorders (p. 139)

Also possible are:
- Arthritis of the hip and shoulder joints
- Chest pain due to inflammation of the sternomanubrial junction
- Pain in the pubic bone due to symphysitis
- Painfully inflamed tendinous attachments of the Achilles tendon, plantar aponeurosis, trochanters, ischium, and pelvic crest
- Inflamed eyes, iritis
- Involvement of internal organs with cardiopathy, aortic valve regurgitation, and kidney involvement

Diagnosis

- Patient history and clinical picture
- HLA typing: 95% of patients are HLA-B27-positive.
- Radiological findings:
  - In the early stages, association of osteolytic and sclerotic changes is typical.
  - In the late stage, bamboo spine is an expression of complete ossification.
- Scintigraphy: In unclear cases, scintigraphy shows isotope concentrations in the iliosacral joints before changes can be detected in the radiograph.

Therapy

Causal treatment is not possible, so consistent physiotherapeutic treatment has the highest priority in the attempt to retard stiffening of the spine and thorax and to allow the patient to become rigid in an upright position.

In inflammatory attacks or where there is pain, NSARs are prescribed.

▦ Reactive Arthritis and Reiter Syndrome

The following infectious diseases of the urogenital or gastrointestinal tract can trigger reactive arthritis in 2%–3% of patients:
- Gonorrhea (p. 282) and nongonorrheal urethritis caused by *Chlamydia* and *Ureaplasma*
- Enteritis caused by *Yersinia*, *Salmonella*, *Shigella*, *Campylobacter*, and other organisms (p. 271)

Eighty percent of affected patients are HLA-B27-positive.

Symptoms

Reactive Arthritis

Joint inflammation develops about 2–6 weeks after a urinary or gastrointestinal infection. It is asymmetrical and usually affects the lower extremities, for example, knees or ankles, and occasionally also affects finger and toe joints.

Reiter Syndrome

Only one-third of patients develop Reiter syndrome, in which at least two of the following signs appear:
- Urethritis
- Eye involvement in the form of conjunctivitis or iritis

- Reiter dermatosis with erythema in the male genital mucosa, lesions in the oral mucosa, weals or pustules on palms of hands and soles of feet, and psoriasis-like skin changes on the body

Accompanying symptoms include fever, sacroiliitis, and inflammation of tendinous attachments; internal organs are only rarely involved.

Diagnosis

Diagnosis is based on the patient's medical history, and clinical criteria. Laboratory studies show elevated inflammation parameters and HLA-B27 in 80% of cases. The urethral or enteric infection has usually subsided by the time of presentation, so that it is only rarely possible to identify the pathogen.

Therapy and Prognosis

If urethritis is still detectable, antibiotic therapy is adapted to the pathogen. Treatment of the patient's partner is also important. In postenteric reactive arthritis, antibiotic treatment is not effective. Symptomatic therapy includes:
- Physical therapy, e.g., cryotherapy in acute arthritis
- Nonsteroidal antirheumatics
- Possibly additional anti-inflammatory substances such as glucocorticosteroids or sulfasalazine in a highly acute or chronic course

Up to 80% of reactive arthritis cases resolve after 12 months. A complete Reiter syndrome has a less favorable prognosis.

Psoriatic Arthritis

About 5%–8% of patients with psoriasis contract psoriatic arthritis. Men and women of all ethnicities are affected.

Symptoms

The finger joints are most frequently affected. In contrast to rheumatoid arthritis, the distal interphalangeal joint and thus the entire finger is affected ("sausage finger"; **Fig. 13.5**). Joint deformities that characterize rheumatoid arthritis occur in only 5% of patients with psoriatic arthritis.

In some cases, there are inflammatory changes in the central pivot points. The clinical picture then resembles that of Bechterew disease.

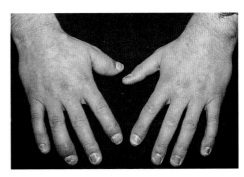
Fig. 13.5 Typical distal-joint involvement in psoriatic arthritis.

Diagnosis

Diagnostic orientation is given by the clinical triad of:
- Skin changes typical of psoriasis with red papules and silver-white scaly plaques, predominantly on the extensor side of the extremities, the sacral and anal regions, and the hairy scalp
- Nail changes typical of psoriasis with pitting, oildrop spots, nail plate crumbling, and loosening of the nail
- Arthritis

Diagnosis is difficult when joint involvement appears before the skin changes.

Therapy

Therapy must be systemic treatment with anti-inflammatory or immunosuppressant drugs. Joint involvement does not improve with local treatment of skin changes.

Collagenosis

Systemic Lupus Erythematosus

Systemic lupus erythematosus (SLE) is also known as disseminated lupus erythematosus. This is a systemic disease based on autoimmune reactions that attack the skin as well as the vascular connective tissue of numerous organs. The cause of this serious disease is unknown. The prevalence is 50/100 000 and women are affected about 10 times as often as men. SLE usually manifests around the age of 30 years.

Consequences and Symptoms

The disease progresses in flares and each case is different. In addition to general symptoms such as fever, weakness, loss of weight, and generalized swelling of lymph nodes, there can be manifestations in almost all organ systems, as summarized in **Table 13.4** (see also **Fig. 13.6**).

Raynaud Syndrome

In Raynaud syndrome, vascular spasms lead to transient malperfusion of the fingers. At first the fingers become cold and pale, then cyanotic and later, as a result of reactive hyperemia, red (p. 43).
- *Primary Raynaud syndrome* is a functional disorder. The vascular spasms are triggered by such things as cold or emotion.
- *Secondary Raynaud syndrome* is organic in nature and can occur in collagenosis or vasculitis.

Diagnosis

The American College of Rheumatology (ACR) has established 11 criteria for diagnosis, consisting of clinical signs and immunological findings (**Table 13.5**). A diagnosis of SLE is probable if 4 of 11 criteria are satisfied.

Therapy

There is no causal treatment. If no internal organ involvement can be found, the following medications will curb the inflammatory process:
- Nonsteroidal antirheumatics
- Hydroxychloroquine
- Glucocorticosteroids during the flare

In organ involvement, high doses of glucocorticosteroids and immunosuppressants are administered.

Prognosis

Course of the disease can vary significantly. The 10-year survival rate is about 90%, where renal failure and cardiac, neurological, and septic complications of immunosuppressant therapy are the chief causes of death.

■ Progressive Systemic Sclerosis

Progressive systemic sclerosis (PSS) or systemic scleroderma is a chronic, systemic connective-tissue disease. Collagen collects in the skin and internal organs and thickening of vessel walls causes skin and organ infarctions. The cause of this rather rare disease in not known. It affects women four times

Table 13.4 Consequences of SLE

Organ (frequency)	Consequences and symptoms
Joints (>80%)	Polyarthritis
Skin (70%–80%)	• Butterfly erythema, i.e., redness on bridge of nose and cheeks (**Fig. 13.6**) • Photosensitivity • Discoid lupus, i.e., disc-shaped scaly redness • Oral and nasal mucosal ulcers • Telangiectasis, i.e., vascular distension • Raynaud syndrome (p. 43)
Kidneys (70%)	• Lupus nephritis, glomerulonephritis (p. 209) • Renal hypertension (p. 117)
Heart (60%–70%)	• Pericarditis with pericardial effusion • Rarely, endocarditis
Lungs (60%)	Pleuritis with pleural effusion
Nervous system (60%)	• Headache • Loss of consciousness • Psychoses • Paresis • Sensation disorders • Epileptic seizures
Muscles (50%)	Myositis
Blood	• Anemia • Leukopenia • Thrombopenia

as often as men and usually manifests between the third and fifth decades of life.

Symptoms

Skin Signs

The Raynaud phenomenon and telangiectases in the nail beds are seen in 60%–90% of patients as early symptoms. The characteristic skin changes usually begin in the hands. The skin first shows doughy-edematous swellings and then becomes taut and shiny. Signs of sclerotic shrinking are:
- Distinctly reduced joint mobility with contractures (**Fig. 13.7**)
- Fingers tapering distally: so-called Madonna fingers
- Reduced facial mobility through to facial rigidity
- Small mouth opening with radial creases ("drawstring purse mouth"; **Fig. 13.8**)

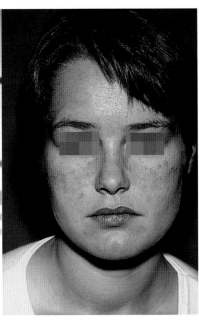

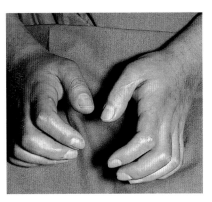

Fig. 13.7 Systemic sclerosis with distinct curving contractures of the fingers. (Jung 1998.)

Fig. 13.6 Butterfly erythema in systemic lupus erythematosus. (Jung 1998.)

Table 13.5 SLE criteria of the American College of Rheumatology (ACR)

Area	Criterion
Skin	• Butterfly erythema • Discoid lupus erythematosus • Photosensitivity • Oral or nasal mucosal ulcers
Other organs	• Arthritis, at least two joints • Serositis (pleuritis, pericarditis) • Kidney involvement • CNS involvement
Laboratory	• Hematological findings – Anemia – Thrombopenia – Leukopenia • Immunological findings – Anti-dsDNA (anti-double stranded DNA) – Anti-Sm (anti-Smith protein) – Anti-phospholipid antibodies – Anti-nuclear antibodies (ANA)

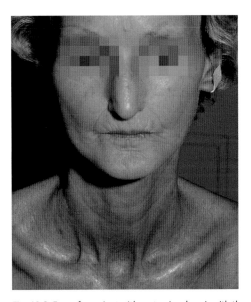

Fig. 13.8 Face of a patient with systemic sclerosis with the typical "drawstring purse mouth." (Gerlach 2000.)

Additional changes in skin and mucosa are:
• Atrophy of the sweat glands with altered sweat secretion
• Hair loss
• Pigmentary changes
• Calcinosis, calcium deposits in the skin
• Necrosis, especially in the fingertips, known as rat bite necroses

• Shortened lingual frenulum, decreased tongue mobility, and dry mouth, since the mucosa and the salivary glands are also affected

Organ Manifestations

• Swallowing disorder due to rigid esophagus
• Pulmonary fibrosis (p. 160)
• Rigid heart wall and cor pulmonale as a result of the pulmonary fibrosis
• Renal involvement with kidney infarction and renal hypertension

Course of the Disease

- Type I is also known as the acral type and mainly affects the hands. Since the organs are not affected, the prognosis is favorable.
- Type II is also called proximal ascending type, since it begins in the hands and progresses toward the trunk. In the course of the disease, the organs become affected.
- Type III is also known as the truncal type, since it begins at the trunk and progresses early into the organs.

Diagnosis

- Clinical picture
- Laboratory studies, especially antinuclear antibodies
- Capillary microscopy, which permits evaluation of the smallest blood vessels in the nail bed
- Biopsy of affected skin
- Possible radiography of the hands to image cutaneous calcification

Therapy

No causal treatment is known. In addition to administration of glucocorticosteroids and immunosuppressants, only symptomatic treatment is available, in which physiotherapy has considerable importance.
- Active and passive measures to retard or treat contractures
- Lymph drainage and connective-tissue massage
- Respiratory therapy for pulmonary fibrosis
- Physical measures such as paraffin and mud baths

Prognosis

The 10-year survival rate is 70%. In half of the deaths, the cause of death is kidney involvement.

▪ Polymyositis and Dermatomyositis

- Polymyositis is an inflammatory systemic disease of the skeletal muscles. Internal organs are sometimes involved.
- In dermatomyositis, there are also typical skin changes.

Both diseases are relatively rare, affect women twice as often as men, and can occur at any age.

Causes

- About 55% of cases are idiopathic.
- About 30% coincide with other collagenoses.
- About 10% occur in association with a malignant disease (paraneoplasia, p. 34).

> Polymyositis or dermatomyositis can be a signal of paraneoplasia.

Symptoms

- Myositis principally affects the proximal muscles of the extremities. Typical disease signs include muscle weakness, particularly when standing up or raising the arms above the horizontal. Many patients also complain of pain like a muscular cramp and some have a fever.
- Skin changes can appear before or after the myositis. The first characteristic sign is lilac-colored erythema in the face and upper trunk (**Fig. 13.9**) that turns into shiny, whitish plaques. This makes facial expression difficult and causes the face to assume a sad expression. The backs of the fingers show similar skin changes and telangiectases.
- There can be accompanying myocarditis (p. 133) or esophageal involvement that makes swallowing difficult.

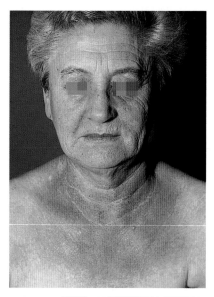

Fig. 13.9 A patient with dermatomyositis. Reddening and swelling of the neck and upper chest. (Jung 1998.)

Diagnosis

The typical symptoms provide the first signs. The suspected diagnosis is confirmed by:
- Elevated creatine kinase (CK)
- Electromyography
- Muscle biopsy

Screening for a tumor is then required.

Therapy and Prognosis

If there is an underlying malignancy, tumor therapy can improve the polymyositis or dermatomyositis. The remaining patients are treated with glucocorticosteroids and possibly immunosuppressants.

After 5 years, 50% of patients are completely asymptomatic, 30% show improvement, and in 20% the disease continues to progress.

▓ Sjögren Syndrome

Sjögren syndrome is the second most frequently occurring disease, after rheumatoid arthritis, in the spectrum of rheumatic disorders. Women are affected 10 times more frequently than men. The disease can occur in isolation or in combination with rheumatoid arthritis or other collagenoses.

Characteristic elements are chronic inflammation of the tear ducts, the salivary ducts, and sometimes other exocrine glands, with the effect of reduced production of their secretions.

Symptoms

The typical complaints are grouped together as the *sicca syndrome*:
- Keratoconjunctivitis sicca (dry eye syndrome): Since insufficient quantities of tears are produced, the patient complains of burning eyes and a feeling of a foreign body in the eye. There is a danger of corneal ulceration.
- Xerostomia: Dry mouth leads first of all to difficulty in swallowing.

Diagnosis

- Patient history and clinical picture
- Laboratory parameters such as elevated ESR, evidence of certain antibodies
- Schirmer test for evidence of decreased tear secretion

Therapy

- Symptomatic therapy such as artificial tears and high fluid intake
- If appropriate, therapy of the underlying disease

▓ Sharp Syndrome

Sharp syndrome is a disease with a favorable prognosis with symptoms that overlap with:
- Rheumatoid arthritis
- Systemic lupus erythematosus
- Progressive systemic sclerosis
- Polymyositis

Synonyms are *mixed collagenosis* or *mixed connective-tissue disease* (MCTD).

Since kidneys, heart, and CNS are only rarely involved, treatment with nonsteroidal antirheumatics and possibly low doses of glucocorticosteroids is usually sufficient.

Vasculitis

Vasculitis is an inflammatory vascular disease triggered by immunological reactions that manifests in various organs. Thus, vasculitis can appear as numerous different syndromes and involve the affected patient with numerous different specialists.

▓ Overview

Classification

Systemic vasculitis is classified according to the Chapel Hill Classification of 1992, depending on the size of the mainly affected vessels (**Table 13.6**).

In addition to the clinical pictures listed in **Table 13.6**, vasculitis can occur with different underlying diseases, for example, in:
- Autoimmune diseases such as rheumatoid arthritis (p. 256) and collagenosis (p. 264)
- Infectious diseases, e.g., HIV infection
- Use of certain medications

Diagnosis and Therapy

Diagnosis is reached on the basis of a mosaic of clinical, pathological, anatomical, and immunological data, presented below as an example for Wegener granulomatosis and giant cell arteritis.

Table 13.6 Classification of vasculitis according to the Chapel Hill Classification (ANCA = anti-neutrophil cytoplasmic antibodies)

Affected vessels	Clinical picture

Small	• ANCA-associated
	  – Wegener granulomatosis (p. 266)
	  – Churg–Strauss syndrome, manifesting chiefly at the lung
	  – Microscopic panarteritis
	• Non-ANCA-associated
	  – Schönlein–Henoch purpura, usually affecting children
	  – Vasculitis in essential cryoglobulinemia, i.e., with immune complexes that are destroyed by cold
	  – Cutaneous leukocytoclastic angiitis, affecting the skin alone

Medium-size	– Classical panarteritis nodosa – Kawasaki disease or mucocutaneous lymph node syndrome that affects small children

Large	• Giant-cell arteritis (p. 266)
	  – Horton temporal arteritis
	  – Polymyalgia rheumatica
	• Takayasu arteritis, frequently affecting young, Asian women

Therapy includes immunosuppression and, where appropriate, special immunotherapy for specific neutralization of the molecules that are taking part in the inflammatory process.

■ Wegener Granulomatosis

This form of vasculitis is associated with ulcerating nodes or granulomas and typically starts locally in the upper respiratory tract, so that the patient usually consults an ENT specialist first.

Symptoms

Typical for the initial stage are:
• Symptoms of chronic rhinitis, sinusitis, and otitis
• Ulcers in the nose, mouth, and pharynx
• Round pulmonary foci

The disease becomes generalized in its course and in the context of a pulmorenal syndrome attacks the lungs and particularly the kidneys. Rapid renal failure and an acute, life-threatening course can develop. Typical symptoms and manifestations in the generalized stage are:

• Fever, weight loss, night sweats
• Hemoptysis resulting from alveolar bleeding
• Arthralgia and myalgia
• Signs of kidney failure (p. 209)
• Signs of CNS involvement

Diagnosis and Therapy

The following are diagnostically helpful:
• ENT examination with mucosal biopsy from the nasopharyngeal space
• Laboratory findings:
  – Inflammation markers such as ESR and leukocytosis
  – Evidence of anti-neutrophilic cytoplasmic antibodies (ANCA)
  – If applicable, evidence of kidney involvement such as elevated serum creatinine or erythrocytes in the urine
• Radiographs showing shadows in the nasal sinuses, infiltrates, and round foci in the lungs
• MRI or CT showing granulomas of the nasal sinuses and possible intracerebral foci
• If applicable, lung or kidney biopsy

Antibiotics such as co-trimoxazole and temporary treatment with glucocorticosteroids are effective in the initial, locally circumscribed stage. In the generalized stage, aggressive treatment with immunosuppressants is required in order to help the patient out of the life-threatening situation. Long-term immunosuppressant maintenance therapy is also required because at present the cause of the illness is still unknown and a cure is not possible.

Prognosis

Without therapy, the prognosis is not favorable. With optimal treatment, the 5-year survival rate is 85%. The extent of kidney involvement determines the prognosis.

■ Giant-Cell Arteritis

Giant-cell arteritis is the most frequently occurring vasculitis with an incidence of about 30/100000. It affects mainly older women.

Vasculitis manifests in the perfusion area of the carotid artery and is symptomatic as *temporal arteritis* or *Horton disease*. Half of affected individuals also suffer from *polymyalgia rheumatica*. The cause is unknown.

Symptoms

Signs of temporal arteritis are:
- Throbbing headaches located in the temples, possible jaw pain while chewing
- Painful eyes, visual disorders, and danger of blindness through involvement of the central artery supplying the retina
- Palpably hardened temporal artery, painful to pressure (**Fig. 13.10**)

The following symptoms additionally occur in polymyalgia rheumatica:
- General symptoms such as fatigue, sweating, weight loss, fever, and depression
- Symmetrical shoulder and pelvic girdle pain, especially at night
- Upper arms painful to pressure
- Morning stiffness
- Possible extracranial manifestation of vasculitis in the aorta and arteries of the extremities

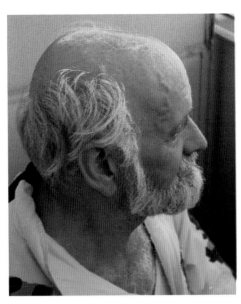

Fig. 13.10 Temporal arteritis. The inflamed temporal artery stands out. (Gerlach 2000.)

Diagnosis

- Patient history and clinical complaints
- Ophthalmological examination
- Elevated inflammatory parameters such as very high ESR and leukocytosis
- Color duplex sonography of the extracranial arteries
- Biopsy and histology of the temporal artery with evidence of giant-cell arteritis

Therapy

The disease improves rapidly on glucocorticosteroids, initially administered at a high dose and after improvement as an obligatory consistent, low-dose maintenance therapy for at least 2 years to prevent relapse.

Without treatment, about 30% of affected individuals become blind.

14   Infectiology

Diseases That Do Not Involve the Respiratory Tract Alone

■ Influenza

Viral infection with *Myxovirus influenzae*	
Infectious pathway	Droplet infection
Incubation time	1–5 days
Infectiousness	Directly before start of illness to 7 days thereafter
Immunization	Where indicated
Obligation to notify	No

Of the three known virus types, A, B, and C, type A is the most frequently occurring. There are several subtypes that can be distinguished by their surface properties. Since these change every few years, a previously contracted influenza produces no permanent protection, so that there are regularly occurring influenza epidemics and pandemics. The seasonal maximal incidence is from December to April. In contrast to a simple cold, influenza can involve life-threatening complications that are particularly dangerous for children, old people who are already sick, and immunocompromised patients.

Symptoms and Complications

Only about 20% of infected individuals present the complete clinical picture with:
- Violent onset of the disease and an intense feeling of sickness
- High fever over a period of 2–3 days; a second febrile peak indicates a bacterial superinfection.
- Pain in head, joints, and muscles
- Rhinitis and coughing, which can be associated with blood-stained sputum

Retarded convalescence, weakness, and fatigue can typically last for weeks. The chief complications are:
- Pneumonia caused by the influenza virus itself or by bacterial superinfection (p. 155)
- Perimyocarditis (p. 113)

- Meningoencephalitis
- Worsening of an existing disease

Diagnosis and Therapy

The symptoms provide diagnostic orientation. During an influenza epidemic, fever and coughing indicate an 80% certainty of influenza. Detection of antigens and antibodies is possible but not significant in practice.

Antiviral therapy with neuraminidase inhibitors is possible, but it must be instituted within the first 24–48 hours. Symptomatic treatment consists chiefly of:
- Sufficient fluid intake
- Measures to reduce fever
- Antibiotic therapy in case of bacterial superinfection

Prophylaxis

Immunization is recommended, especially for individuals over the age of 60 years with existing diseases, for immunocompromised patients, and medical personnel. The viral strains of the previous year are taken into account in the manufacture of the vaccine, but since the pathogen is constantly changing, immunization provides only 50%–70% protection.

■ Tuberculosis

Bacterial infection with *Mycobacterium tuberculosis*	
Infectious pathway	Droplet infection
Incubation time	4–12 weeks
Infectiousness	Open TB, i.e., as long as pathogens can be identified
Immunization	Where indicated
Obligation to notify	Yes

Tuberculosis (TB) can take many forms, the commonest form is infection of the lungs. It is also called consumption or Koch disease, since Robert Koch identified the pathogen in 1882. The microorganism has some special characteristics:

- It has a capsule that makes it particularly resistant to various substances, e.g., acid.
- The long generation time of about 20 hours has consequences for incubation time, diagnosis, and duration of antibiotic therapy.
- Antibiotic resistances have been identified in the meantime.

One-third of the world's population is infected, i.e., is tuberculin positive. Of the infected individuals, up to 10%, especially in the developing world, become ill with active TB and every year about 3 million people die as a result of the disease, which has a two-stage course:
- Primary tuberculosis
- Postprimary tuberculosis

Primary Tuberculosis

Tuberculosis is usually transmitted by droplet infection. In infection with tuberculosis for the first time, the *primary complex* is formed, consisting of a pulmonary focus and the associated lymph node. This phase of the infection is usually asymptomatic.

Postprimary Tuberculosis

The pathogens survive intracellularly for many years. Factors that lower resistance can trigger *active TB*.

> Most cases of tuberculosis arise through endogenous self-reinfection.

Factors that Decrease Resistance

- Malnutrition
- Old age
- Alcohol and drug abuse
- Diabetes mellitus
- Long-term glucocorticosteroid and immunosuppressant therapy
- HIV infection and AIDS as well as other causes of weakened immunity
- Malignancies

Manifestations

In 85% of cases, postprimary TB affects the lungs, but it can also affect other organs by blood-borne dissemination:
- Bone TB (Pott disease)
- Skin TB (lupus vulgaris, **Fig. 14.1**)

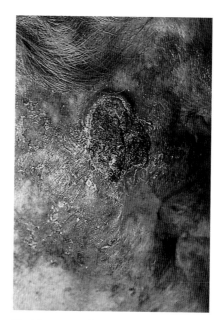

Fig. 14.1 Lupus vulgaris, a form of skin tuberculosis.

- Urogenital TB
- Tuberculous meningitis

Symptoms of Pulmonary Tuberculosis

Noncharacteristic, general symptoms are decreased physical capacity, fatigue, subfebrile temperatures, night sweats, and weight loss ("consumption"). Persistent cough possibly with blood-stained sputum is typical for pulmonary TB.

Diagnosis of Pulmonary TB

Detection of the Pathogen

Sputum, fasting gastric juice, and bronchial secretions obtained by bronchoscopy can be examined.
- Direct microscopic examination for pathogens in the specimens is not reliable.
- Because of the long generation time, culturing the pathogen on nutrient medium can require up to 4 weeks.

> If the bacteriological test shows the presence of Mycobacterium tuberculosis, the patient has contagious open TB and must be isolated.

Tuberculin Test

Components of the tubercle bacillus are injected intracutaneously (Mantoux test, patch test). If the patient's immune system has already encountered the pathogen, a coarse swelling is formed at the injection site within 72 hours.

> A positive tuberculin test indicates contact with tubercle bacilli, through either injection or vaccination; it does not indicate active tuberculosis.

Chest Radiography

In primary TB, the radiograph shows the primary complex. This is usually an incidental finding or a finding in a person who has had contact with a patient with contagious TB.

In postprimary pulmonary tuberculosis, cavernae may be visible. These are circumscribed hollow spaces resulting from tissue disintegration and constitute an expression of contagious TB. There may be associated pleural effusion.

Therapy

Any active TB must be treated. Therapy is begun with the hospitalized patient and continued on an outpatient basis as soon as the pathogen can no longer be detected. This therapy consists of a combination of up to four tuberculostatics and lasts for 6–9 months. The long duration of the therapy is necessary because of the long generation time of the mycobacteria.

■ Legionellosis

Bacterial infection with *Legionella pneumophila*	
Infectious pathway	Aerosols from air conditioners and water supplies
Incubation time	2–10 days
Infectiousness	No transmission from person to person
Immunization	No
Obligation to notify	Yes

Legionellosis was first diagnosed in 1976, in Philadelphia, in a group of war veterans who met in a hotel and were infected by aerosols escaping from an air handling system.

Courses of the Disease

Which form of the disease infected persons will develop depends especially on their immune status.

- About 90% of infected individuals remain asymptomatic.
- About 7% develop the so-called Pontiac fever with flulike symptoms and without pneumonia. The prognosis is good.
- About 3% develop *Legionella* pneumonia which, for historical reasons, is known as Legionnaires' disease. This is an atypical pneumonia (p. 155) that can also be associated with kidney failure. In previously healthy persons, lethality is about 15%; in patients with existing underlying illnesses, it is up to 80%.

Diagnosis and Therapy

After the patient's history and physical examination have provided the first indications, the diagnosis is confirmed by detection of the pathogen in sputum, bronchial secretions, or urine as well as in the suspected source. Antibiotic therapy must be started even on the basis of suspicion.

Prophylaxis

Hot water supplies and air-conditioning systems must be regularly serviced and maintained. Water temperatures above 70 °C kill the pathogen.

■ Diphtheria

Bacterial infection with *Corynebacterium diphtheriae*	
Infectious pathway	Usually droplet infection
Incubation time	2–5 days
Infectiousness	As long as bacteria can be identified, i.e.: • Up to 4 days after start of antibiotic treatment • Untreated, 4 weeks
Immunization • Active • Passive	 Yes Yes
Obligation to notify	Yes

Since the introduction of immunization, diphtheria has become rare. However, it continues to be imported, especially from Eastern Europe. Diphtheria toxin is the chief factor in the high lethality of 5%–10%.

Symptoms

A *local infection* arises at the pathogen's point of entry. The most frequent form of this infection is pharyngeal and laryngeal diphtheria. Other possible infection sites are the nose, skin, wound, and navel.

- A characteristic of *pharyngeal diphtheria* is infected tonsils with a thick, greasy pseudomembrane and a sweetish-stale breath odor.
- A sign of *laryngeal diphtheria* is muffled speech, barking cough, distinct dyspnea with fear of suffocation, and inspiratory stridor caused by narrowed airways. Laryngeal diphtheria is also known as *genuine croup.*

In the second week of illness, high fever and vomiting indicate *systemic intoxication.* Diphtheria toxin leads to life-threatening complications such as:

- Myocarditis, which is the most frequent cause of death (p. 113)
- Polyneuritis
- Nephritis

Diagnosis and Therapy

The diagnosis is confirmed through the clinical picture and detection of the pathogen in the pharyngeal smear. Patients are hospitalized and isolated. Since the prognosis depends on prompt institution of therapy, the patient is given diphtheria antitoxin without waiting for the results of the bacteriological examination. Antibiotics are simultaneously administered to eliminate the pathogen and prevent further production of the toxin. Contact persons also receive a prophylactic antibiotic.

Prophylaxis

> Basic immunization begins at 3 months of age, with a booster every 10 years.

Infectious Diarrheal Diseases

■ Overview

Pathogens

Countless microorganisms can cause diarrheal diseases.

Bacteria

- *Salmonella:* Salmonella infections are frequent and are described in detail below.
- *Escherichia coli:* The four different groups are responsible for about 40% of travel diarrheas and enteritis in infants.
- *Staphylococcus aureus* and *Clostridium perfringens:* The toxin of these bacteria cause so-called food poisoning. Vomiting and diarrhea begin after a short incubation period of only a few hours.
- *Yersinia enterocolitica:* This bacterium causes colicky abdominal pain often misdiagnosed as appendicitis. It can also cause joint and skin involvement.
- *Clostridium difficile:* All antibiotics can trigger diarrhea by disturbing the physiological intestinal flora and promote lavish growth of clostridia and other bacteria; antibiotic-associated diarrhea is often caused by the toxin of *Clostridium difficile.*
- Other responsible organisms are *Campylobacter jejuni*, *Shigella*, and *Vibrio cholerae.*

Viruses

Examples of viral pathogens causing diarrheal diseases:

- *Rotavirus*, mainly affecting children
- *Norovirus*, the most frequent pathogen in acute gastroenteritis

Protozoa and Fungi

- *Entamoeba histolytica* is the pathogen for amoebic dysentery.
- *Cryptosporidia* infect mainly immunosuppressed patients.
- *Candida* and *Aspergillus* species. They can act as pathogens in immunocompromised patients, though yeasts are present in the intestine in the majority of healthy persons.

Complications

In all diarrheal diseases, the consequences of dehydration and loss of electrolytes are a threat, particularly of:
- Circulatory failure
- Acute kidney failure
- Thrombosis

▌ *Beware of dehydration!*

Diagnosis

- Patient history, e.g., travel and medication history
- Screening of stool for pathogens

Therapeutic Principles

Symptomatic therapy

▌ *Fluid and electrolyte replacement is the most important, possibly life-saving, measure.*

Other possibilities are:
- Dietary restriction
- Constipating medications that inhibit intestinal peristalsis. However, this retards elimination of pathogens.
- Spasmolytics in paroxysmal abdominal pain

Causal Treatment

Antibiotics are indicated only in the rarest cases. They are prescribed in a targeted manner after stool diagnosis, for example, for:
- Patients with bloody diarrhea
- Infants
- Old people

■   *Salmonella* Infections

More than 2000 species of *Salmonella* are known worldwide. They cause two different clinical pictures:
- *Salmonella* gastroenteritis
- Typhoid fever

Salmonella Gastroenteritis

Bacterial infection with, e.g., *Salmonella enteritidis* or *Salmonella typhimurium*	
Infectious pathway	▪ Usually via animals and animal products, e.g. chicken and eggs ▪ In rare cases, smear infection
Incubation time	5–72 h depending on the infectious dose
Contagiousness	As long as the pathogen can be detected
Immunization	No
Obligation to notify	Yes

Symptoms and Complications

After a short incubation period, the toxin produces the typical symptoms:
- Diarrhea and vomiting
- Paroxysmal abdominal pain
- Fever
- Headache

In addition to the consequences of dehydration and electrolyte loss (see above), septic complications are possible as the bacteria spread to endocardium, meninges, bones, and joints, especially in patients with impaired immunity. One in 1000 infected individuals remains a chronic carrier, without symptoms but acting as a source of infection for others.

Diagnosis and Therapy

After the pathogen has been detected in the stool, symptomatic therapy is instituted with the main objective of correcting the fluid and electrolyte balance. Usually antibiotics are not indicated since they do not have a positive effect on the course of the disease and simply retard the elimination of salmonellae. An exception is made if the course of the disease is severe and if the patient is an infant, or an immunosuppressed or old person.

Prophylaxis

- Personal hygiene
- Food hygiene, e.g., sufficient heating of potentially infected food
- Exclusion of carriers from working in the food industry and gastronomy

Typhoid Fever

Bacterial infection with *Salmonella typhi*	
Infectious pathway	• Smear infection • Drinking water or contaminated food
Incubation time	On average 10 days (3–60 days)
Infectiousness	As long as pathogens can be found in stool
Immunization	Yes
Obligation to notify	Yes

Frequency

Worldwide, more than 30 million people contract typhoid fever every year, especially in India and Nepal. In the United States, there are about 400 new cases every year.

Symptoms and Complications

In contrast to *Salmonella* gastroenteritis, typhoid fever begins insidiously with:
- Headache
- Stupor (typhus means "haze" in Greek)
- Fever
- Grayish-white coating on the tongue
- Red spots, so-called rose spots, on the abdomen
- Constipation

■ *Diarrhea does not appear until the second week.*

In addition to the consequences of dehydration and electrolyte loss (see above), there is a threat of:
- Septic complications with spread of bacteria to the endocardium, meninges, bones, and joints
- Intestinal bleeding
- Intestinal perforation

About 4% of infected individuals remain chronic carriers, without symptoms but acting as a source of infection for others.

Diagnosis and Therapy

At the start of the illness, the pathogen can be detected in the blood. Salmonellae are only found in the stool with the onset of diarrhea. In addition to symptomatic measures, antibiotics are indicated in typhoid fever.

Prophylaxis

- Personal hygiene
- Hygienic handling of food and drinking water
- Monitoring of (chronic) carriers by health departments
- Active immunization before traveling to high-risk regions

Staphylococcal and Streptococcal Diseases

■ Overview

Cocci are small, spherical bacteria. When the cocci gather together in bunches, they are called staphylococci; streptococci line up in chains (p. 21). Both bacteria are found among the normal body flora but they are also pathogens for purulent inflammations.

Staphylococci

Staphylococcus epidermidis

Staphylococcus epidermidis is found among physiological human flora. It causes infectious diseases only in exceptional cases and is therefore considered a facultative pathogen (p. 19).

Staphylococcus aureus

Examples of Diseases Caused by Staphylococcus aureus:
- Infections of the hair roots (folliculitis, furuncles or carbuncles, depending on their extent)
- Abscesses, i.e., localized accumulations of pus creating a new encapsulated cavity (p. 5)
- Empyema, i.e., a collection of pus in a preexisting body cavity such as the pleural space, gallbladder, or joint capsule (p. 5)
- Postoperative wound infections
- Mastitis, an infection of breast tissue, usually occurring during nursing
- Osteomyelitis, a dreaded infection of bones and bone marrow
- Food poisoning through bacterial toxins (p. 271)

MRSA

Increasingly, staphylococci are developing resistances to antibiotics. MRSA is a pathogen feared in hospitals. The abbreviation stands for methicillin-resistant *Staphylococcus aureus* or more simply, multiresistant *Staphylococcus aureus*. MRSA can cause postoperative wound infections and pneumonia. Since hardly any antibiotic is effective, these infections can develop into sepsis. Affected patients must be isolated. Medical personnel are not themselves endangered but they can transmit the bacteria to other patients.

> Patients colonized or infected by MRSA must be protectively isolated.

Streptococci

There are numerous species of *Streptococcus*, classified according to their ability to break up hemoglobin as α, β, and γ hemolytic streptococci. Most infectious diseases are caused by β-hemolytic streptococci, which are further subdivided into groups.
   Examples of streptococcal infections are:
- Erysipelas (p. 274)
- Scarlet fever (p. 275)
- Tonsillitis, a purulent infection of the tonsils
- Phlegmon or cellulitis, a diffuse inflammation of the skin and connective tissue (p. 5)
- The most serious soft-tissue infection, necrotizing fasciitis, which can be lethal in spite of amputation

Secondary Streptococcal Diseases

> Secondary streptococcal diseases are also called post-streptococcal diseases and represent a dangerous late complication after streptococcal infection. They occur when the antibodies formed attack not only the infectious agent but also the body's own structures. The diseases involved are rheumatic fever, in which the antibodies attack cardiac structures in particular (p. 110), and glomerulonephritis, where kidney tissue is affected (p. 209).

■ Erysipelas

Definition

Erysipelas, also called "holy fire" or "St. Anthony's fire," is an acute inflammation of the dermis by group A β-hemolytic streptococci and more rarely other streptococci or staphylococci. The infectious agent enters the skin through portals such as wounds or athlete's foot and spreads along the lymphatic vessels.

Symptoms

- The disease begins suddenly with general symptoms such as headache, fever, and chills.
- Locally a broad, usually sharply defined and very red erythema with tongue-shaped extensions can be seen (**Fig. 14.2**).
- The skin changes are accompanied by edema, unusual warmth, and pain, the typical signs of inflammation.
- Sometimes vesicles form.
- The local lymph nodes are enlarged.

Complications

- When it is impossible to clean up the entry portal, there is a threat of relapse.
- Adhesions in the lymphatic vessels can lead to lymphedema.
- Following erysipelas, glomerulonephritis is a more frequent secondary disease than rheumatic fever (p. 273).

Diagnosis and Therapy

The diagnosis is based on the clinical picture.
- Antibiotic treatment requires at least 10 days.
- At the same time, the affected area is cooled and kept at rest, e.g., with bed rest and elevation of an affected leg or abstinence from speaking and chewing if the face is affected.
- In case of bed rest, there is a need for thrombosis prophylaxis.
- In addition, the portal of entry must be cleansed.

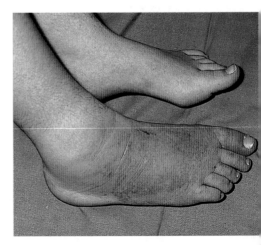

Fig. 14.2 Beginning erysipelas on the right foot. (Jung 1998.)

■ Scarlet Fever

Bacterial infection with Group A β-hemolytic streptococci	
Infectious pathway	Droplet infection
Incubation time	2–4 days
Contagiousness	Up to 24 hours after start of antibiotic therapy
Immunization	No
Obligation to notify	Yes

The β-hemolytic streptococci cause a purulent inflammation of the tonsils. The bacterial toxin, of which three variants are known, causes the characteristic skin changes The infection results only in antitoxic immunity, so that it is possible to contract scarlet fever up to three times.

Symptoms

Violent onset with:
- High fever
- Sore throat and headache
- Cough
- Enlarged tonsils with a purulent coating
- Enlarged lymph nodes
- Abdominal pain and vomiting

After about 3 days, skin and mucosal changes set in:
- Dark red enanthema on the gums
- Raspberry tongue (**Fig. 14.3a**)
- Exanthema, starting in the groin and armpits, consisting of small, densely scattered red spots (**Fig. 14.3b**). It spreads quickly over the entire surface of the body, except for the mouth–chin triangle.

At the end of the first week of illness, the rash resolves and small scales form on the skin. The skin falls from the palms and soles in large flakes.

Complications

Early Complications

- Toxic course with bleeding from skin and mucosa, myocarditis, altered states of consciousness, and cerebral convulsions (rare)
- Septic course with meningitis and cerebral sinus vein thrombosis

Late Complications

As in all streptococcal diseases, secondary complications can arise in scarlet fever as well (p. 273):
- Rheumatic fever (p. 110)
- More rarely glomerulonephritis (p. 209)

Diagnosis and Therapy

The following are diagnostically helpful:
- Detection of the pathogen in a throat smear
- Detection of antibodies (antistreptolysin)

The bacterial infection is treated with penicillin and, if there is a penicillin allergy, with erythromycin.

Herpes Virus Diseases

There are about 100 different herpes viruses, of which only a few are human pathogens:
- Herpes simplex virus (HSV), which causes the well-known blisters on the mouth (Type 1) or in the genital areas (Type 2)
- Varicella zoster virus (VZV; p. 276)

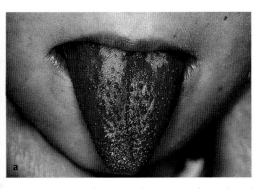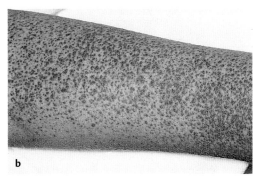

Fig. 14.3a, b Scarlet fever. **a** Raspberry tongue. **b** Macular rash. (Sitzmann 2002.)

- Epstein–Barr virus (EBV), which causes infectious mononucleosis (p. 277) and the following malignancies:
  - B cell lymphoma in immunosuppressed patients (p. 250)
  - Burkitt lymphoma, occurring mainly in central Africa
  - Carcinoma in the nasopharyngeal space, found mainly in Asia
- Cytomegalovirus (CMV) (p. 278)
- Kaposi sarcoma herpes virus, which principally causes Kaposi sarcoma on the skin and internal organs in AIDS patients

■ Varicella Zoster Virus Infection

The varicella zoster virus (VZV) is highly infectious and causes chickenpox (varicella) in children. In more than 90% of 14-year-olds, antibodies indicate that they have had the infection. The viruses persist in the spinal ganglia and with reduced immune defenses can become active again: an endogenous reinfection can cause shingles (herpes zoster) in about 20% of affected individuals.

> - *The first infection causes varicella (chickenpox).*
> - *Endogenous reinfection causes herpes zoster (shingles).*

Varicella (Chickenpox)

Infection with varicella zoster virus	
Infectious pathway	Droplet infection
Incubation time	14–16 days (in rare cases 28 days)
Contagiousness	2 days before to 7 days after onset of exanthema
Immunization	
• Active	Yes
• Passive	Yes
Obligation to notify	Yes

Symptoms and Complications

Chickenpox is associated with exanthema and a strong itch, whereas the general condition is not severely impaired. Red spots form on the body surface in flares and turn into itchy blisters and finally crusts that fall off after 2–3 weeks (**Fig. 14.4**). With mechanical irritation or bacterial superinfection, typical scars remain that give the impression of

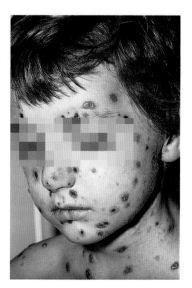

Fig. 14.4 A small child with chickenpox. (Sitzmann 2002.)

Table 14.1 Possible complications of chickenpox

Patient group	*Possible complications*
Immunocompetent individuals	• Cerebellitis, a rare inflammation of the cerebellum
Immunosuppressed individuals	• Pneumonia • Encephalitis • Hepatitis • Pancreatitis
Pregnant women with first infection during pregnancy	Congenital varicella syndrome with: • Severe skin changes • Dwarfism • Cataract • Cerebral atrophy with convulsive disorder

being embossed. Possible complications are summarized in **Table 14.1**.

Diagnosis and Therapy

The diagnosis is based on the clinical picture. Symptomatic therapy alleviates the itch and prevents bacterial superinfection. Virostatic treatment with acyclovir is only indicated for immunosuppressed patients.

Prophylaxis

In 2006, the Centers for Disease Control in the United States recommended a routine two-dose vaccination against chickenpox for all children, adolescents,

Herpes Zoster (Shingles)

Definition and Risk Factors

Shingles (herpes zoster) presents a segmental disease picture caused by reactivation of the dormant chickenpox virus. The shingles can be an expression of a reduced immune status. The disease occurs preferably in:
- Old people
- Patients with immune deficiencies or those undergoing immunosuppressant therapy
- Patients with malignancies
- Stress and trauma

Symptoms and Complications

Every dermatome can be affected. However, shingles appears most frequently in a thoracic or lumbar nerve segment. Shingles progresses in three stages, each of which lasts about 7 days.
- In the prodromal phase, there are severe, neuralgiform pains in the affected segment without visible skin changes.
- After about 7 days, the affected segment becomes red and groups of blisters with watery or even blood-stained contents are formed (**Fig. 14.5**).
- During the healing stage, the blisters dry up.

Of possible concern are:
- Involvement of the eye or inner ear, if the first branch of the trigeminal nerve is affected
- Postshingles neuralgia, i.e., continuous pain in the affected segment that can still torment the patient months or years after the infection
- Generalized zoster, i.e., involvement of several segments where there is severely reduced resistance to infection
- Zoster encephalitis

Diagnosis and Therapy

The typical clinical picture leads to the diagnosis. In addition, there must be screening for the causes of the endogenous reinfection, for example, a malignancy.
Treatment:
- Systemic virostatic therapy with acyclovir
- Local therapy to prevent bacterial superinfection

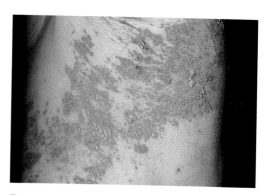

Fig. 14.5 Shingles with typical zonal manifestation in segments T2–T4. (Jung 1998.)

■ Infectious Mononucleosis

Infection with Epstein–Barr virus	
Infectious pathway	Via contact with infected saliva ("kissing disease")
Incubation time	8–21 days (in rare cases 50 days)
Immunization	No
Obligation to notify	No

In 90% of adults, antibodies indicate that the individual has had mononucleosis, which is called glandular fever because of the symptoms or *kissing disease* because of the pathway of infection.

Symptoms and Complications

Usually infectious mononucleosis in infants and small children is asymptomatic, whereas schoolchildren and adults show the full disease picture. In addition to fever up to 40 °C, the lymphatic glands are affected:
- Generalized swelling of the lymph nodes, especially in the neck
- Tonsillitis
- Enlarged spleen
- Possible liver involvement with hepatitis

One patient in five also presents with exanthema resembling the skin changes in German measles. In children, the disease lasts about 10 days; in adults, it lasts 20 days or longer.
The most frequently occurring complication is bacterial superinfection of the tonsils. In rare cases, the myocardium, lungs, kidneys, or nervous system are involved.

Diagnosis and Therapy

Clinical and laboratory data showing the typical blood changes and specific antibodies aid in diagnosis. Since this is a viral infection, patients are treated symptomatically. An antibiotic is only indicated in bacterial superinfection of the tonsils.

■ Cytomegalovirus Infection

Infection with cytomegalovirus (CMV)	
Infectious pathway	• Via the placenta, during birth or nursing • Droplet and smear infection • Contact with blood • Sexual intercourse • Organ transplantation
Incubation time	Unclear, probably 3–6 weeks
Immunization	No
Obligation to notify	No

Most people contract a CMV infection in their lifetime. CMV antibodies can be found in 50% of adults in the United States. In immunocompetent individuals, the infection is usually asymptomatic and creates lifelong immunity, whereas there is a danger for immunosuppressed patients with bone marrow or organ transplants, AIDS patients, and developing fetuses.

CMV Infections in Pregnancy

Cytomegalovirus infection is the most frequently occurring prenatal and perinatal infection that occurs only when the mother suffers a primary infection during pregnancy. In the first trimester, it usually causes miscarriage; in the second and third trimesters, it causes fetopathy with CNS involvement, pneumonia, liver and spleen enlargement, anemia, and deafness. These complications can be combated with immunoglobulins.

CMV Infection in Immunosuppressed Patients

In immunosuppressed patients, CMV produces a clinical picture resembling infectious mononucleosis (p. 277). The principal symptoms are fever, enlarged lymph nodes, swelling of the spleen and liver as well as muscle and joint complaints. Some important complications are:

- Retinitis (inflammation of the retina), which is the most frequent manifestation of CMV in AIDS patients
- Interstitial pneumonia (p. 155), with a lethality of 50%
- Encephalitis, etc.

Immunosuppressed patients are treated with virostatics and immunoglobulins.

Tetanus (Lockjaw)

Bacterial infection with *Clostridium tetani*	
Infectious pathway	Wound infection
Incubation time	4–16 days
Immunization	
• Active	Yes
• Passive	Yes
Obligation to notify	Yes

Clostridium tetani occurs everywhere, but chiefly in soil. Since the pathogen forms spores, it is enormously resistant. It can penetrate even the smallest wounds, multiply, and form the neurotoxin tetanospasmin that is carried by the bloodstream to the anterior horn cells of the spinal cord, where its principal action is to block the inhibitory impulses and thus cause tetanic spasms.

> Every wound is potentially at risk of infection with tetanus.

Symptoms

The patient first notices nonspecific signs such as generalized weakness, headache, vertigo, and sweating. The toxin causes muscle tone to increase from cranial to caudal, resulting in:

- Difficulty in swallowing
- Tense chewing and facial muscles that lead to risus sardonicus (sardonic grin, lockjaw, **Fig. 14.6**)
- Increasing stiffness in the neck
- Later, opisthotonus (rigidity and severe arching of the back) with massive overextension of the trunk and involvement of respiratory muscles

In spite of severe symptoms, patients are fully conscious.

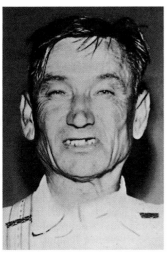

Fig. 14.6 The face of a tetanus patient with risus sardonicus (sardonic grin, lockjaw). (Kuner and Schlosser 1995.)

Diagnosis

The clinical picture and the patient's medical history of injuries with no immunization provide a suspected diagnosis. It is often difficult to detect the pathogen.

Therapy

- Administration of tetanus hyperimmunoglobulin, to inactivate the toxin
- Excision of the wound and administration of penicillin, to eliminate bacteria
- Symptomatic measures such as sedation and ventilation

Prophylaxis

Active Immunization

- *Start of basic immunization with tetanus toxoid at 3 months*
- *A booster vaccine every 10 years*

Passive Immunization

Patients must be asked about their immunization status with every wound. Any patient with a puncture wound who is uncertain of when he or she was last vaccinated receives a passive immunization with human anti-tetanospasmin immunoglobulins. Simultaneously, a booster vaccine is applied.

Tick-Borne Diseases

Various tick species are known as vectors that transmit a number of pathogens and thus can cause different tick-borne diseases (**Table 14.2**). Ticks lie in wait in wooded areas and areas with high grass and bushes. They tend to be more active during warmer seasons. Every pathogen has its own endemic region, and the geographic areas in which they are found are expanding. The incidence of tick-borne illnesses is increasing.

Symptoms

Symptoms range from asymptomatic to severe and sometimes lethal courses. Persons bitten by an infected tick usually experience symptoms such as fever, weakness, joint pain, and rashes. An overview of the major pathogens and the resulting diseases can be found in **Table 14.2**.

Prophylaxis

The following prophylactic measures can be useful to avoid tick bites:
- Wearing light-colored clothing with long pants, long sleeves, and headgear
- Tucking pant legs into socks
- Using insect repellents that contain DEET
- Checking for ticks frequently
- Carefully removing ticks
- Washing and drying clothes in a hot dryer

■ Lyme Disease

Bacterial infection with *Borrelia burgdorferi*, among others	
Infectious pathway	Tick as vector
Incubation time	1–6 weeks (on average 9 days) until stage I
Immunization	No
Obligation to notify	Yes

The percentage of infected ticks varies markedly from region to region in the United States. For example, fewer than 5% of adult ticks south of Maryland are infected, while up to 50% are infected in hyperendemic areas (areas with a high tick infection rate) of the northeast. The tick infection rate in Pacific

Table 14.2 Overview of tick-borne diseases

Disease	Pathogen	Endemic to	Major symptoms	Therapy
Lyme Disease	*Borrelia burgdorferi* (bacterium)	North America; Eurasia	• Flulike illness with fever, arthritis • Erythema migrans • Neuroborreliosis • Carditis	Antibiotics
Relapsing fever	*Borrelia species* (bacterium)	US West	• Recurring high fevers • Headaches • Muscular pain • Altered mental status • Rash	Antibiotics
Ehrlichiosis	*Ehrlichia* or *Anaplasma* (bacterium)	US South-Atlantic, South Central	• Flulike illness with fever, arthritis • Rash • Sometimes immunosuppression	Antibiotics
Rocky Mountain Spotted Fever	*Rickettsia rickettsii* (bacterium)	US East, South West; Brazil	• Fever • Myalgia • Headache • Altered mental status • Rash	Antibiotics
Tick-borne meningoen-cephalitis (TBE)	*Flavivirus*	Europe, Northern Asia	• 70%–90% asymptomatic • Flulike symptoms • Meningitis or encephalitis • Relapse of fever • Late neurological complications in 10% • Lethality of 1%–2%	Symptomatic treatment; immunization is available
Colorado tick fever or American mountain tick fever	Colorado tick fever virus	US West, Canada West	• Fever, chills • Headaches • Light sensitivity • Muscular pain • Abdominal pain • Nausea and vomiting • Rash • Rarely meningitis	Symptomatic treatment
Babesiosis, "The Malaria of the Northeast"	*Babesia microti* (protozoon)	US Northeast, West Coast	• Mostly asymptomatic • Light cases with mild fever, anemia • Severe cases with high fevers, chills, hemolytic anemia, organ failure	Antibiotics

coastal states is between 2% and 4%. With a bite from an infected tick, the infection rate is about 10% and the illness rate is about 4%.

Symptoms

The typical three stages of the disease do not necessarily occur in every case.

Stage I

About 9 days after the tick bite, redness develops at the site, extending centrifugally and becoming pale centrally. A spreading rash results that is called chronic migrating erythema (**Fig. 14.7**). This skin change recedes spontaneously.

Stage II

Without treatment, the following complications can develop within a year:
• Joint involvement, especially in the knees and ankles
• Cardiac manifestation such as myocarditis (p. 113) and typically AV block (p. 107)
• Neurological manifestations such as meningitis, encephalitis, and meningoradiculitis (Bannwarth syndrome)

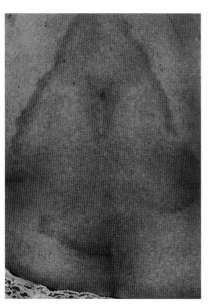

Fig. 14.7 Erythema migrans in Stage I of Lyme disease.

Stage III

Years and decades after the tick bite, typical skin changes and neurological symptoms can arise:
- The skin becomes parchment-thin, so that blood vessels can be seen through it. This change is called acrodermatitis chronica atrophicans.
- Polyneuropathy and chronic progressing encephalomyelitis are neurological manifestations of the late stage.

Diagnosis and Therapy

The patient's history and clinical picture lead to a suspected diagnosis. The diagnosis is confirmed by evidence of antibodies, which are only detectable after the third week. This requires antibiotic therapy. The antibiotic used and the length of the treatment depend on the disease stage. No immunization is available.

Prophylaxis

- Protect against tick bites.
- After a bite, remove the tick from the skin and disinfect the site. Do not use oil, adhesives, or similar materials.
- No immunization is available.

Sexually Transmitted Diseases (STD)

A synonymous designation is venereal infections (from *Venus*, the goddess of love).

According to the WHO, 1 million people are infected every day with the most frequently occurring sexually transmitted pathogens. The most important prophylactic measures are education about the spread of infection and avoidance of infection by the use of condoms.

Of the more than 20 STDs, syphilis, gonorrhea, and HIV infection will be presented here.

■ Syphilis

Bacterial infection with *Treponema pallidum*	
Infectious pathway	• Via the placenta • Sexual intercourse
Incubation time	2–3 weeks until stage I
Contagiousness	All stages
Immunization	No
Obligation to notify	Yes

Syphilis is also known as lues or hard chancre and is a serous sexually transmitted disease caused by the spirochete *Treponema pallidum*. It can be congenital or acquired. Here we will discuss acquired syphilis; the symptoms of congenital syphilis, connatal lues, are summarized in Chapter 2, page 16.

Symptoms

The clinical picture is very diverse and individually variable. Without therapy, the disease progresses over decades in three stages.

Primary Stage (Lues I)

After 2–3 weeks a painless, weeping, highly infectious hard sore appears at the pathogen's entry point. The related lymph nodes are swollen. After a few days to weeks, the ulcer heals with a scar, even without treatment.

Secondary Stage (Lues II)

The bacteria (treponemes) generalize and 3–4 months after the infection the following symptoms show:

- Fever and joint pain
- Generalized skin changes that can imitate a number of skin diseases
- Generalized lymph node enlargement
- Sometimes patchy hair loss occurs
- Organ involvement in the form of mild hepatitis, nephritis, or meningitis

The secondary stage can last about 3 months, after which the patient can become completely free of symptoms.

Tertiary Stage (Lues III)

From 5 to 50 years after the infection, about 30% of untreated patients develop Lues III, which is characterized by granulomatous tissue reactions. The granulomas are also called gummas. They can affect skin, mucosa, or all organ systems, and may disintegrate and leave a structural defect. There is a particular threat of cardiovascular and cerebral syphilis. Thanks to persistent antibiotic therapy, the third stage of the disease rarely occurs today.

Diagnosis

- Patient history and physical examination
- Screening for the pathogen
- Detection of antibodies, which will succeed 3–4 weeks after infection

Therapy

Penicillin is the therapy of choice in all stages.

■ Gonorrhea

Bacterial infection with *Neisseria gonorrhoeae*	
Infectious pathway	• Sexual intercourse • Birth
Incubation time	2–10 days
Contagiousness	Until a control smear is negative
Immunization	No
Obligation to notify	Yes

Neisseria are very sensitive to temperature fluctuations and drying, so that they are only transferred through direct mucosal contact, usually in sexual intercourse.

It is believed that worldwide 60 million people are infected yearly.

Symptoms and Complications

Men

Twenty percent of infected individuals are asymptomatic but potential transmitters of gonorrhea. In the rest, the disease leads to a purulent inflammation of the urinary tract. This urethritis causes:
- Purulent discharge from the penis, especially in the morning
- Dysuria, i.e., massive pain on urination

Possible complications are accompanying arthritis and infertility.

Women

In women, the disease is often unrecognized. Possible signs are:
- Cervicitis with flux, since the bacteria predominantly infect the cervix uteri
- Urethritis with dysuria

In women, too, gonorrhea can cause arthritis. In addition, the infection can travel upward to the fallopian tubes and cause infertility when adhesions in the tubes develop after adnexitis.

Newborns

Newborns that have become infected during birth develop a purulent conjunctivitis that can lead to blindness. This complication has become rare since pregnant women are examined and treated if necessary. Some obstetric hospitals even today treat every newborn by putting silver nitrate solution into their eyes (Credé method) to prevent gonococcal conjunctivitis.

Diagnosis and Therapy

Screening for the pathogen is done as follows:
- In men, with a urethral smear
- In women, with a cervical smear

The success of antibiotic therapy, which includes treating the partner, should be checked with a control smear after 10 days.

HIV Infection and AIDS

Infection with the human immunodeficiency virus: HIV-1, HIV-2, and subtypes

Infectious pathway	• Sexual intercourse • Contact with blood • Birth • In rare cases via the placenta and during nursing
Incubation time:	
Serologically, i.e., until antibodies are detected	• 1–3 months; in rare cases 6 months
Clinically, i.e., until onset of AIDS	• About 10 years in industrialized countries, otherwise shorter
Contagiousness	Depending on the virus load
Immunization	No
Obligation to notify	Yes

Significance

Acquired immune deficiency syndrome (AIDS) caused by the human immunodeficiency virus, is one of the five leading causes of death through infection worldwide. Every year there are:

- Five million new cases
- Three million deaths

Africa is most severely affected, where 70% of all AIDS patients are found. HIV infection is also increasingly spreading in Southeast Asia, South America, and Eastern Europe. In the United States over 43 000 people were infected with HIV in 2009. About 1 000 000 people are living with HIV in the United States.

> It is a very dangerous situation that in the industrialized world, awareness of the human immunodeficiency virus and its infectious pathways is decreasing and sometimes even nonexistent among the younger population in spite of educational campaigns.

Pathogenesis and Course of the Disease

The human immunodeficiency virus is a lymphocytotropic and neurotropic retrovirus, that is, the immune system and the nervous system are directly damaged. Target cells are all cells with the CD4 surface antigen, especially the T lymphocytes. These CD4 cells play an important role in defense against nonbacterial pathogens and tumor cells. Although persons with HIV infections form antibodies against the virus, the organism is not capable of eliminating it. The virus-induced immune deficiency and the resulting disease pictures are continuously progressive.

> In each of the following phases, the affected person is contagious.

HIV Primary Disease

Six days to 6 weeks after the infection, some of the infected persons develop a disease picture resembling acute mononucleosis (p. 277) with:

- Fever
- Swollen lymph nodes
- Skin rash
- Painful difficulty in swallowing

These symptoms last 1–2 weeks and are usually not recognized as HIV primary disease.

Asymptomatic Stage

The asymptomatic dormant phase can last from months to many years. In clinically healthy carriers of the virus, the detection of HIV-specific antibodies is often the only indication of existing infection. The further progress is individually very varied; clinical symptoms can be followed by a period free of symptoms. On the other hand, complications caused by immunodeficiency can develop in apparently completely healthy individuals. Often there are nonspecific signs such as:

- Decline of general wellbeing
- Changes in skin and mucosa
- Swollen lymph nodes
- Gastrointestinal symptoms
- Neurological complaints such as HIV-associated polyneuropathies and encephalopathy

AIDS

Without prophylactic measures, the complete picture of the full-blown disease generally manifests in the form of the life-threatening opportunistic infections that define AIDS, for example:

- Pneumonia caused by *Pneumocystis jiroveci* (PCP, p. 155)
- Esophagitis caused by *Candida albicans* (p. 177)
- Cytomegalovirus infection (p. 278)
- Toxoplasmosis (p. 284)
- Tuberculosis, which is the cause of death in 30% of all AIDS deaths (p. 268)

Certain malignancies are characteristic in AIDS:
- Kaposi sarcoma in skin and internal organs
- Lymphomas (p. 250)
- Cervical cancer in women

Diagnosis

Diagnostic indications are provided by the onset of clinical symptoms and by the risks of infection revealed by the patient's history. Important laboratory parameters for diagnosis, therapy, and monitoring of the course as well as for making prognoses are:
- Detection of antibodies: HIV-specific antibodies can be detected in the serum about 6 weeks after infection.
- Quantification of viruses: The viral load, i.e., the number of HIV genome copies in the plasma, gives an indication of the prognosis and is used as a parameter for therapy and course monitoring.
- The CD4 cell count is a measure of the immune deficiency.

Therapy and Prognosis

No cure is possible, but the therapeutic possibilities have improved the prognosis considerably in wealthy nations.
- Affected persons should live a healthy life and avoid factors that decrease resistance.
- Antiretroviral therapy inhibits virus multiplication, allowing CD4 cells and the immune system to regenerate. In order to avoid emergence of resistant viruses, combinations are used, the so-called HAART (highly active antiretroviral therapy). This therapy is individually adapted and continues to be developed. For patients, this therapy improves quality and expectancy of life. However, the medications produce side-effects of a magnitude that will become understood with increasing experience through use. Without retroviral therapy, about 50% of HIV-infected persons will have fallen ill 10 years later with severe immune deficiencies. The chief causes of death are uncontrollable infections.
- Prophylaxis and therapy of opportunistic infections and other complications
- Psychosocial help

Prophylaxis

The most important prophylactic measures are education about the pathways of infection and avoidance of infection by:
- Using condoms
- Screening of all blood donors for HIV infection
- Minimizing blood transfusions from non-self donors, and preferring autologous blood donation, e.g., in nonemergency surgery
- Careful handling of blood products, especially using protective gloves and, if appropriate, face masks or protective goggles when infectious aerosols may be present
- Secure disposal of needles, syringes, sharp instruments
- Provision of relevant information by infected patients to treating physicians and dentists

If a needle stick occurs despite these safety precautions, the risk of infection can be decreased by taking the following immediate measures:
- Encourage bleeding
- Disinfect the wound
- Consult a physician
- Where appropriate, institute antiviral postexposure prophylaxis at the latest within 2 hours

Protozoan Diseases

■ Toxoplasmosis

Protozoan infection with *Toxoplasma gondii*	
Infectious pathway	· Eating raw meat from infected animals · Contact with oocyte-containing cat feces · Via the placenta
Incubation time	Days to weeks
Immunization	No
Obligation to notify	No

Most people become infected during the course of their life. In immunocompetent individuals, the infection is usually asymptomatic and creates lifelong immunity, whereas there is a danger for immunosuppressed patients such as AIDS patients and developing fetuses.

Toxoplasmosis in Pregnancy

If a woman is infected for the first time during pregnancy, toxoplasmas can be transmitted across the placenta, while the mother remains asymptomatic. The consequences for the fetus depend on the time of the infection (**Table 14.3**).

A fetopathy (p. 16) causes encephalitis with:
• Intracerebral calcifications
• Hydrocephalus, i.e., accumulation of an excessive quantity of fluid in the brain, due to inflammatory obstruction of the cerebrospinal fluid circulation
• Chorioretinitis, i.e., inflammation of the retina and choroid

Additional possible complications are:
• Hepatosplenomegaly, i.e., enlargement of liver and spleen
• Myocarditis (p. 113)
• Interstitial pneumonia (p. 155)
• Sometimes miscarriage or stillbirth

If no antibodies can be detected in the blood of a pregnant woman, she is advised to avoid raw meat and contact with cats. In addition, antibody screening should be repeated every two months so that antibiotic therapy can be started if infection is observed.

Toxoplasmosis in Immunosuppressed Patients

The main threats in immunosuppressed patients are:
• Cerebral toxoplasmosis that can end in death
• Septic dissemination, especially into heart, liver, and spleen

Once the diagnosis is confirmed by evidence of antibodies and pathogens, as well as of cerebral lesions visualized by CT or MRI, antibiotic therapy is instituted.

Table 14.3 Risk of transmission and consequences of toxoplasmosis, depending on stage of pregnancy

Trimester	Risk of infection (%)	Consequences
First	15	Usually miscarriage
Second	30	Usually serious damage or miscarriage
Third	60	Usually slight damage

▨ Malaria

Protozoan infection with plasmodia	
Infectious pathway	*Anopheles* mosquito as vector
Incubation time	1–5 weeks (up to 2 years)
Immunization	No
Obligation to notify	Yes

Malaria, which is also known as paludism or intermittent fever, is the second most frequently occurring infectious disease in the world after tuberculosis. It is believed that there are 500 million humans infected with malaria; 90% of them live in Africa, where 2 million children die of the consequences of this protozoan infection every year. In the United States there are 1200–1400 imported cases every year.

Pathomechanism

During its blood meal, the female *Anopheles* mosquito takes in certain developmental stages of the plasmodia from infected humans. The plasmodia undergo sexual multiplication inside the mosquito and sporozoites emerge from the eggs, which are then re-transmitted to human beings.

The maturation process begins in the human liver. The sporozoites develop unnoticed into merozoites, and these enter the erythrocytes, where they undergo asexual reproduction. The infected erythrocytes burst simultaneously and release merozoites, which can again be taken up by mosquitoes. The expression of this synchronous hemolysis is intermittent fever, which occurs in a specific rhythm, depending on the developmental time of the plasmodium species (**Table 14.4**).

Table 14.4 Fever cycles in different types of plasmodia and malaria forms

Plasmodium	Malaria	Fever cycle
P. vivax P. ovale	Tertian malaria	Every 48 h, i.e., fever on "Day 3"[a]
P. malariae	Quartan malaria	Every 72 h
P. falciparum	Tropical malaria (malaria maligna)	Irregular

[a] *The system of this nomenclature goes back to the Roman custom of declaring today "Day 1".*

Symptoms and Complications

- Headaches and limb pain
- Fever up to 40 °C in a typical rhythm. However, this rhythm is not seen in tropical malaria or infection with several generations of plasmodia
- Signs of anemia (p. 246)
- Enlargement of liver and spleen

The most frequent incorrect diagnosis is influenza.

In tropical malaria, which affects two-thirds of all patients, severe complications are possible, such as acute kidney failure, encephalitis, acute pulmonary failure, shock, and spontaneous bleeding. For this reason, it is designated as malignant malaria and is associated with a 4% mortality.

Diagnosis and Therapy

In febrile patients with the appropriate travel history, malaria must always be considered. Plasmodia are found in erythrocytes in stained blood smears under microscopic examination.

The choice of medication is determined by the geographic region in which the patient became infected, since there is increasing resistance to chloroquine and other substances.

Prophylaxis

Since the disease produces only partial immunity, an immunization is not possible. Prevention is sought through:

- Protection against exposure, i.e., protection against mosquitoes, e.g., by the use of protective clothing, insect repellent on bare portions of the body, and mosquito nets
- Chemical prophylaxis, about which one should be informed before traveling

Study Questions on Internal Medicine

Review the text and increase your understanding of it to prepare for the examination. (The page numbers in parentheses indicate where the answers can be found.)

1. Describe the symptoms of left heart failure. (p. 88)

2. Describe the symptoms of right heart failure. (p. 88)

3. What are the degrees of clinical severity of chronic heart failure? (p. 90)

4. What mechanisms does the organism use to compensate for heart failure and what are the consequences? (p. 89)

5. Which heart murmur occurs in mitral regurgitation? (p. 90)

6. Sketch and interpret the basic leads of an ECG. (p. 92)

7. What is the importance of a chest radiograph in cardiological diagnosis? (p. 94)

8. What must a patient look out for after left heart catheterization? (p. 95)

9. Which medications are used in symptomatic treatment of chronic heart failure? (p. 96)

10. You are treating a patient with a heart transplant. What must you take into account? (p. 97)

11. What is the cardinal symptom of CAD? (p. 98)

12. Describe the therapy for stable angina pectoris. (p. 100)

13. What is a "silent infarction"? (p. 102)

14. How is a myocardial infarction diagnosed? (p. 102)

15. When does a patient receive a cardiac pacemaker and when does he or she receive an implantable cardioverter-defibrillator? (p. 106)

16. What complications threaten a patient with atrial fibrillation? (p. 107)

17. What action do you take after you have observed circulatory arrest in a patient? (p. 108)

18. Name the causes and consequences of endocarditis. (p. 110)

19. For what kind of a risk patient is endocarditis prophylaxis indicated? (p. 110)

20. What is the difference between stenosis and regurgitation of a heart valve? (p. 111)

21. How can myocarditis manifest itself? (p. 113)

22. When is arterial hypertension present? (p. 117)

23. Name the forms and causes of arterial hypertension. (p. 118)

24. What complications threaten a patient with arterial hypertension? (p. 118)

25. Name the clinical stages of PAD according to Fontaine–Ratschow. (p. 123)

26. What findings do you expect in the physical examination of a PAD patient? (p. 123)

27. How is PAD treated? (p. 125)

28. What causes acute occlusion of an artery in the extremities? (p. 126)

29. Differentiate between thrombophlebitis and phlebothrombosis. (p. 132)

30. What are the causes of a DVT? (p. 132)

31. What are the symptoms of a DVT? (p. 133)

32. How is a DVT prevented? (p. 134)

33. Describe the stages of CVI. (p. 135)

34. Differentiate between obstructive and restrictive ventilation disorders. (p. 139)

35. What is the difference between partial respiratory insufficiency and global respiratory insufficiency? (p. 141)

36. What causes cor pulmonale? (p. 142)

37. What are the forms and causes of atelectases? (p. 142)

38. What are bronchiectases? (p. 143)

39. Define lung volumes and lung capacities. (p. 145)

40. What is the purpose of the Tiffeneau test? (p. 145)

41. Define chronic bronchitis. (p. 148)

42. What are the causes of pulmonary emphysema? (p. 149)

43. What are the clinical signs that suggest abnormal accumulation of air in the alveoli of the lungs? (p. 150)

44. Describe an asthma attack. (p. 153)

45. What medications are indicated for asthma patients? (p. 154)

46. What actions should you take if your patient suffers an asthma attack? (p. 155)

47. What is the difference between typical and atypical pneumonia? (p. 156)

48. What are the pulmonary and intestinal manifestations of mucoviscidosis (cystic fibrosis)? (p. 161)

49. How is CF treated? (p. 162)

50. What symptoms may indicate a pulmonary embolism? (p. 164)

51. Why is a tension pneumothorax so dangerous? (p. 166)

52. What are the causes and symptoms of upper gastrointestinal bleeding? (p. 172)

53. What is the difference between maldigestion and malabsorption? (p. 173)

54. What are the consequences of malassimilation? (p. 173)

55. What complications are possible in gastritis? (p. 179)

56. What factors promote a gastric ulcer and a duodenal ulcer? (p. 180)

57. Describe the pathomechanism of gluten sensitive enteropathy. (p. 182)

58. What is the difference between Crohn disease and ulcerative colitis? (p. 183)

59. What factors promote the development of colorectal cancer? (p. 186)

60. What measures are suggested for early detection of colorectal cancer? (p. 186)

61. What are the causes of mechanical ileus? (p. 188)

62. How is hepatitis B transmitted? (p. 193)

63. What causes cirrhosis of the liver? (p. 192)

64. What are dangerous complications for patients with cirrhosis of the liver? (p. 194)

65. Define the nephrotic syndrome. (p. 205)

66. What factors lead to acute renal failure? (p. 209)

67. What are the most frequent causes of chronic kidney disease? (p. 209)

68. Describe the symptoms of advanced chronic kidney disease. (p. 210)

69. What factors promote urinary tract infections? (p. 211)

70. How do Type 1 and Type 2 diabetes develop? (p. 215-216)

71. Which acute metabolic disorders are threats in diabetes mellitus? (p. 216)

72. What are frequent complications in long-term diabetes mellitus? (p. 217)

73. What constitutes the metabolic syndrome? (p. 223)

74. What factors promote primary osteoporosis? Which diseases lead to secondary osteoporosis? (p. 226)

75. How does osteoporosis manifest itself? (p. 226)

76. What are the causes of osteomalacia? (p. 228)

77. What are the symptoms of hyperthyroidism? (p. 236)

78. Describe the symptoms of hypothyroidism. (p. 236)

79. How does Cushing disease or Cushing syndrome develop? (p. 239)

80. What is the Conn syndrome? (p. 240)

81. What symptoms are produced by adrenocortical insufficiency? (p. 241)

82. What information can be gained from the blood count? (p. 245)

83. Which laboratory parameters are used to evaluate hemostasis and coagulation? (p. 245)

84. What are the causes of anemia? (p. 246)

85. How is acute leukemia treated? (p. 249)

86. What are the consequences of a plasmocytoma? (p. 252)

87. What causes thrombocytopenia? (p. 252)

88. Why do only boys and men suffer from hemophilia? (p. 253)

89. What is the most frequently occurring coagulopathy? (p. 254)

90. Describe the typical deformities in RA. (p. 257)

91. What organ manifestations are possible in RA? (p. 258)

92. Name the ACR criteria for RA. (p. 258)

93. What is the rheumatoid factor? (p. 258)

94. What symptoms constitute the Reiter syndrome? (p. 260)

95. Describe the Raynaud syndrome. (p. 262)

96. What are significant skin and organ manifestations of progressive systemic scleroderma? (p. 263)

97. What characterizes Sjögren syndrome? (p. 265)

98. What factors promote tuberculosis? (p. 269)

99. What is "open tuberculosis?" What are the consequences of this condition? (p. 269)

100. How is a positive tuberculin test interpreted? (p. 270)

101. What are the possible consequences of (infectious) diarrheal diseases? (p. 272)

102. What does the abbreviation MRSA stand for? (p. 273)

103. What is a secondary streptococcal disease? (p. 274)

104. What diseases are caused by the varicella zoster virus? (p. 276)

105. How often should a tetanus immunization be repeated? (p. 279)

106. What are the usual manifestations of Stage I Lyme disease? (p. 280)

107. How is HIV transmitted? (p. 283)

108. What are characteristic diseases in AIDS? (p. 283)

109. Who is endangered by toxoplasmosis? (p. 285)

Glossary of Terminology

(For a list of abbreviations, please see p. IX–X)

Ablation: Removal of a tissue or organ

Abscess: A localized collection of pus enclosed in a tissue cavity formed by cell destruction

Acarbose: An oral antidiabetic drug

ACE inhibitor: An inhibitor of the angiotensin-converting enzyme that transforms angiotensin I into angiotensin II in the renin–angiotensin–aldosterone system. ACE inhibitors are mainly prescribed for arterial hypertension and heart failure.

Acetylsalicylic acid: Pain medication and inhibitor of platelet aggregation

Achalasia: Esophageal motility disorder that affects the ability of the esophagus to move food to the stomach

Acidosis: Disorder of the acid–base balance with a decline of blood pH values below 7.36

Acromegaly: Distinct enlargement of the extremities after the age of growth as a result of overproduction of growth hormone by the pituitary gland

Actinic: Resulting from radiation

Activated protein C resistance: A congenital clotting disorder with elevated tendency to thromboses

Acute: Having a rapid onset and short but severe course

Addison disease: Primary adrenocortical insufficiency

Adenoma: Benign tumor arising from glandular tissue

Adequate: Appropriate, proportionate, reasonable

Adjuvant: Furnishing added support

Adynamia: Lack of strength or vigor due to a pathological condition

Aerobic: Depending on oxygen

Air hunger: Dyspnea

Air trapping: Overinflation of the lungs

Aldosterone: Steroid hormone produced in the adrenal cortex with an effect on electrolyte balance

Alguria: Pain and burning on urination

Alkalosis: Disorder of the acid–base balance with blood pH values rising to over 7.44

Allogenic transplantation: Donor and recipient belong to the same species

Alpha-fetoprotein: Most highly concentrated in fetal tissue. An elevated blood level in adults is found in liver and testicular cancer (tumor marker).

Amenorrhea: Absence of menstrual flow

Amniocentesis: Extraction of amniotic fluid for diagnostic purposes

Amyloidosis: A rare disease in which extracellular protein deposits in organs lead to organ enlargement and impairment of function; the kidneys are often involved.

Anaerobic: Active in the absence of oxygen

Anamnesis: Memory, recall; the case history of a medical patient as recalled by the patient

Androgens: Male sex hormones

Anemia: Lowered hemoglobin concentration; hematocrit or erythrocyte count below normal

Aneurysm: Widening of a portion of an artery or the heart

Angina: Pain, constriction

Angiography: Contrast radiography of arteries

Ankylosing spondylitis: Bechterew disease

Antibiogram: The result of a laboratory test for the sensitivity of an isolated bacterial strain to different antibiotics

Anticoagulation: Inhibition of blood clotting with drugs

Antineutrophil cytoplasmic antibodies: A laboratory parameter for diagnosis of vasculitis

Antinuclear antibodies: A laboratory parameter in systemic lupus erythematosus

Antithrombin III: A physiological inhibitor of blood clotting

Antitussive: Cough-suppressant medication

Anuria: Urine output of less than 200 mL per day

Aortic dissection: A tear in the wall of the aorta that causes blood to flow between the layers of the wall of the aorta and force the layers apart

Apnea: A cessation of breathing

Appendicitis: Inflammation of the vermiform appendix

Application: The use of something for a particular (medical) purpose

Arthritis: Inflammation of the joints

Arthrodesis: Stiffening of the joints

Asbestosis: Interstitial pulmonary disease caused by inhalation of asbestos

Ascites: Abnormal accumulation of fluid in the abdominal cavity

Asystole: Cardiac arrest where the heart has stopped beating

Atelectasis: Absence of air in the alveoli with collapse of the affected areas of the lung

Atopy: A genetic predisposition toward the development of immediate hypersensitivity reactions against common environmental antigens

Atrophy: A wasting or decrease in size of a body organ, tissue, or part owing to disease, injury, or lack of use

Auscultation: Listening to acoustic phenomena within the body (usually with a stethoscope)

Autogenous transplantation: Transplantation using one's own tissue

Autologous transplantation: Transplantation using one's own tissue

Autosomes: All chromosomes that are not sex chromosomes (human chromosomes 1–22)

AV block: Disorder of atrioventricular conduction

Azathioprine: An immunosuppressant, cytostatic drug; for treatment of autoimmune diseases and prevention of transplant rejection

Barrett syndrome: Tissue changes in the lower esophagus as a result of many years of reflux esophagitis; a precancerosis

Basedow disease: An autoimmune disease that leads to, among other things, hyperactivity of the thyroid gland

Benign: Not malignant

Beta blocker: Drugs that inhibit the effects of the sympathetic nervous system

Biguanide: An oral antidiabetic drug

Blumberg sign: A clinical sign of appendicitis; pain in the lower right abdomen after sudden release of the depressed abdomen on the left side

Body mass index: A ratio of weight to height-squared used as a diagnostic tool

Boeck disease: Synonym for sarcoidosis

Booster effect: Faster and stronger immune response after a second antigen contact; an effect used in active vaccination

Borreliosis: Lyme disease; an infectious disease transmitted by ticks

Bradycardia: Decrease in heart rate to below 60 beats per minute at rest

Bronchiectasis: Irreversible expansion of bronchi or bronchial branches caused by weakness of the walls

B symptoms: Fever, night sweats, and weight loss that can accompany a malignant disease

Bypass surgery: Surgical formation of collateral vessels to bypass arteriosclerotic narrowing

Cachexia: Weight loss, wasting of muscle, loss of appetite, that can occur during a chronic disease

Calcinosis cutis: Calcium deposits in the skin

Calcitonin: A hormone that acts to reduce blood calcium levels

Candida: A type of yeast

Caput medusae: Medusa head; engorgement and tangling of the vessels of the abdominal wall as a result of shunting from the portal vein region, e.g., in cirrhosis of the liver or portal vein thrombosis

Carcinogen: Any substance that produces cancer

Carcinoma: A malignant tumor arising from epithelial tissue

Carcinoma in situ: A cluster of malignant cells that has not yet invaded the deeper epithelial tissue or spread to other parts of the body

Carcinomatous lymphangiosis: Spread of cancer along the lymph vessels

Cardiac glycosides: Glycosides, obtained from *Digitalis* species and other plants, that increase the contractile power of the heart muscle

Cardiology: Specialty that studies diseases of the heart and the large vessels

Cardiomyopathy: Disease of the heart muscle associated with a functional disorder

Cardioversion: Normalization of the heart rhythm by means of drugs or electric current

Carrier: An individual who has a gene for a disease without suffering from the disease himself/herself

Catecholamines: Naturally produced stress hormones

Catheter: A hose or tube-shaped instrument to be introduced into hollow organs or blood vessels

Causal: Being at the root of a given effect

Celiac disease: Congenital intolerance for gluten and the gliadins contained in it, with damage to the mucosa of the small intestine and malabsorption

Child stages: Degrees of severity in cirrhosis of the liver

Chloroquine: Drug used for prophylaxis and treatment of malaria and in systemic lupus erythematosus and rheumatoid arthritis

Cholangitis: Inflammation of the bile ducts

Cholecystitis: Inflammation of the gallbladder

Cholecystolithiasis: Gallstones within the gallbladder

Choledocholithiasis: Gallstones within the bile ducts

Cholelithiasis: The presence of gallstones

Cholestasis: Blockage of bile flow

Cholesterols: A group of plasma lipids vital for the structure of cell membranes and steroid hormones; also subgroups are a significant risk factor for the development of arteriosclerosis

Chromosomal aberration: Any change in the normal structure or number of chromosomes; it often results in physical or mental abnormalities

Chronic: Lasting a long time or marked by frequent recurrence

Churg–Strauss syndrome: Autoimmune vasculitis of the small vessels

Cirrhosis of the liver: Chronic scarring transformation of liver tissue with loss of function

Clostridium: A bacterial genus

Coagulopathy: Inborn or acquired blood clotting disorder

Cocci: Spherical bacteria

Coffee grounds vomiting: A form of blood vomiting in which the blood is decomposed by contact with gastric juices

Colic: Intermittent, spasmodic pain in a (hollow) organ

Collagenosis: Collective term for systemic connective tissue diseases

Coma: A state of deep and often prolonged unconsciousness; usually the result of disease or injury

Compensation: Equilibration

Compliance:
1. Patients' willingness to collaborate and cooperate
2. Distensibility of hollow organs or hollow spaces
3. Distensibility of lungs and thorax

Congenital: Inborn

Conjunctivitis: Inflammation of the conjunctiva

Conn syndrome: Primary hyperaldosteronism caused by aldosterone-producing adenomas of the adrenal cortex

Conservative therapy: Nonsurgical treatment

Contamination: Deposition of undesirable substances or microorganisms

Contraindication: Circumstances that prohibit the application of a diagnostic or therapeutic measure

Cor pulmonale: Enlargement of the right ventricle of the heart as a response to increased resistance or high blood pressure in the lungs

Corona phlebectatica: A noticeable wreath of veins on the edge of the foot in chronic venous insufficiency

Courvoisier sign: Painless obstructive icterus with palpably enlarged gallbladder, e.g., in pancreas head carcinoma

C-reactive protein: An inflammation parameter

Creatine kinase: An intracellular enzyme

Creatinine: The breakdown product of creatine phosphate in muscle metabolism; a marker for kidney function

Crohn disease: Chronic inflammatory intestinal disease

Croup: Inflammation of the larynx

Curative: Tending to overcome disease and promote recovery

Cushing syndrome: A syndrome caused by elevated levels of glucocorticosteroids in the body

Cyanosis: Bluish color of the skin and the mucous membranes due to insufficient oxygen

Cyclosporin A: An immunosuppressant used for treatment of autoimmune diseases and prevention of transplant rejection

Cyst: An encapsulated, liquid-filled, hollow space

Cystitis: Inflammation of the urinary bladder

D hormone: Vitamin D; a hormone that chiefly affects calcium and phosphate metabolism

D-dimers: Fibrin degradation products released into the blood when a clot is degraded by fibrinolysis

Defibrillation: An electrical emergency measure for treatment of ventricular fibrillation

Dermatomyositis: Inflammatory systemic disease of the skeletal muscles with associated skin changes

Desmopressin: Medication that releases clotting Factor VIII and von Willebrand factor from the endothelium and is used in hemophilia A and von Willebrand syndrome

Deviation: Abnormality

Dexamethasone: Highly effective synthetic glucocorticosteroid used as an anti-inflammatory and immunosuppressant drug

Diabetes insipidus: A disorder of water metabolism with excessively increased urination

Diabetes mellitus: A metabolic disease involving high blood glucose levels and increased urination

Dialysis: An extracorporeal blood cleansing procedure to compensate for insufficient renal function

Diaplacental: Passing through the placenta

Diarrhea: A condition where a patient frequently passes liquid feces

Diastole: Phase of the cardiac cycle in which the ventricular muscles relax and the blood flows from the atria into the ventricles

Diastolic murmur: Heart murmur during the relaxation phase of the heart

Dilatation: A state of distension

Diphtheria: Infectious bacterial disease caused by *Corynebacterium diphtheriae* with manifestation in the pharynx and larynx

Diploid chromosome set: Having a pair of each type of chromosome, so that the basic chromosome number is doubled

Disposition: A tendency to become ill; susceptibility to an illness

Disseminated: Spread over a wide area of the body or an organ

Diuresis: Urine production

Diuretic: Medication that encourages production and excretion of urine

Diverticulum: A bulge in the intestinal wall

Dressler syndrome: Postmyocardial infarction syndrome; inflammation of the pericardium days to weeks after a myocardial infarction

Dukes classification: The staging of colon cancer

Duplex sonography: An ultrasound procedure for imaging blood vessels

Dysphagia: Swallowing disorder

Dysplasia: Abnormal development or growth of tissues, organs, or cells

Dyspnea: Uncomfortable awareness of breathing; shortness of breath

Dysuria:
1. Difficulty in urination
2. Pain and burning on urination

Ecchymosis: The skin discoloration caused by the escape of blood into the tissues from ruptured blood vessels, large hematoma

Echocardiography: Ultrasound examination of the heart

-ectomy: A word-forming element meaning "removal"

Edema: The swelling of soft tissues as a result of fluid accumulation

Effusion: Escape of fluid into an anatomically defined body cavity

Ejection fraction: Ejection capacity of the heart: the portion of the available blood that is ejected from the left ventricle

Electrocardiogram: A recording of electrical potentials of the heart

Embolism: Sudden obstruction of a blood vessel by an embolus

Embolus: A structure, not soluble in blood, that has been carried into the bloodstream and causes an embolism; most frequently a detached thrombus, fat droplets, air or gas bubbles, tumor cells, or foreign bodies

Embryo: The organism in the early stages of growth and differentiation, from fertilization up to the third month of pregnancy in humans

Embryopathy: A developmental abnormality of an embryo especially when caused by a disease; damage during first trimester of pregnancy

Emphysema:
1. Collection of air or gas in tissues that are normally free of air, e.g., skin emphysema
2. Excessive accumulation of air or gas in an air-containing tissue or organ, e.g., pulmonary emphysema

Empyema: Collection of pus in an anatomically defined cavity

Enanthema: Rash on a mucous membrane, as in measles or chickenpox

Encephalopathy: A general term for any noninflammatory brain disease or damage of the brain with neurological or psychiatric symptoms

Endemic: A disease prevalent in or peculiar to a particular locality, region, or people

Endocarditis: Inflammation of the inner lining of the heart that usually also affects the heart valves

Endocrine glands: Ductless glands that secrete hormones directly into the bloodstream

Endogenous: Originating or produced within an organism, tissue, or cell

Endoscopy: Examination of a hollow organ with optical systems

Enophthalmos: Sunken eyeballs

Epidemic: A widespread outbreak of an infectious disease

Epidemiology: The study of the causes, distribution, and control of diseases in populations

Eradication: Destruction of a pathogen, e.g., of *Helicobacter pylori*, by a combination of drugs

ery-: A word-forming element meaning 'red'

Erysipelas: An acute streptococcal skin infection most frequent in the elderly, infants, and children

Erythema: Abnormal redness of a limited area of the skin

Erythrocytes: Red blood corpuscles

Erythroderma: A skin condition in which the whole body surface is marked by redness due to inflammation

Esophagitis: Inflammation of the esophagus

Estrogens: Female sex hormones

Etiology: Study of the underlying cause of diseases

eu-: A word-forming element meaning "good" or "normal"

Eukaryote: One-celled or multiple-celled organism with a true cell nucleus and cell organelles

Euthyroidism: Normal thyroid function

Event recorder: A device that records the heart rhythm and helps in detecting arrhythmias

Exanthema: Skin rash

Excretion: Elimination of metabolic waste products

Exogenous: Arising outside the body

Exophthalmos: Protruding eyeballs

Expiration: Exhalation

Exsiccosis: Drying out; decrease in body water

Extirpation: Surgical removal of a structure, (e.g., tumor, cyst) or organ

Extracorporeal shock wave lithotripsy: Externally controlled shattering of kidney or ureteral stones by means of sonographically controlled shock waves

Extrasystole: Heartbeats that occur outside the basic rhythm

Extrinsic asthma: Allergic asthma

Exudate: A fluid rich in protein and cellular elements that oozes out of blood and lymph vessels

Exudative pleuritis: Inflammation of the pleura with formation of effusions

Fallot tetralogy: A complex, congenital heart defect

Felty syndrome: A severe form of rheumatoid arthritis

Fetopathy: Disease before birth caused by damage in the second or third trimester of pregnancy

Fetor: Bad smell

Fetus: An unborn child from the beginning of the fourth month of pregnancy until birth

Fibrates: Drugs that lower lipids

Fibrin: An insoluble protein formed in response to bleeding; the major component of a blood clot

Fibrinogen: Blood clotting factor formed in the liver, dependent on vitamin K; fibrin precursor

Fibrinolysis: Degradation of fibrin and fibrin clots, the products of blood coagulation

Fibrosis: Transformation into connective tissue with loss of function, e.g., pulmonary fibrosis

Fissure: A crack or tear in tissue

Fistula: A pathological connection between two hollow organs or hollow organ and skin

Focal nodular hyperplasia: A benign liver tumor

Forced expiratory volume in one second: The amount of air that can be exhaled in 1 second after taking a deep breath; FEV_1, measured by the Tiffeneau test

Fragile: Constitutionally delicate, lacking in vigor

Fructosamine: A substance formed from blood proteins that can be measured to determine the plasma glucose concentration over a period such as the previous 14 days

Fulminant: Appearing and progressing suddenly

Functional complaints: Complaints without objective findings in the organs

Functional residual capacity: The mount of air that remains in the lungs after an unforced expiration

Fungoid mycosis: A type of lymphoma originating in malignantly changed T-lymphocytes

Galactorrhea: Escape of milk from the breast

Galactose: A simple sugar occurring in milk

Gastritis: Inflammation of the gastric mucosa

Gastroenteritis: Inflammation of the gastrointestinal tract

Gestational diabetes: Diabetes during pregnancy

GI bleeding: Gastrointestinal bleeding

Giant-cell arteritis: Vasculitis of the large vessels; Horton temporal arteritis

Gliadin: A protein present in cereals, a component of gluten; trigger for celiac disease

Glomerular filtration rate: A measure of kidney function

Glucagon: A pancreatic hormone that raises blood glucose levels; antagonist of insulin

Glucagonoma: A rare pancreatic tumor that autonomously produces glucagon and causes hyperglycemia

Glucocorticosteroid: Steroid hormone produced in the adrenal cortex, e.g., cortisol

Gluconeogenesis: Formation of glucose

Glucosuria: Glucose excretion in the urine

Gluten: A cohesive, elastic protein in wheat, barley, oats, and rye

Glycogenesis: The process by which glucose is converted into glycogen, a type of starch

Glycogenolysis: The process by which glycogen is broken down from glucose

Gonads: Glands (testes and ovaries) that produce the reproductive cells (ova and spermatozoa)

Gonorrhea: Infectious sexually transmitted disease caused by *Neisseria gonorrhoeae*

Gonosomes: Sex chromosomes

Gout: Disease resulting from deposition of uric acid crystals in joints and kidneys, with inflammatory reaction and gout arthropathy or nephropathy

Grading: A description of a tumor based on how differentiated the cancer cells are

Granulation tissue: The precursor of scar tissue in wound healing

Granulocytes: Subgroup of white blood corpuscles

Granuloma: Nodules of immune cells surrounding foreign materials the body cannot get rid of, e.g., pathogens of tuberculosis, the nodules of sarcoidosis, or foreign bodies that are hard to decompose (seen in silicosis, asbestosis)

Haploid chromosome set: Having the same number of sets of chromosomes as a germ cell or half as many as a somatic cell

Helicobacter pylori: A bacterium that causes chronic inflammation of the gastric mucosa and contributes to formation of ulcers in stomach and duodenum

Hemangioma: Strawberry mark, benign vascular tumor

Hematemesis: Vomiting of blood, usually in upper gastrointestinal bleeding

Hematochezia: Stool stained with light to dark red blood

Hematocrit: The proportion of solid components in the blood

Hematogenous:
1. Producing blood;
2. Originating in or spread by the blood

Hematuria: Blood in the urine

Hemoccult test: A stool test for the detection of occult (i.e., nonvisible) blood lost through the gastrointestinal tract

Hemodialysis: A procedure for removing waste products and free water from the blood; renal replacement therapy

Hemofiltration: A renal replacement therapy similar to hemodialysis, used mainly in an intensive care setting

Hemoglobin A1c (HbA1c): Serves as a parameter for monitoring therapy in diabetes mellitus.

Hemolysis: Abnormally increased breakdown of erythrocytes

Hemophilia A: A hereditary blood disease with inactive or missing clotting Factor VIII

Hemophilia B: Hereditary blood disease with inactive or missing clotting Factor IX; Christmas disease

Hemorrhage: Excessive discharge of blood from the blood vessels; profuse bleeding

Hemostasis: Arrest of bleeding; clotting

Heparins: A group of substances that inhibit coagulation

Hepatitis: Inflammation of the liver tissue

Hepatosplenomegaly: Enlargement of liver and spleen

Hernia: Protrusion of an organ through the wall of the cavity that normally contains it

Herpes zoster: Shingles; a painful, blistering skin rash caused by reactivation of the varicella zoster virus

Heterologous transplantation: Donor and recipient belong to different species

Heterotopic: Referring to an abnormal anatomical location

Heterozygote: Possessing two different forms of a particular gene

Histocompatibility: A state or condition in which the absence of immunological interference permits the transplantation of an organ or tissue

Hodgkin disease: Lymphogranulomatosis; malignant lymph node disease that develops into a systemic disease and can also attack extralymphatic organs

Holter ECG: Electrocardiogram recording for a long-term period of usually 24 hours

Homans sign: Clinical sign of thrombosis; in dorsal extension of the foot the patient reports pain in the calf

Homologous transplantation: Donor and recipient are genetically different but of the same species

Homozygote: Possessing two identical forms of a particular gene, one obtained from each parent

Horner syndrome: Damage to the neck sympathetic nerve due to a tumor on the apex of the lung (Pancoast tumor) with the triad of narrowed pupil, drooping upper lid, and apparently sunken eyeball

Horton temporal arteritis: Giant-cell arteritis; vasculitis in the perfusion area of the carotid artery

Human leukocyte antigens: Distinctive membrane properties of white blood cells, e.g., almost all patients with spondylarthropathy have HLA-B27

Hypercapnia: Elevated arterial carbon dioxide level

Hypercholesterolemia: Elevated blood cholesterol level

Hyperglycemia: Elevated blood glucose level

Hyperlipidemia: Elevated blood lipid level

Hyperosmolar: Having elevated osmolarity, i.e., an increased number of dissolved particles per liter of liquid

Hyperparathyroidism: Excessive secretion of parathyroid hormone (PTH) by the parathyroid glands

Hyperplasia: Enlargement of an organ through cell proliferation

Hypertension, arterial: Elevated blood pressure in the systemic circulation

Hypertension, pulmonary: Elevated blood pressure in the pulmonary circulation

Hypertriglyceridemia: Elevated blood level of triglycerides

Hypertrophy: Enlargement or overgrowth of an organ or part of the body due to an increased size of the constituent cells

Hyperuricemia: Elevated blood level of uric acid

Hypocapnia: Decreased arterial carbon dioxide level

Hypoglycemia: Decreased blood glucose level

Hypogonadism: Decreased function of the reproductive glands

Hypophysis: Pituitary gland

Hypotension, arterial: Decreased blood pressure in the systemic circulation

Hypoxemia: Decreased oxygen content in the arterial blood

Hypoxia: Decreased oxygen content in body tissues

Iatrogenic: An adverse condition caused by the action of a physician

Icterus: A yellow tint in skin, tissues, bodily fluids caused by an accumulation of bile pigment in the blood

Idiopathic thrombocytopenic purpura: A disease with increased breakdown of platelets and tendency to bleeding

Ileitis terminalis: Synonym of Crohn disease

Ileus: Obstruction in the intestine

Immunity: The ability of the organism to recognize and fight pathogens

Immunocytoma: A type of lymphoma originating in B-lymphocytes with malignant transformation

Immunoglobulins: Antibodies

Immunosuppression: Inhibition of defensive reactions

Incidence: The number of new cases of a specific disease in a defined period of time

Incretion: Internal secretion, direct delivery into the blood

Incubation time: The time between infection and the appearance of the first signs of a disease

Indication: A generally recognized reason for application of a specific therapy or measure

Infarction: Necrosis as a result of ischemia

Infection: Transfer and adhesion of microorganisms to an organism and multiplication inside the organism

Infectious mononucleosis: Pfeiffer glandular fever, "kissing disease"; a disease resulting from infection with Epstein–Barr virus

Influenza: Grippe, flu

Inspiration: Inhalation

Inspiratory reserve volume: The amount of air that can be additionally inhaled after an unforced respiration

Insufficiency: Weak functioning of an organ or part of an organ

Insulin: A pancreatic hormone that regulates carbohydrate and fat metabolism

Insulinoma: The most frequent endocrine pancreatic tumor with autonomous insulin production and severe hypoglycemia

Intermittent claudication: Walking-related pain in peripheral arterial disease

Intermittent: With interruptions, arising periodically, progressing in flares

Interstitium: Space between organs, tissues or cells

Intestinal: Having to do with the intestines

Intrinsic asthma: Nonallergic asthma

Irradiation: Use of radiation to treat patients

Irreversible: Applied to a condition that cannot be cured

Ischemia: Lack of oxygen due to insufficient arterial blood supply to a tissue

Isologous transplantation: Donor and recipient are genetically identical

ISWL: Intracorporeal shock wave lithotripsy; endoscopically controlled shattering of ureteral stones by means of shock wave

Juvenile: Having to do with youth

Kawasaki disease: Mucocutaneous lymph node syndrome; a type of vasculitis in small children

Ketoacidosis: Hyperglycemic metabolic disorder with uninhibited lipolysis

Korotkow sound: Arterial sounds synchronous with the pulse during blood pressure measurement

Lactase: An enzyme that splits milk sugar

Lactose: Milk sugar

Lanz point: A painful pressure point in the right lower abdomen in appendicitis

Laparoscopy: Minimally invasive examination of abdominal organs with an optical system

Legionellosis: Infection with *Legionella pneumophila* with chief manifestations in the lungs

Lethality: The percentage of patients dying from a specific disease compared with the total number of patients suffering from the disease

Leukemia: Malignant disease of the blood-forming system with uncontrolled formation of white blood cells

leuko-: A word-forming element meaning "white"

Leukocytes: White blood cells

Leukocytopenia: Decrease in white blood cell count

Leukocytosis: Increase in white blood cell count

Leukocyturia: Excretion of more than four leukocytes per mL urine

LH: Luteinizing hormone

Lipogenesis: Formation of fat deposits

Lipolysis: Breakdown of lipids to glycerol and free fatty acids

Lipoproteins: Lipids coated with proteins

Livid: Bluish pale, wan

Low-density lipoprotein: A lipoprotein high in cholesterol

Lues: Syphilis

Lupus: Wolf

Lymphatic: Connected with the lymphvessels and the lymphatic glands or lymph nodes

Lymphocytes: Subgroup of white blood cells

Lymphoma: Malignant disease of the lymphatic system

Lysis: Dispersal, dissolution

Macroangiopathy: Disease of the large arteries; arteriosclerosis

Madonna fingers: Distally tapering fingers, typical in progressive systemic sclerosis

Malabsorption: Digestive disorder in which nutrient components cannot be absorbed

Malaria: A disease resulting from infection with plasmodia; intermittent fever

Malassimilation: Digestive disorder in which nutrient components cannot be taken up in the intestine, due either to malabsorption or to maldigestion

Maldigestion: Digestive disorder in which nutrient components cannot be adequately broken down

Malignant: Characterized by progressive and uncontrolled growth (especially of a tumor), not benign

Manifestation: Emergence of the recognizable signs of a disease

Mayr sign: A clinical sign of thrombosis; the patient complains of pain when the calf is compressed

McBurney point: A painful pressure point on the right lower abdomen in appendicitis

Meiosis: The type of cell division by which germ cells (eggs and sperm) are produced

Melena: Tarry stool; black stool in gastrointestinal bleeding

Mesothelioma: Tumor originating in the mesothelium, usually the pleural mesothelium, and usually caused by exposure to asbestos

Metabolic syndrome: A combination of medical disorders that increase the risk of cardiovascular disease and diabetes

Metaplasia: Tissue transformation in which a differentiated tissue becomes a different differentiated tissue

Methotrexate: An immunosuppressant medication; a basic therapeutic drug in treatment of rheumatoid arthritis

Microangiopathy: Disease of the small vessels

Micturition: Urination

Mineralocorticosteroids: Steroid hormones, especially aldosterone, formed in the adrenal cortex, having an influence on electrolyte balance

Miosis: Contraction of the pupil

Monogenic: Determined by a single gene

Monosomy: A chromosomal anomaly in which one chromosome of a pair is missing

Morbidity: The number of persons suffering from a certain disease out of 100 000 inhabitants at a certain point in time

Mortality: The death rate from a specific disease. It reports how many individuals out of 100 000 inhabitants in a specific population have died as a result of a specific disease within a certain period of time

Mucoviscidosis: Cystic fibrosis; a hereditary metabolic disease with manifestation in airways and intestine

Multiple myeloma: Plasmocytoma; a malignant systemic disease originating in the plasma cells in the bone marrow

Mydriasis: Expansion of the pupil

Myeloproliferation: Increased production of a certain cell line in the bone marrow

Myocarditis: Inflammation of the heart muscle

Myxedema: Doughy swelling of the tissues caused by deposition of mucopolysaccharides in hypothyroidism

Necrosis: Death of cells or tissues through injury or disease in the living body

Neoplasia: The process of abnormal and uncontrolled growth of cells

Nephrolithiasis: Presence of kidney stones

Nephropathy: Generalized term for any noninflammatory kidney disease

Neuropathy: Noninflammatory nerve disease

Nitroglycerin: A vessel-dilating medication

Nocturia: Increased urination at night

Nosocomial: Acquired in the hospital

Noxa: Something that exerts a harmful effect on the body

Obesity: A condition with excessive accumulation of body fat

Obstipation: Constipation

Occult: Hidden, chronically unnoticed

oligo-: A word-forming element meaning "little" or "scant"

Oliguria: Urine volume of less than 500 mL per day

Oncology: The branch of medicine concerned with the study and treatment of malignant tumors

Organogenesis: Formation and development of organs

Orthopnea: Shortness of breath that occurs when the patient is in a supine position and disappears when the patient is sitting up; typical for heart failure

Orthotopic: In the normal position

Osteomalacia: Disease with insufficiently mineralized bone tissue, usually as a result of a vitamin D deficiency

Osteomyelosclerosis: Disease in which the blood-forming bone marrow fibroses and loses its function

Osteopathy: Noninflammatory bone disease

Osteoporosis: Degradation of bone, disappearance of bony mass

Oxygenation: Supply of oxygen

Oxytocin: A hormone released by the posterior lobe of the pituitary gland

Palliative: Offering relief

Palpation: Obtaining findings by feeling with the hands

Panarteritis nodosa: Vasculitis of the small or medium-sized vessels

Pancoast syndrome: Carcinoma of the apex of the lung that can grow into the first rib, the body of the first thoracic vertebra, the brachial plexus, and the subclavian vein and lead to Horner syndrome

Pancreatitis: Inflammation of the pancreas

Pandemic: Spread of an infectious disease beyond local boundaries, i.e. over countries and continents

Papilloma: Benign tumor originating in epithelial tissue

Paraneoplasia: Systemic pathological clinical and biological disturbances associated with a malignant neoplasm

Parasympatholytics: Medications that inhibit the action of the parasympathetic nervous system

Parasympathomimetics: Medications that promote the action of the parasympathetic nervous system

Parathyroid hormone: A hormone affecting calcium and phosphate metabolism

Paroxysmal: Suddenly appearing symptoms of a disease

Partial thromboplastin time: A coagulation parameter

Pathogenesis: Origin and development of a disease

Payr sign: Clinical sign of thrombosis; the patient experiences pain from pressure on the sole of the foot

Peak flow: Maximal speed of expiration measured with a peak flow meter

Percussion: Striking a body part and evaluating the resulting sound

Percutaneous transluminal coronary angioplasty: Distension of narrowed coronary vessels by means of a balloon catheter

Perfusion:
1. Circulation
2. The delivery of a liquid to an organ or tissue

Pericarditis: Inflammation of the sac around the heart (pericardium)

Peritoneal dialysis: Dialysis across the peritoneum; a renal replacement therapy

Peritonitis: Inflammation of the tissue that lines the wall of the abdomen and covers the abdominal organs

Petechia: A small red or purple spot caused by hemorrhage under the skin

Pfeiffer glandular fever: Infectious mononucleosis; "kissing disease"; disease caused by infection with the Epstein–Barr virus

Pheochromocytoma: A tumor usually originating in the medulla of the adrenal cortex and producing excessive amounts of epinephrine and norepinephrine

Phlebothrombosis: Occlusion of a deep vein by a blood clot

Phlegmon: Purulent inflammation, diffusely spread throughout the skin and connective tissue

Plasmid: An extrachromosomal ring of DNA

Plasmin: A protein-splitting enzyme that degrades fibrin clots in the bloodstream (fibrinolysis)

Plasminogen: Precursor of the enzyme plasmin

Plasmocytoma: Multiple myeloma; a malignant systemic disease that originates in the plasma cells of the bone marrow

Pleural mesothelioma: A primary tumor of the pleura, usually caused by asbestos

Pleuritis sicca: Dry pleural inflammation, i.e., without formation of effusions

Pneumoconiosis: An interstitial lung disease resulting from inhalation of inorganic dust

Pneumonia: Inflammation of the lungs

Pneumothorax: Accumulation of air in the pleural space with partial or complete collapse of the lung

Podagra: Gout attack in the basal joint of the great toe

Pollakiuria: Frequent urge to urinate although the urinary bladder is not full

Polymyalgia rheumatica: a disease involving muscle pain; a possible associated manifestation in giant cell arteritis

Polymyositis: Systemic inflammatory disease of the skeletal muscles

Polyp: A swelling consisting of mucous tissue

poly-: A word-forming element meaning "many" or "much"

Polyuria: Excretion of more than 3000 mL urine per day

Precancerosis: Tissue changes that have a statistically elevated risk of becoming malignant; cancer precursor

Prevalence: The proportion of a population with a disease at a particular time or within a specific time period

Prick test: A skin test for allergies

Progress: The course of a disease

Progression: The worsening of a disease

Prokaryotes: Unicellular organisms without a membrane-bound nucleus

Prolactin: A hormone of the anterior lobe of the pituitary gland

Prolactinoma: Pituitary adenoma that produces prolactin autonomously

Protein C: A physiological inhibitor of blood clotting

Protein S: A physiological inhibitor of blood clotting; cofactor of protein C

Proteinuria: Excretion of more than 150 mg protein per day in the urine

Prothrombin time: A blood test that measures how long it takes the blood to clot. Synonyms: thromboplastin time, Quick value

Protozoon: A unicellular animal organism (plural: protozoa)

Psoriasis: A skin condition that causes redness, itching, and scaly flaking

Ptosis:
1. Drooping of the upper lid
2. Dropping of organs

Purines: Components of nucleic acids

Purpura: Redness of skin and mucosa caused by spotty bleeding that cannot be pressed away with a glass spatula

Pyelonephritis: Infection of the ureters and the pelvis of the kidney

Pyrogen: A substance that produces a fever

Pyuria: Milky, pus-filled cloudy urine

Quick value: Thromboplastin time; a clotting parameter

Radiation therapy: Use of radiation to treat patients; see also irradiation

Raynaud syndrome: Vascular spasms lead to short-term malperfusion in the fingers, so that they become pale, then cyanotic, and later red because of hyperemia

Recurrence: Relapse

Reflux: Back flow

Regeneration: Healing, regrowth of lost tissue

Reiter syndrome: Reactive arthritis associated with urethritis, eye involvement, and skin and mucosal involvement

Remission: Complete disappearance of all manifestations of a disease

Renal: Relating to the kidneys; originating in the kidneys; affecting the kidneys

Reperfusion: Restoration of blood flow

Resection: Complete or partial surgical removal of an organ or structure

Residual volume: The amount of air that still remains in the lungs after maximal expiration

Resistance: The ability to withstand

Revascularization: Restoration of circulation

Reversible: Applied to a condition that can be cured

Rhagades: Skin tears or fissures

Rheumatic fever: Autoimmune process after streptococcal disease that chiefly affects the heart

Rheumatoid factor: Autoantibody of the IgM type against the body's own IgG

Rickets: Childhood disease with insufficient mineralization of the epiphysis as a result of vitamin D deficiency

Rovsing sign: A clinical sign of appendicitis; the patient experiences pain from retrograde palpation of the colon

Salmonella: A genus of bacteria; a pathogen of infectious diarrheal diseases

Salutogenesis: The study of maintaining and restoring health

Sarcoidosis: Systemic disease with disrupted T-lymphocyte function and formation of granulomas on the skin, in internal organs, and in lymph nodes; the involvement of the lungs determines the clinical picture and the prognosis

Sarcoma: Malignant tumor not originating in epithelial tissue

Scarlet fever: A disease resulting from infection with streptococci with purulent tonsillitis and characteristic skin changes

Schönlein–Henoch purpura: Vasculitis of the small vessels

Scleroderma: Systemic scleroderma, progressive systemic sclerosis; chronic connective-tissue disease with hardening of skin and internal organs

Sclerosis: Hardening

Septicemia: Blood poisoning

Septum: Separating wall between two parts of an organ

Serology: The scientific study of blood serum and other body fluids to find and characterize antibodies, antigens, and other immunological substances

Sharp syndrome: Mixed collagenosis with symptoms of rheumatoid arthritis, systemic lupus erythematosus, progressive systemic sclerosis, and polymyositis

Shunt: A short-circuit connection

Sicca syndrome: Chronic inflammation of the exocrine glands with reduced secretion; Sjögren syndrome

Silicosis: Interstitial lung disease caused by inhalation of quartz dust

Sjögren syndrome: Chronic inflammation of the exocrine glands with reduced secretion; sicca syndrome

Somatotropin: Growth hormone

Somnolence: Drowsiness, sleepiness

Sonography: A technique that uses the reflections of high-frequency sound waves to construct an image of a body organ

Sopor: An abnormally deep sleep from which the patient can no longer be fully awakened by external stimuli

Spider nevi: Star nevus, vascular spider; pinhead-sized red spots appearing primarily in the face with fine radial extensions; frequent in liver disease

Spirometry: Measurement of lung volumes and ventilation volumes

Splenomegaly: Enlargement of the spleen

Spondylarthropathies: Chronic inflammatory diseases that involve the spinal column, large joints, tendon attachments, and ligaments as well as occasionally other organs, e.g., Bechterew disease, reactive arthritis, psoriasis arthritis, arthritis in chronic inflammatory intestinal diseases

Spore:
1. A small, bacterial reproductive body that is highly resistant to drying and heat and is capable of growing into a new organism.
2. The sexual and/or asexual reproductive forms of fungi

Sputum: Matter expelled from the respiratory tract, such as mucus or phlegm

Staging: Determination of the local and systemic spread of a tumor

Staphylococcus: A genus of bacteria; a pathogen for purulent infections

Statins: Cholesterol synthesis inhibitors

Steatorrhea: Increased fat excretion in the stool

Stenosis: Narrowing

Stent: A support structure to keep vessels or hollow organs open

Sternotomy: Surgical measure to cut through the breast bone

Still syndrome: A systemic form of juvenile rheumatoid arthritis with pronounced organ involvement

Stoma: Mouth, opening

Streptococcus: A genus of bacteria; a pathogen for purulent infections

Stridor: Whistling breath sound occurring when the airways are constricted

Struma: Enlarged thyroid gland, goiter

Stupor: A state of mental numbness without recognizable mental or physical activity, but without loss of consciousness

Sulfasalazine: An anti-inflammatory medication; used for treatment of rheumatoid arthritis and chronic inflammatory intestinal diseases

Sulfonylurea: Oral antidiabetic medication

Supraventricular: Located or originating above the ventricle, in the atria of the heart

Surfactant: A surface-active substance in the alveoli of the lungs that lowers the surface tension and thus prevents collapse of the alveoli at the end of expiration

Sympatholytics: Medications that inhibit the action of the sympathetic nervous system

Sympathomimetics: Medications that promote the action of the sympathetic nervous system

Symptom: Any sensation or change in bodily function that is experienced by a patient

Syncope: A sudden, transient loss of consciousness with loss of muscle tonus and spontaneous, complete recovery

Syphilis: A sexually transmitted disease caused by the bacterium *Treponema pallidum*

Systole: Phase of the cardiac cycle in which the muscles of the ventricle contract and pump blood out of the heart

Systolic murmur: Heart murmur during the contraction phase of the heart

Tachycardia: Accelerated heart beat above 100 beats per minute

Tachypnea: Accelerated breathing

Telangiectases: Permanently expanded and tangled smallest vessels that are visible through the skin

Teratogen: An agent that interferes with normal embryonic development

Terminal:
1. referring to the end, being at the end of something;
2. incurable, referring to the last stage of a fatal illness

Tetanus: Lockjaw, a medical condition characterized by muscle spasms, caused by infection with the bacterium *Clostridium tetani*

Thrombocytopathy: Functional disorder of the blood platelets

Thrombocytopenia: Decreased number of platelets in the blood

Thrombocytosis: Increased number of platelets in the blood

Thrombophlebitis: Inflammation of a surface vein with vascular obstruction

Thromboplastin time: Quick value; prothrombin time, coagulation parameter

Thrombus: A blood clot arising in a blood vessel

Tick-borne encephalitis: An infectious disease spread by ticks

Tidal volume: The amount of air that is breathed in and out with every resting breath

Tiffeneau test: Test to determine the amount of air that can be exhaled in one second after a deep inspiration

Total capacity: The amount of air in the lungs after maximal inspiration

Toxoplasmosis: Infectious disease caused by *Toxoplasma gondii*

Transposition: Tissue or organ displacement, e.g., transposition of the large vessels as a congenital heart defect

Transudate: Noninflammatory effusion low in protein

Treponema pallidum: A species of bacteria; a pathogen for syphilis

Triad: Medically, a complex of three major symptoms

Trigger: An event that precipitates other events

Trimester: 3-month period (in pregnancy)

Trisomy: The presence of three copies of a chromosome rather than the normal two

Troponin: A protein contained in the thin filaments of muscle cells; the heart muscle-specific troponins I and T are of diagnostic importance for myocardial infarctions

Tumor: Swelling, formation of abnormal new tissue

Typhoid fever: Infectious disease caused by certain species of *Salmonella*

Ulcerative colitis: A chronic inflammatory intestinal disease

Ulcus: Ulcer

Urea: A nitrogenous end product of protein metabolism

Urethritis: Inflammation of the urethra

Uric acid: A product of purine breakdown

Urinary incontinence: Involuntary urination

Urolithiasis: Nephrolithiasis, Calculi formation in the urinary tract

Varicella: Chickenpox

Varicosis: Varicose vein disease

Varicosity: A varicose vein

Vascular medicine: Study of blood vessels and their diseases

Vasculitis: Inflammatory vascular disease

Venerology: Study of sexually transmitted diseases

Venous stasis: Engorgement due to slow or impaired blood flow

Ventilation: Artificial respiration

Vertigo: Dizziness

Vipoma: A usually malignant pancreatic tumor that autonomously produces vasoactive intestinal polypeptides and causes watery diarrhea

Virchow triad: Name for the triad, proposed by Rudolf Virchow, of factors that promote thrombosis: slowed blood circulation, changes in the vessel walls, and changed blood composition

Vital capacity: The maximal amount of air that can be exhaled after maximal inspiration

Vital signs: Collective term for arterial blood pressure, heart rate, and respiration rate

von Willebrand syndrome: The most frequent congenital coagulopathy

Waterhouse–Friderichsen syndrome: Meningococcal sepsis

Wegener granulomatosis: Vasculitis of the small vessels

White atrophy: Depigmented, atrophied areas of the skin over the malleoli in chronic venous insufficiency

Xanthelasma: Xanthomas on the eyelids

Xanthoma: Skin changes in the form of yellowish fat-containing nodules

Xenogenic transplantation: Donor and recipient belong to different species

Xerostomy: Dry mouth

Further Reading

■ Visceral Anatomy, Physiology

Faller A, Schünke M. The Human Body. Stuttgart–New York: Thieme Publishers; 2004.

Fritsch H, Kühnel W. Color Atlas of Human Anatomy. Vol 2: Internal Organs. 5th ed. Stuttgart–New York: Thieme Publishers; 2007.

Huppelsberg J, Walter K. Kurzlehrbuch Physiologie. Stuttgart: Thieme; 2005.

Klinke R, Pape HC, Silbernagl S. Lehrbuch der Physiologie. 5th completely revised edition. Stuttgart: Thieme; 2005.

Lippert H. Lehrbuch Anatomie. Munich: Urban & Fischer; 2003.

Sadler TW, Langman J. Medizinische Embryologie. Die normale menschliche Entwicklung und ihre Fehlbildungen. Stuttgart: Thieme; 2003.

Schiebler, TH. Anatomie. Heideldelberg: Springer; 2004.

Schmidt RF, Lang F, Thews G. Physiologie des Menschen mit Pathophysiologie. Heidelberg: Springer; 2004.

Schünke M, Schulte E, Schumacher U. Thieme Atlas of Anatomy. Vol 1: General Anatomy and Musculoskeletal System. 2nd ed. Stuttgart–New York: Thieme Publishers; 2010.

Silbernagl S, Despopoulos, A. Color Atlas of Physiology. 6th ed. Stuttgart–New York: Thieme Publishers; 2008.

Thews G, Mutschler E, Vaupel P. Anatomie, Physiologie, Pathophysiologie des Menschen. Stuttgart: Wissenschaftliche Verlagsgesellschaft; 1999.

Van den Berg F. Angewandte Physiologie. Bd. 2. Organsysteme verstehen und beeinflussen. 2nd revised edition. Stuttgart: Thieme; 2005.

Zalpour C. Anatomie, Physiologie. Munich: Urban & Fischer; 2002.

■ Pathology

Böcker W, Denk H, Heitz PU. Pathologie. Stuttgart: Urban & Fischer; 2004.

Riede UN, Werner M, Schaefer HE. Allgemeine und spezielle Pathologie. 5th completely revised edition. Stuttgart: Thieme; 2004.

Silbernagl S, Lang F. Color Atlas of Pathophysiology. 2nd ed. Stuttgart–New York: Thieme Publishers; 2009.

■ Internal Medicine

Baenkler HW, Fritze D, Füeßl HS. Duale Reihe Innere Medizin. Stuttgart: Thieme; 2001.

Dietel M, Suttorp N, Zeitz M, Harrison TR. Harrison's Innere Medizin. Berlin: ABW Wissenschaftsverlag; 2005.

Greten H. Innere Medizin Verstehen, Lernen, Anwenden. 12th completely revised edition. Stuttgart: Thieme; 2005.

Herold G. Innere Medizin. Cologne: Dr. Gerd Herold; 2010.

Longo D, Fauci A, Kasper D, Hauser S, Jameson J, Loscalzo J. Harrison's Principles of Internal Medicine. 18th ed. Philadelphia: McGraw-Hill; 2011.

Renz-Polster H, Krautzig S, Braun J. Basislehrbuch Innere Medizin. Munich: Urban & Fischer; 2004.

Siegenthaler W. Differential Diagnosis in Internal Medicine. Stuttgart–New York: Thieme Publishers; 2007.

■ Surgery

Bruch HP, Trentz O, Berchtold R. Chirurgie. Munich: Urban & Fischer; 2005.

Henne-Bruns D, Dürig M, Kremer B. Duale Reihe Chirurgie. Stuttgart: Thieme; 2003.

Schumpelick V, Bleese NM, Mommsen U. Kurzlehrbuch Chirurgie. 6th ed. Stuttgart: Thieme; 2004.

Schumpelick V. Atlas of General Surgery. Stuttgart–New York: Thieme Publishers; 2009.

Siewert JR. Chirurgie. Heidelberg: Springer; 2006.

■ Pharmacology

Aktories K, Förstermann U, Hofmann F, Forth W. Allgemeine und spezielle Pharmakologie und Toxikologie. Munich: Urban & Fischer; 2004.

Lüllmann H, Mohr K, Hein L. Pocket Atlas of Pharmacology. 4th revised edition. Stuttgart–New York: Thieme Pubslihers; 2011.

Mutschler E, Geisslinger G, Kroemer HK. Arzneimittelwirkungen kompakt. Basiswissen Pharmakologie/Toxikologie. Stuttgart: Wissenschaftliche Verlagsgesellschaft; 2005.

Figure Sources

Baenkler H-W, Fritze D, Füeßl HS. Duale Reihe innere Medizin. Stuttgart: Thieme; 2001.

Baenkler H-W. Duale Reihe Innere Medizin. Stuttgart: Thieme; 1999.

Epstein O. Bild-Lehrbuch der klinischen Untersuchung. Stuttgart: Thieme; 1994.

Flachskampf FA. Echookardiographie. 2nd ed. Stuttgart: Thieme; 2004.

Füeßl H, Middeke M. Duale Reihe Anamnese und Klinische Untersuchung. Stuttgart: Thieme; 2005.

Gerlach U. Innere Medizin für Pflegeberufe. 5th ed. Stuttgart: Thieme; 2000.

Greten H. Innere Medizin. 12th ed. Stuttgart: Thieme; 2005.

Jung EG. Dermatologie. 4th ed. Stuttgart: Hippokrates; 1998.

Kellnhauser E. THIEMEs Pflege. 10th ed. Stuttgart: Thieme 2004.

Kuner E-H, Schlosser V. Traumatologie. 5th ed. Stuttgart: Thieme; 1995.

Niethard FU, Pfeil J. Duale Reihe Orthopädie. 5th ed. Stuttgart: Thieme; 2005.

Riede U-N. Color Atlas of Pathology. Stuttgart–New York: Thieme; 2004.

Sitzmann FC. Duale Reihe Pädiatrie. 2nd ed. Stuttgart: Thieme; 2002.

Index

Page references in *italic* refer to illustrations.